Schuster, Daniel B
  Clinical supervision of the psychiatric resident, by Daniel
B. Schuster, John J. Sandt, and Otto F. Thaler.   New
York, Brunner/Mazel [1972]

  xv, 334 p.   24 cm. $10.00

  Includes bibliographical references.

  1. Psychiatry—Study and teaching.   I. Sandt, John J., joint author.   II. Thaler, Otto F., joint author.   III. Title.

RC336.S38   616.8'9'007   76–190077
ISBN 0–87630–057–3   MARC

Library of Congress   72 [4]

CLINICAL SUPERVISION OF THE PSYCHIATRIC RESIDENT

Clinical Supervision of the Psychiatric Resident

By

DANIEL B. SCHUSTER, M.D.

*Professor of Psychiatry, University of Rochester
School of Medicine and Dentistry*

JOHN J. SANDT, M.D.

*Assistant Professor of Psychiatry, University of Rochester
School of Medicine and Dentistry*

and

OTTO F. THALER, M.D.

*Professor of Psychiatry, University of Rochester
School of Medicine and Dentistry*

BRUNNER/MAZEL • New York
BUTTERWORTHS • London

Introduction

Perhaps above all else, that which has characterized the training of the aspiring psychiatrists in the residency training programs of our country during the past quarter century has been the clinical supervision provided for the students. In several respects it has differed from that elsewhere throughout the world. Firstly, there became available for such instruction increasing numbers of psychiatrists who had undertaken psychoanalytic training and had evolved an extensive knowledge of psychodynamics, both in theory and through clinical practice. Secondly, the leaders in the academic field, whether in the university centers or the major hospital residency training programs, had an open and accepting attitude toward provision of clinical supervision by psychoanalytically trained psychiatrists. In this respect they differed from their many peers elsewhere in the world who remained aloof and frequently rejected the offers of the psychoanalytically trained psychiatrists to contribute to their educational programs.

As time went on, this close clinical supervision of the psychiatric resident in his clinical diagnostic and therapeutic work by experienced and highly skilled dynamic psychiatrists expanded from the urban centers of its origin. More such educators were trained and were sought out by the medical schools and hospitals throughout the land. Some psychiatric institutes supplied clinical supervision of this type to teach the residents in training even in remote state hospitals. Within a decade, many of the psychiatric residency training programs in the United States were graduating psychiatrists with supervised clinical experience equal or equivalent to that of psychoanalysts entering practice from their training in the European and American institutes prior to and even after World War I. One may state with assurance that this country has been blessed with an increasing number of psychiatrists entering practice who have acquired the knowledge not only of psychopathology and the somatic therapies but also of the psychodynamics of personality, along with the capacity to use this knowledge in their treatment of the ill.

Knowledge in depth of the motivating forces determining much of psychopathology becomes both a much demanded but equally a much dispensed and recognizable characteristic of the American-trained psychiatrist. It has had much to do with the vast changes which have occurred in the new patterns of service given to the needy public, in practices as related to preventive programs, and perhaps even in the changing phenomenology of some forms of mental illness.

To be sure, not all psychiatric residency training programs in the country acquired this cadre of able clinical supervisors—nor have all welcomed them. Yet the desire for such educational experience brought many students from the less well staffed programs to seek privately that which they missed in their formal training programs.

Over the years, those involved in clinical supervision, both in the psychoanalytic institutes and in the psychiatric residency training programs, have reported in writing and in discussions their observations and experiences in an extensive literature. Drs. Schuster, Sandt and Thaler have given us an outstanding review of the earlier written reports. But they have gone much further. Describing their own experience with the developmental processes of the psychiatric residents in training, they have noted them in the initial years of training, as well as the changes emergent in later years of clinical training. Their clinical and educational sophistication shines through these discussions of the supervisory process. They discuss at length the problems created in the field by pressures to evolve a psychiatric physician to meet the demands of a burgeoning clamor for service for the many, as well as the danger of the potential erosion of the quality of the practitioner that may ensue if the unique in the present training program is lost. Their point of view is one with which I fully agree. Perhaps the most unusual section of this book is that on the supervisory conference, in which the writers report verbatim their discussions over their work with their resident trainees. This chapter and that preceding it on the supervisory process will grasp the attention of all those psychiatric educators participating in or involved in the supervision of residents. Their book is recommended reading for all engaged in this work—not only those engaged in training of psychiatrists but also those concerned with training of psychotherapists amongst the other mental health professions.

LAWRENCE C. KOLB, M.D.
Director, New York State Psychiatric Institute

Table of Contents

Preface

As a consequence of many years of supervision of the clinical work of psychiatric residents, the authors have realized that there is as yet no comprehensive description of this fundamental area of teaching. We believe that clinical supervision is by all odds the paramount aspect of a resident's training. Nonetheless, there is a sparse literature on this subject, much of it concerned with the more specific topic of supervision of psychotherapy. Our focus here is upon a broader field than psychotherapy: it is concerned with the supervision of the resident's contact with his patients from the first days of his psychiatric service to the conclusion of his formal graduate education. From these encounters the developing psychiatrist gradually acquires the skills of interviewing, the capacity to gather adequate and pertinent historical information and the ability to make sophisticated behavioral observations and clinical deductions—ultimately synthesizing these skills into the work of a humane clinician.

We feel particularly concerned about this aspect of training, because in recent years we have sensed a decreasing emphasis on traditional attention to clinical detail and diagnosis. We are convinced that only through rigorous training can a resident come to understand and adequately treat his patients. He must have the time, encouragement, and precept to study individual patients in some depth. The ability to make sound clinical observations and accurate evaluation of patients cannot be learned easily, nor quickly. This capacity takes years of development, requiring constant attention to primary clinical observations. Too often the resident may be encumbered with theoretical notions, many of them inaccurate or misapplied, before he has an opportunity to make his own observations of disordered human behavior. All of us need to be reminded that only through such observations can the resident gain conviction about concepts of the human personality and mental functioning.

Recent shifts in psychiatric emphasis distract the resident from the careful evaluation of individual problems which we regard as essential to his education. There is today a growing concern with large scale problems, emphasizing group approaches, and concomitantly a decline of interest in individual psychotherapy. Some of these methods de-emphasize the cognitive, rational and verbal aspects of traditional group therapy, venturing into highly charged areas including nonverbal body contact, stimulation and expression of impulse. These adventures puzzle and distress serious clinicians who have devoted their lives to the principle of careful and reasoned study of patients and their problems, as they struggle at close range with the powerful conflicts and instincts of man, maintaining the traditionally appropriate boundaries between patient and physician.

In addition, psychiatry itself is having an "identity crisis" and is under attack from many quarters, including its own ranks. Many question our function and purpose; some even challenge the necessity for our existence. Herbert C. Modlin in a recent paper[1] begins by quoting a colleague who asked, "Can you psychiatrists really justify your existence?" Arnold J. Mandel[2] states that psychiatrists don't know what they're supposed to be doing and charges that psychiatry "is going through an adolescent 'identity crisis.'" This ambience of doubt and confusion inevitably influences a psychiatric resident's resolution of his future role in life. Our answer to such challenges is simple and direct. We believe that a psychiatrist is *first* a physician. In spite of loose and pejorative comments about the "medical model" current today, we feel it imperative to reaffirm our interest in and loyalty to the general ranks of medicine and rededicate ourselves to the model of the clinician. No matter how much our field changes,

---

[1] "What Is a Psychiatrist?" *Psychiatry Digest,* February, 1971, pp. 19-26.
[2] *Roche Report,* Vol. 1, January 15, 1971. pp. 1-2.

what demands are made upon us, or what professional or para-professional groups are involved in psychiatric care, the psychiatric clinician will always play a primary role in the care of patients, in the teaching of professionals and in the conduct of research.

Another powerful force upon psychiatry today is community pressure for "delivery of service" to wider segments of the population perceived as not now served or inadequately served, with a tendency to derogate "one-to-one psychotherapy" as an ineffectual or unnecessary luxury. As a consequence, the resident's attention seems to be drawn to the care of groups before he understands, in any profound sense, individual psychodynamics. This seems to us to be basically unsound. Despite the social pressures of "a sick society," the *sine qua non* of a psychiatric clinician is his understanding and judgment of the unique individual psyche.

Our experience over the years leads us to believe in the importance of a substantial clinical exposure, first in the study and care of in-patients, many of whom have complicated combinations of physical and emotional difficulty, and who can be observed intensively over a period of time in a supervised setting; and second, in the supervised study of ambulatory patients, where the opportunity to observe the patient is inherently limited compared with the 24-hour-a-day status of the in-patient.

It is only through guided and careful investigation of a number of individual patients, embracing a wide spectrum of psychopathological states, that the psychiatrist in training begins to develop clinical acumen and judgment, and attains a basic perspective of "the psychiatric patient." Once he has attained this view, he can apply his perception to wider fields: to groups, to organizations, to the community, and finally to cultural and trans-cultural issues. We are concerned that the young psychiatrist achieve this balance so that he is able to continue his clinical maturation progressing from training to practice.

Our concern is for the survival of the clinician!

Acknowledgments

We wish to thank and give proper credit to the members of the supervisory conference which consolidated many of our ideas concerning supervision. In addition to Rodney J. Shapiro, Ph.D., who played a special part in initiating this conference, the following colleagues participated with the authors: G. Raymond Babineau, M.D., Leon J. Canapary, M.D., Gertrude E. Flynn, M.S., Lutrelle P. Gearhart, M.S.W., G. Porter Perham, M.D., and Leonard B. Salzman, Ph.D. It should also be noted that Dr. Otto F. Thaler assumed the role of chairman of our conference and took responsibility for taping our sessions.

We thank the Editor of the *Archives of General Psychiatry* for permission to use material previously published in an article by one of the authors ("Supervision of the Resident's Initial Interview," Vol. 23, December, 1970 by Daniel B. Schuster, M.D. and Edwin N. Freeman, M.D.) in Chapter IV of this book.

Last, but not least, we wish to thank our secretary, (Mrs.) Marcia Wallace, for her untiring efforts in typing this manuscript. She remained faithful and cheerful throughout the months required to complete this book.

CLINICAL SUPERVISION OF THE PSYCHIATRIC RESIDENT

1

The Psychiatric Clinician

The clinician's role today is as complex, as problematic, as conflicted, as is the society within which, and as part of which, he practices his profession. The very concept of professionalism is embattled. Its aridities and rigidities are exposed and decried. Its profound and subtle passion, its austere ethos, its aesthetics, its practical indispensability are devalued, disregarded, suspected.

The clinician does profess—must profess—i.e., must commit himself. He professes the role of informed, of expertly skilled helper, the role of practicing behavioral scientist, the role of the life-long student of individual human behavior.

The word "clinician" comes from the Greek *Khĭνη*, the word for bed, actually the couch in the temple of Aesculapius, where Greeks went to find a cure for their ills. The clinician's primary data, the data which inform his actions, are gathered at the bedside, directly from *a* patient. With this patient the clinician has a unique relationship, a one-to-one relationship, which has been the single most important, indispensable and unchanging condition for the clinician's therapeutic effectiveness since classical antiquity and before. Today's clinicians are a saving remnant of experts. The core of their expertness consists of an understanding of the two-person field, of the knowledge, the skill, the insight, the subtlety, the compassionate rationality with which the clinician can approach, can contact one other human being, beneficially. Departments of psychiatry have many tasks,

1

which grow in number each year. Their primary, basic task is the essential, crucial task of educating professional psychiatric clinicians —experts in the evaluation of individual human beings, in their behavior, their pathology, their therapeutic needs.

The role of the professionally skilled, participating observer with therapeutic intent, in a one-to-one relationship—that is the clinician's identity.

Man, viewed as a biological organism, can be studied from and understood at many different levels of organization, from the ecosystem to the level of intracellular biochemistry. Each student of human biology neglects at his peril levels of organization other than the one of his central interest and concern. But he contributes most by using as his vantage point *one* level where he takes his stand and from which he views the other levels—upward to greater, downward to lesser complexity—and how these other levels interact with and influence the area of his primary concern. The vantage point of the psychiatric clinician is that of the single individual as he moves within the fabric of his internal and external environment. The level of complexity from which the psychiatric clinician views human behavior will be that of the psychological level of organization of individual human beings. To utilize, to understand, to evaluate the data available from this vantage point he must become engaged with the objects of his study—who are at the same time his patients.

That term, too, has a long history: a patient—from the Latin "a person who undergoes action, a sufferer" (1). The passive mode in this definition is significant—it points to the most profound aspects of the patient-physician relationship. The patient's enforced passivity, his dependency on the physician, represents the most intractable problem, the most constant and provocatively demanding stress for the clinician and for the ethos he has had to create for his profession.

The clinical therapeutic tradition is old. It has diverse roots which have come together to inform the role of the clinician today. There are roots in magic, in religion, in shamanism—irrational roots; there are roots in the Hippocratic tradition of rational observation, based on the rejection of a concept of disease due to other than natural causes.

The healer's, the shaman's, the witch doctor's role is a central one in primitive cultures. It is often combined with that of political and/or religious leader. His potent therapeutic influence depends on his personal qualities, on his personal interaction with those who seek his help, in the role prescribed for him by his culture. "He may be the leader of the community, who functions as a safety valve and as a regulator of the psychic life of the clan. He lives under the permanent feeling of bearing a great responsibility." Since he is possessed by potent spirits over whom he also exerts a measure of control "the shaman is always careful when finding himself with other people . . . very often he becomes more or less isolated . . . he cannot refuse to assist his clansmen . . . the person attended by the shaman must not seek assistance from other shamans unless the shaman recommends it himself. So that the shaman gradually forms around himself a group of permanent clients. . . ." The shaman experiences a "call" early in life. His initiation, his training, engender great hardship and personal turmoil. "The preparatory period is compared to a long severe illness, the acquisition of inspiration to a recovery." "A good shaman ought to possess many unusual qualities but the chief is the power acquired by tact and knowledge to influence people around him" (2).

Modern psychiatry has as one of its tasks studying, understanding, teaching about, utilizing therapeutically the complementary interaction between this essential aspect of the clinician's role and his activities as a rational, scientific, consciously skillful practitioner of the healing arts.

This attitude of objectivity, knowledgeability, scholarliness and dedication to truth no less than his magical attributes maintained the physician's prestige and therapeutic effectiveness in Western society for 2500 or more years—in spite of his almost total lack of an effective technological or pharmaceutical armamentarium and his nearly total ignorance of human biology till the middle of the 19th century.

Hippocrates demands of the clinician:

1. "Hard, persistent, intelligent, responsible, unremitting labor in the sickroom, not in the library.
2. Accurate observation of things and events, selection guided by judgment born of familiarity and experience of the salient and the recurrent phenomena and their classification and methodical exploitation.
3. The judicious construction of a theory." (3)

Henderson sums it up: "The physician must have intimate, habitual, intuitive familiarity with things; he must have systematic knowledge of things and he must have an effective way of thinking about things" (3).

Aesculapius is a God. Hygeia (prevention) and Panacea (treatment) are his daughters—mythological figures, both. But, the service of Aesculapius, the wooing of his daughters, demands of us, as Hippocrates tells us, a commitment to rationality and to a concept of medicine that is based on our knowledge of the natural sciences— an ideal stated 2500 years ago and only beginning to be realized since less than 100 years ago.

The Hippocratic tenets of medical science continue to be applicable today:

1. Well-being is influenced by all environmental factors.
2. Health is the harmony between environment, ways of life and man's nature.
3. There is a constant reciprocal influence between mind and body.
4. When the organism's equilibrium is disturbed use rational remedies.
5. Reverence for man and a strict code of ethics are basic requirements for the effective practice of medicine. (5)

The last point can be expanded further and leads us back to the affective, interpersonal, extra-rational roots of the clinician's role, without which even today the clinician lacks one of his most potent tools.

Hard work, correct observation, clear thinking, a devotion to the natural sciences—all necessary but not altogether sufficient. We add: involvement, availability, and the capacity to take action (6).

Involvement: The clinician's involvement is with one other individual. It requires closeness, a personal affective quality, and its control—its rationally determined timing and dosage, based not only on the patient's overt demands but on an understanding also of the patent's often contradictory, covert, actual needs.

A severely depressed, severely agitated woman, hospitalized, on first meeting you, who is to be her physician, says in a loud voice and with intense feeling: "It's you who are sick, not me. You're the crazy one who needs a psychiatrist."

Involvement—closeness and control—how to involve yourself with this? What does closeness mean for you, for her? What to control in her, within yourself? What does she want, what need that you can know and gratify—with words? "It hurts to be in need of help." "Right now, it would be easier to talk of me than of yourself." "It makes you mad to sit where you are sitting and me in the doctor's chair, in charge." "You're scared of your own thoughts and feelings, a little less so if you can see them in me—but what a bind you're in to need to see your helper as a mad man!" There are many other choices of response. All represent degrees of closeness and degrees of control—each choice determined by the patient's tolerance and your capacity for involvement and by your skill and experience in calculating and evaluating both.

Availability—some of this is obvious—to be there on time and at all times when you're needed, at odd times, too, when necessary, in spite of the conflict, the necessary compromise with your own needs, with the scale weighing just a little heavier on the side of the needs of the other. But availability has a more inward meaning, too—it refers to aspects of yourself being available to, open to the patient, without interference from your needs or wants or lacks. Your perceptions, your intuitions, your feelings to be accessible, flexibly available for the work of listening, of looking, of understanding, of responding—without reciprocation, without reward in kind.

And the capacity for action: to know that inaction is intervention, too! The capacity then to tolerate the knowledge that by virtue of your role, your professed role, you are in interaction—always acting, influencing, intervening, and almost always on the basis of insufficient, inadequate, incomplete, sometimes erroneous data. This you must learn to bear, and your developing skills, your accumulating knowledge, your accretion of clinical experience above all, help you to bear the stress of uncertainty and of imperfection, and gradually increase the level of your feeling of mastery. Your patients and the unending novelty of human misery, will surely keep you humble whenever you feel over-confident or excessively comfortable in the performance of your tasks.

Thus, then, the stance of the clinician: he works hard at the bedside. There he finds his primary data. He observes, accurately, carefully. So he can think about them he orders the phenomena. He uses, he exploits himself. He becomes involved, with a closeness which he controls for the patient's benefit, is available realistically, readily, punctually, with physical presence, and open perceptions, and with focused attention—and he acts with judgment born of experience and tempered by the constant presence of uncertainty.

The study of human behavior is what differentiates most clearly the study of human biology from the study of animal biology. J. Z. Young (7), an anatomist, states: "The biologist's question about man is, how does he get his living on the earth? . . . eating and walking are not the really important features of man . . . it is far more significant that he is a thinking creature . . . just these traits of what we commonly call man's mind are also his most peculiar and important biological characteristics. These are the features by which he gets his living. They are the very ones that should most attract our attention as biologists." To be a human biologist one "must be an accomplished interpreter of the human species, its mental physiology, cultural accomplishments, faculties of symbolic expression, genetic makeup, adaptive potential, psychological endowments and sociobiological situation" (8).

While no one can fulfill all these criteria, it is possible to strive towards them as an ideal, by adopting the attitude of a "Common Reader" in human biology, an attitude happily fostered by and able to flourish in the setting of medical education. Virginia Woolf borrows the idea of the common reader from Samuel Johnson. One can borrow it from her and rephrase it (9):

"The Common Reader in human biology is guided by an instinct to create for himself, out of whatever diverse insights he may come by, some kind of whole—a portrait of man, a sketch of his evolution, a theory of his species-specific behavior. Often with haste, often superficially, he snatches now at this review of the latest in genetics, now at that compendium of current theories of mind—so long as his purpose is served: to round out his search for a synthesis of that bewildering multitude of scientific fragments which some day may bring us closer to a more useful understanding of ourselves."

To be a physician, a practicing clinical psychiatrist, a psychoanalyst, and a clinical teacher: these combined roles define the limits of one kind of Common Readership. They point to the likely peaks in the profile of a literary diet as well as to its likely deficiencies. These roles also imply a firm basis of "uncommon" readership from which to survey the broader field, and in terms of which a teacher, a supervisor, can order his perceptions.

The psychiatric clinician who studies the data of human biology at the levels of complexity found at the psychological level of organization and beyond finds, aside from his intellectual limitations, another kind of limitation imposed on his objective understanding, even on his selection or identification of the data of human behavior. He shares this problem with all other behavioral scientists. For the clinician, especially, this problem is his cross and his special reward, his most intractable variable and his focus of interest, his most insidious source of practical and theoretical error and his most potentially powerful therapeutic weapon. It is his most potent stimulus for learning about himself and about the other; it is the problem of the participant observer.

Being a participant, therapeutically active observer in a human interaction adds other problems to the problems of methodology: problems of morality and of ethics and problems which are intensely personal. These affect the interaction itself, its form, its possibilities, its outcome. They affect also our understanding, our ordering of the data, our very capacity for perceiving the data, our modes of perception and our interpretations of what we see, hear and do.

The history of the behavioral and social sciences reflects these problems. Both supervisor and supervisee are well advised to keep in mind the historical perspective (10).

"The relation between facts and theories in discussing social problems was roughly the same for 2000 years. . . . One will find history and existing social life considered as simply a storehouse of examples to illustrate presumed truths" (11). The major social changes of the 19th century produced new ways of perceiving and theorizing about man's social behavior. "In no period of human knowledge has man ever become more problematic to himself than in our own days" (Scheler, cited by Cassirer) (12).

Increased physical mobility needed to be accompanied by greater psychological flexibility (14). This led to major changes in man's self-image and in his views about and perceptions of both the human and non-human environment. An unprecedented self-consciousness produced startling new beliefs, organized and articulated in the new sciences of society.

The definition of the essence of man ceased to be substantial and fixed and became instead functional (12). Man's outstanding characteristic now is not his physical or metaphysical nature but his work—or his works. "Humanity" is defined and determined by that system of human activities of which language, myth, religion, art, science and history are the constituents, all equally open for study and examination. These new views of man introduce— with delayed explosive, side-effects—the possibility of the compara- tive study and evaluation of cultures. We are confronted suddenly with the relativity of all standards of behavior. Humanity is not explained by man, but man by humanity (Comte)—in its utter variety and variability. A startling new insight: the social world of man is not known and, even more startling perhaps: nor is the private world of the individual. The doubts arising from such insights are not even primarily about established truths. They are even more ba- sic. The doubts are about facts, facts which so far had been taken for granted: the very facts of human existence and its organization. Hence, the intense need for the collection of more facts, *all* the rele- vant facts about social phenomena, about individual human beings. Our concern with facts, with data-gathering, remains our preoccupa- tion, at times our curse; our doubts about whether anyone is really telling it how it is, or even knows how, or whether it is even possible to do so, such doubts continue to plague us. The assertion so often heard today: "I'm telling it how it is," tries to hide the uncertainty we feel about the possibility of ever apprehending social reality.

The social sciences began to develop empirical, quantitative, policy- related methods of inquiry and a tradition of frank, comprehensive observation regardless of the subject matter studied. Terence's "Noth- ing human is alien to me" became the motto of professionals in- volved in the study of human behavior. It is a noble motto and is often cited as the basic tenet of the ethos of the behavioral scientist. It is curious that the context in which Terence uses the phrase is not so well remembered. In one of his comedies he puts it into the mouth of an old lecher who uses it to brag about his personal acquaintance with the practice of all varieties of human depravity— a fine example of the importance of context for the understanding of ascribed quotation and a somber hint at the potential problems involved in living and working by this motto.

For us, in the context of the study of human behavior, the motto remains valid as a prescription of attitude: all manifestations of human behavior are appropriate objects of study, of our honest and dispassionate scrutiny. Our main motive is understanding, our emo- tional set in this context, nonjudgmental and accepting. As the inscription reads above the door of Rabelais' Abbey of Theleme: "Let nothing be unknown to you."

The new social sciences and that branch of medicine which was to become modern psychiatry, though stemming from different traditions, have found much in common in their perceptions of mankind. Significant differences also remain—not only in subject matter but also in basic attitudes.

Brandishing their new tool, statistics, the social sciences began to focus with fascination on the study of population groups perceived as so different, so deviant from the group of observers as to appear at first hardly human. The new class of industrial workers was "discovered" to live under incredibly destitute conditions in the new industrial slums of the 19th century. At first these poor—and other population groups hitherto ignored—were seen as frightening, as exotic, as foreign, alien. But the data-gathering of the new sciences demanded contact, contact on a level much more holistic than did the techniques of the physical sciences. Contact was needed at the level of feeling, of behavior, of experience and this was possible only through human involvement with the objects of study. For these scientific and methodological demands a new set of professional attitudes had to emerge. These had to include the new political ethos emerging from the American and French revolutions: the rights of individuals—indeed the existence of individuals—and the belief-system of egalitarianism (10).

Sociology aspired to be "value-free" (in terms of the data collected) and it aimed for acts of "pure" perception. Society is to be understood in a disciplined way, clearly, objectively and without any attempt to judge what is or should be normative (13). The sociologist is "endlessly, shamelessly interested in the doing of men"—all kinds of men. Nothing is too sacred or too distasteful for his dispassionate inquiry. A value system that emphasizes basic scientific honesty, a non-judgmental, expectant, accepting attitude, openness of mind and catholicity of vision—these are common features of all the behavioral sciences, including psychiatry (13).

For a long time (and to some degree this is still so today) the major concern of the psychiatric physician was the problem of madness. During the Middle Ages madness was considered a vice (14). As such it led the procession of all the other human weaknesses—self-love, flattery, forgetfulness, sloth, sensuality, stupidity, indolence. (There are, incidentally, for all of these, today, cognate terms of diagnostic significance—narcissism for self-love, submissiveness for flattery, dementia for forgetfulness, psychomotor retardation for sloth, impulse disorder for sensuality, mental deficiency for stupidity, anhedonia for indolence.) In the middle ages, then, madness reigned supreme over all that is bad in man. The great era of confinement for the mad commenced in the 17th century when one out of every 100 Parisians was at one time or other incarcerated in what was called "L'Hôpital Général." This institution was, however, not devoted to medicine but to "order" and its director had quasi-absolute powers over the inmates. The great sin of the 17th century was sloth—"mendicancy and idleness are the source of all disorders"—hence, also of madness. Little distinction was made between the mad and the unemployed (15).

Since the mad were not perceived as sick, their condition was seen as evidence of the residue of animality in man which can be contained only through the use of discipline and brutality (15).

By mid-18th Century the concept of disease became attached to the phenomenon of madness but this is now coupled with the fear of sickness, that is, of contagion, of taint and of corruption. The physician became the guardian of the mad to protect others from infection, not to heal the mentally ill. Not until the late 19th Century do we locate the roots of madness in the individual life experience of the afflicted person. At this time, too, we cease to make a sharp, categorical distinction between the mad and the sane. The seeds of madness are in all of us it seems. A broad spectrum of idiosyncratically determined adaptive capacities to a complex social set is matched by an equally broad spectrum of possible maladaptive outcomes, now subsumed under the heading of psychiatric disorders (15). The mad are readmitted to the ranks of common humanity—with the result of unmasking the illusion of sanity among the rest of us: "Methinks everyone is a little mad, except me and thee," says the Quaker lady to her friend, "and sometimes I doubt a little about thee." "To behave as if we were in control is our most precious delusion" (15a). The realization that perhaps we are not the masters even in the house of our own mind was as traumatic a blow to man's self-image as were the insights of Copernicus who robbed us of our central place in the solar system and those of Darwin who deprived us of our biological uniqueness. Such was Freud's conception of the impact of his work.

Realization of the kinship between the mentally disturbed and the sane, the lack of any absolute distinction between them, required of the physician a new elaboration of the Hippocratic ethic.

If the exotic, the bizarre, the mad, the deviant are indeed not only like the rest of mankind but if even the physician is their conspecific ... The relationship, then, between such patients and those who would understand, serve, help them, this relationship would necessarily reflect their kinship. Do unto others ... becomes a therapeutic maxim!

It follows further that such a relationship needs to be voluntary and deliberate, and that the rule of confidentiality is basic, mandatory ethically, and indispensable therapeutically (16). The individuality and the autonomy of the other must be respected as if it were one's own—because it is entirely like one's own. Individuality, however, arouses curiosity, secrecy stimulates the desire for intrusion, confidentiality produces the temptation for startling disclosure. In all these areas the patient entrusts his vulnerability to the physician's restraint and the physician's therapeutic intent. The medium of the unifying factor for trust on the one hand, restraint on the other, is the therapeutic contract. This is the most important difference between the work of the physician and that of the social scientist who is not working as a physician.

Like the social scientist the physician is *dispassionate,* dispassionate in his search for truth, in his acceptance of all data of human behavior, in his contributions to man's knowledge about his own biology. Unlike the social scientist the physician is also *compassionate,* compassionate in his relationship to another and in his recognition of the other's needs which he must meet. And the physician is *passionate* in his fulfillment and his defense of the therapeutic contract. Here his extra-scientific ancestors must play a complementary role to his scientific forebears. The shamans, the witch doctors, the priests of Aesculapius, sometimes usefully, sometimes inappropriately, still speak through the physician of today. And if he does not let them speak—the patient may hear them anyway. Especially the psychiatrist of today offers equivalents for ancient, traditional relationships and rituals which have either disappeared in their ancient form or in that form have lost their efficacy (17). He involves himself in family concerns, in marriage, in divorce, in parent-child relationships, in madness and in deviancy. He is becoming more publicly visible, more vocal, more in demand and more involved. Public acclaim and personal ambition tempt him to confound his therapeutic role within the doctor-patient relationship with that of social engineer. He analogizes from the sick individual to the sick society and sees himself as the self- or community-appointed therapist for all. He allows himself to be viewed as *the* "expert" in all matters relating to manners, to mores, and to morals.

With the rest of his vocal colleagues in the behavioral sciences, indeed, in competition with them, he eagerly ranges, in his pronouncements, from drugs to sexual intercourse to the role of violence in our society and prescribes where he should, at most, inform. The physician, by virtue of his training, of his therapeutic intent and contract, is uniquely equipped to explore areas of behavior which arouse feelings of horror, terror, disgust, of guilt and shame, of pity and dismay in the general public. He is obliged to share his knowledge and his insights, and to use his privilege of entering into these forbidden regions to fashion new therapeutic tools with which to increase and expand for our times the potency of the ancient ethos of Hippocrates. But as a physician, to arrogate to himself the role of healer and saviour of society puts him in danger of losing his physicianhood and of turning into a mountebank.

If there is a dialectic tension between the disciplines of medicine and psychiatry on the one hand and those of the other behavioral sciences on the other, an equally strongly felt tension exists between the natural sciences and the behavioral sciences (which include medicine and psychiatry). The basic differences between these two large areas of human knowledge (18)—both aspects of human biology—call for different methods in the search for knowledge and for different criteria of evaluation of the results of that search. The major difference is in the different levels of complexity of the events under scrutiny.

The social and psychological sciences deal with highly complex constellations of highly complex events occurring in systems which are poorly or not at all isolated. Nor can they be isolated for study without altering the results of the study by destroying the system. In addition, such systems often display an infinite variability. The natural sciences, by contrast, can deal with isolated systems where controllable variables can be chosen for observation. None of the social sciences yet knows precisely which variables must be chosen and which can be safely neglected. If science "is nature refracted through human nature," social science is doubly so refracted. What may be a sufficient kind of explanation in a natural science world would be labeled as oversimplification in the behavioral sciences where explanation must be synthetic and multifactorial. Occam's razor tends to cut too deeply in the behavioral sciences. Here reductionism may not only threaten truth but life itself. Here scientific parsimony must always be leavened with a concern for the sufficiency or adequacy of reasons adduced for complex events. And who is to define what is adequate? Beck, in 1949, concludes that it is too soon to expect or even to be impatient for a Newton of the Behavioral Sciences. Twenty years later it is still too soon (18).

According to Warren Weaver (19), 17th Century science dealt with problems of organized simplicity, 19th Century science with problems of disorganized complexity. Our present century is preoccupied with problems of organized complexity requiring pattern vision and comparative techniques for their solution. And the solution will be worth nothing if we forget the human, the individual, the ideographic dimension, in its articulation.

The social scientist, uniquely, has as his mandate the study of the society which gave him this mandate and of which he is a member (20). Analogously, the psychiatrist has as his mandate the study of a member of that society, of which he is a *fellow*-member. His mandate is twofold—from the side of society and from the side of the patient—so his responsibility is twofold. Both the social scientist and the psychiatrist in all their activities inevitably intervene in, interfere with, the social process in which they are involved as participant observers. In turn each is himself changed by what he does. The broader social relation as much as the one-to-one interpersonal relation is altered by the very attempt to even define it. The very recognition and the identification of a human situation as a problem at once alters the situation—even before any intervention is attempted. In choosing what to describe and how to describe it we exercise not only clinical judgment but a judicial function—we are engaged in a moral as well as in an intellectual act. "Description is like taxation: the right to describe absolutely is the right to destroy absolutely." All human, indeed all biological events are multiply caused. Yet the limitations of our cognitive functions force us to select only one or a few of the multiple determinants for scrutiny. In multiply caused, patterned events the act of selecting for attention one cause before others is a matter of judgment (in the legal sense) since it implies the need for action aimed at that one cause. The "solution" found, the theoretical framework created on the basis of the finding, about human behavior changes the situation one attempts to understand, to order and to predict. Furthermore, the results of the explaining, ordering, theorizing, depend on the observer's own perceptual set, cultural background, life experience and unconscious needs. These in turn are altered by the outcome of one's investigations involving as they do the confrontation with other human beings—and so on in an infinite regress of reciprocal feedback. The construction of a theory of human behavior, then, subject as it is to scientific and intellectual rigor and the teaching of its application, also becomes an act of self-exploration and self-revelation. The communication of theory and technique and the acceptance of such communication, therefore, involve trust, love and the building of an interpersonal relationship between those who would teach such a theory and those who would be taught:

Those who teach—the supervisors, those who would be taught—the psychiatric resident

The psychiatric residency has changed in a number of major ways over the past 15 years. These changes have significantly, and detrimentally, affected the teaching and the learning of psychotherapy. The changes involve a number of complexly interrelated factors.

First of all, the resident population appears to be different. The quality of residents has not changed but both their preparation for and their anticipation of psychiatric training are different than they were a decade or two ago. Psychiatric undergraduate instruction in medical schools not only continues to be deficient generally, but appears to have deteriorated with the advent of greater emphasis on elective time in many schools. Psychiatric instruction seems to be increasingly perfunctory at the undergraduate level and many new residents, when they first arrive in a training program, are totally unsophisticated with regard to the psychological aspects of medicine. Repeated informal surveys indicate, for instance, that hardly any of them have ever read any of Freud's writings by the time they

start their training nor—in most instances—have they read anything else in the field of psychiatry. The new resident's view on and
expectations of what is essential in psychiatric training are exceed-
ingly vague and he confronts the increasingly sumptuous and varied
menu which is offered to him in the curriculum with little notion as
to what are the essential and basic nutrients. I fear that the con-
tinuously kaleidoscopically changing curriculum and a faculty highly
competitive for the resident's time don't help in making this matter
any clearer to the hapless beginner.

Because the field of psychiatry itself has changed and is continuing
to change with bewildering rapidity, a large number of topics and
subspecialties which were either minor or peripheral, which were side
issues or which did not even exist 15 years ago, have today become
full-fledged competing focal professional fields in their own right and
are squeezing out the last open hours of the residency curriculum.
"They have to have an adequate exposure to the courts," "I insist
on an adequate block of time in the community," "We are dreadfully
negligent in our instruction in psychopharmacology"—these are the
increasingly urgent, sometimes strident but usually valid battle
cries heard at meetings of curriculum committees.

How, in this clamor, to preserve, to foster the teaching of psychotherapy, to identify what is basic in such teaching, becomes a vexing
problem in curricular planning. This is a central issue in the preserva-
tion and furtherance of what entitles psychiatry to claim a distinct,
unique and essential place among the other medical disciplines.

Not only has the field of psychiatry expanded enormously in
recent years, the field of psychotherapy has done so also. A vast
array of psychotherapeutic modalities is available in each of which
a psychiatric resident, after his crammed three years, is supposed
to have some expertise: long term, short term, supportive, analytic-
ally-oriented, behavior, relaxation, hypnotic, active, reality, group,
family, role playing, psychodrama, encounter, sensitivity, marathon,
existential, etc., etc. Each has its advocate, each advocacy ranges
from "some experience is necessary in this technique" to "it's the
new thing, the best thing, the only thing."

Among all these therapeutic modalities one-to-one psychotherapy
is the core and essential one. Furthermore, the teaching, learning,
studying about and practicing of this modality in all its ramifications
are the most central, unique, essential and urgent concerns of a depart-

ment of psychiatry both in terms of its own discipline as well as in terms of its impact on the medical profession at large. "All its ramifications" includes such facets as attention to diagnostic evaluation of both pathology and strengths in their clinical, dynamic and ontogenic parameters. It includes the role of the psychotherapeutic ethos in all the other multiple and varied activities of the psychiatrist and the physician. It includes the understanding and the skillful use of intervention at the psychological level of organization in any and all medical situations.

To acknowledge that the curative potential of one-to-one psychotherapy, though often extremely potent, is equally often limited, uncertain, questionable, does not weaken this position: the psychiatrist is the logical custodian of the Hippocratic clinician's ancient concern with the ideographic approach to human behavior. The understanding of, the attention to, the individual, to the unique human being, his behavior, and his suffering is best and most uniquely advanced by the opportunity afforded the psychiatric physician, through the one-to-one psychotherapeutic situation, to study, to involve himself with, to help a fellow human being in his distress and to do so in a more than common sense manner. The psychiatric physician's insistence on his role as a saving remnant in this area may help prevent the increasing dehumanization of medicine, and may serve as a needed counterweight to the increasingly simplistic, shallow, mechanistic and reductionistic views of human behavior and the possibilities for its modification pervading our culture.

As psychiatric curricula over the last number of years have staggered through multiple changes, deletions, additions, corrections and painful re-examinations, focal attention to the teaching of one-to-one psychotherapy has diminished. Residents, however, express renewed interest in this area of their training and demand that faculty again perform its duties in this area more thoughtfully and less diffidently. The one-to-one tutorial continues to be among the most prized teaching experiences in the residency. It behooves us to attend once again, painstakingly, deliberately and with the knowledge that this is one of our basic, essential tasks, to the design and organization of a both didactic and practical, as well as a graduated teaching program in individual psychotherapy throughout the three years of the residency, a program which can serve as a core discipline for psychiatry in the 1970's. The backbone of such a program is one-to-one supervision of the resident's clinical work.

REFERENCES

1. The American College Dictionary, Random House, N. Y. 1947.
2. G. ROHEIM, *The Origin and Function of Culture.* Nervous and Mental Disease Monographs #69, N. Y. 1943.
3. L. J. HENDERSON, *The Study of Man.* Univ. of Penn. Press, 1941.
4. ——, *The Fitness of the Environment,* Beacon Press, Paperback, 1958.
5. R. DUBOS, *Man, Medicine and Environment.* F. A. Praeger, N. Y. 1968.
6. M. L. ADLAND, personal communication.
7. J. Z. YOUNG, *Doubt and Certainty in Science.* Oxford, 1951.
8. P. RITTERBUSH, Review of Adler, Von Bertalanffy. *Science,* 160:57, 1968.
9. VIRGINIA WOOLF, *The Common Reader,* Vol. 2, p. 1, Harcourt, Brace & Co., N. Y. Harvest Paperback, 1953.
10. H. D. LASSWELL, *The Human Meaning of the Social Sciences,* Ed. D. Lerner, Meridian Books, Inc. 1959.
11. D. GLAZER, *The Rise of Social Research in Europe,* in *Human Meaning of Social Sciences,* Ed. D. Lerner, Meridian Books, Inc. 1959.
12. E. CASSIRER, *An Essay on Man.* Doubleday Anchor, 1953.
13. BERGER, *Invitation to Sociology.* Humanistic Perspective, Anchor Doubleday, 1963.
14. D. LERNER, *Social Science: When-Whither,* in *Human Meaning of Social Sciences,* Ed. D. Lerner, Meridian Books, Inc. 1959.
15. M. FOUCAULT, *Madness and Civilization,* Mentor, November, 1967.
15a. HERBERT BLAU, *Relevance: The Shadow of a Magnitude,* Daedalus, Summer, 1969.
16. E. A. SHILS, *Social Inquiry and the Autonomy of the Individual,* in *Human Meaning of Social Sciences,* Ed. D. Lerner, Meridian Books, Inc., 1959.
17. L. L. FRANK, *Psychology and the Social Order,* in *Human Meaning of Social Sciences,* Ed. D. Lerner, Meridian Books, Inc., 1959.
18. L. W. BECK, The Natural Science Ideal in the Social Sciences. *The Scientific Monthly,* Vol. XLVIII: 386-394, 1949.
19. C. KLUCKHOHN, *Common Humanity and Diverse Cultures,* in *Human Meaning of Social Sciences,* Ed. D. Lerner, Meridian Books, Inc., 1959.
20. J. SEELEY, *The Americanization of the Unconscious,* Int. Sci. Press, 1967.

2
Philosophy of Supervision: A Critical Review

   . . . we need not take every desire to learn at its conscious face value. It is good to be wise as it is to be healthy and wealthy. But we must remember that there exists a very widespread fantasy that heaven lay about us in our infancy and that then we were omnipotent and omniscient. The world and our knowledge of it was intuitively *a priori* graspable, finite, though unbounded. When we are proved otherwise than omnipotent and omniscient, there is resentment, followed by an effort through magical, real, or part-magical part-real, means to restore and to repair the gaps and lesions in this primal feeling. Freud had this in mind when he remarked on the three blows delivered to narcissism by Copernicus, Darwin and himself; and Alexander has pointed out that all three led to the efforts at repair which we know as scientific method.

                                     —*Bertram D. Lewin* (1)

   L'art, c'est moi; la science, c'est nous.
                                       —*Claude Bernard*

   Forsan et haec olim meminisse iuvabit.
                                           —*Vergil*

   The psychiatrist's identity—his appropriate skills and functions—is beleaguered today from many quarters, both within and without the field of psychiatry. Despite the disparity of the conflicting views regarding the proper role of the modern psychiatrist, there remains a consistent opinion, shared even by the most dissident, that the "core" of the psychiatrist's identity is his work as an individual psychotherapist (2, 3, 4, 5, 6, 7, 8). There is equally unusual unanimity in the opinion that the cornerstone of the education of the psychiatrist is his clinical supervision: "To all workers in the field, the supervisory phase occupies a central position" (9). "Clinical supervision is the keystone of graduate psychiatric training. Upon the clinical supervisor rests the heavy responsibility of coordinating and integrating the cumulative experiences of the resident into a useful whole . . . dynamically oriented training in psychiatry requires emphasis upon supervision as a cardinal teaching method" (10).

The GAP report of 1955 reflects the traditional tripartite categorization of supervisory focus: "Focus in teaching dynamic psychiatry may be patient-centered, process-centered, or therapist-centered. . . . The following factors may determine the choice of supervisory methods: (1) The beliefs and abilities of the supervisor. (2) The role or function the supervisor fills. (3) The needs and purposes of the hospital. (4) Personality differences of residents. (5) The place of each resident in the training program" (10).

This chapter reviews the literature primarily devoted to the supervision of psychiatric residents, including discussions of psychoanalytic supervision whenever these are relevant. Also, various issues in supervision are surveyed, as they are focused upon the basic elements of the supervisory situation: (a) therapist; (b) supervisor; (c) context (including patient). Several programs and innovations in supervision are reviewed, and a rationale for the supervisory program in psychiatric education is proposed.

I.   MAJOR REVIEWS AND STUDIES

Among the training centers and individuals who have made exceptional contributions to the literature on supervision, pre-eminent reference must be given to Ekstein and Wallerstein at the Menninger Foundation; Fleming and Benedek at Michael Reese in Chicago; Semrad and his colleagues at Boston; Tarachow, in New York; and Rosenbaum, Levine, and Ornstein at Cincinnati.

A. *Reviews*

In 1966, Nathan Schlessinger (11) reviewed the literature on supervision of psychotherapy, focusing on four "essential" issues: "(1) What kind of data are most suitable for supervision? (2) Is supervision a didactic or a therapeutic experience? (3) What is the nature of the supervisory process? (4) What are the countertransference problems in supervision?" Regarding the issue of data, he remarked the distinction in points of view espoused by Kubie—in which the accurate tape recording of the interview is perceived as the primary data—as opposed to Ekstein and Wallerstein's position that "teaching methods based on mechanical recordings do not lend themselves as well to a dynamic learning relationship." Schlessinger agrees with DeBell that there is room for compromise between these positions, depending upon differential needs, and upon various purposes in supervision. The major focus of Schlessinger's review is a consideration of the classical controversy in the literature regarding supervision perceived as "teaching or therapy." He contrasts the position taken by Ekstein and Wallerstein with that of Tarachow (12, 13), and describes the Ekstein-Wallerstein position as "the opinion that supervision is a teaching-learning experience and must be distinguished from therapy." Their emphasis is on learning process and self awareness as they relate to therapy, and they focus on the resident's problems with the patient and the supervisor. They point out that what the resident sees and presents about the patient often parallels comparable problems he experiences in supervision. In contrast, Tarachow "proposes as his basic rule of supervision that it should be instruction in terms of the needs and problems of the patient as expressed in the specific clinical phenomenon of the patient. . . . Tarachow emphasizes the greatest caution in openly focusing on any problem of the resident." Schlessinger proposes a resolution of these "two extreme views"; however, he later modulates this polarization, recognizing that "the extreme positions presented here are somewhat compromised if one examines the case examples offered by the authors, for in practice the methods are not so pure."

Schlessinger adopts Fleming and Benedek's compromise, "First, by viewing supervision as a hierarchy of supervisory tasks over an extended time, and two, by viewing the supervisor not as a teacher or therapist, but as a person in whom the qualities entering into the two roles are fused and used according to the specifics of the situation, i.e. supervisory skill" (14). Schlessinger feels that the listing of supervisory tasks in hierarchical form by Fleming and Benedek is "self sorting" in that "some tasks lend themselves more to a didactic approach, while some approach therapy in the delicate effort to encourage self knowledge and self observation as a means of understanding the patient's productions and the therapeutic process. That these tasks or the relative emphasis placed upon them may be spread over a period of time according to the needs of a particular resident is apparent."

In his discussion of "a special feature of the supervisory process," Schlessinger remarks upon the phenomenon which has been noted by many supervisors, i.e., "that the resident often enacts some behavior of the patient in the supervisory session." He feels that "there is a range of behavior from transient identification to more chronic manifestations stirred up by the patient's conflicts and enacted in the supervisory relationship. . . . The attitudes toward the phenomenon range from helping the resident with reality testing . . . to confrontation where a shared problem interferes with appropriate therapy, to regarding the identification as a necessary ingredient in the therapy. Perhaps this element of the process may also be denied or deliberately disregarded in an approach like Tarachow's." Next, Schlessinger reviews the issue of countertransference in the supervisor, recognizing that there is also in this regard a spectrum of attitudes on the part of supervisors, in some cases even where the process may be promoted as a conscious goal." Again, Schlessinger emphasizes the necessity for awareness on the part of the supervisor of the variety of factors impinging upon the supervision, including his own reactions, and cites the work of Kapp and Ross (15) who "experimented with imagery in response to dreams reported by a patient in order to gain insight into countertransference reactions when the therapy was blocked."

Daryl E. DeBell (16) categorizes his review of the psychoanalytic supervisory literature into eight major areas:

1. The purpose and function of supervision
2. The controversy over therapy versus teaching
3. Methods and procedures
4. When to start supervision

5. Selection of cases for supervision
6. Special problems and dangers of supervision
7. Study of the supervisory process (research)
8. Selection and training of supervisory analysts

DeBell raises several incisive questions, in his discussion, about specific themes in the literature. Of particular interest are his questions about the source and selection of patients, and whether or not cases should be "tailored to fit the candidate's problems." Also, related to selection, is the issue "whether or not it was desirable for the patient to know that his analyst was being supervised. It appears to me to be inconceivable that it would be desirable as a routine invariable procedure." (In view of the oft mentioned importance of the establishment of an explicit "contract" between therapist and patient, it would also appear self contradictory that the patient is not party to the important fact of supervision as a dimension of his treatment situation. This is not to say that the issue needs to be any more emphasized in the original contract with the patient (nor any less) than would be references to tape recording and/or video taping. At our clinic, the supervisor's presence at the initial interview communicates the fact of supervision to the patient.)

Among the other issues which DeBell discusses in his section "Selection of Cases" is the difficulty in deciding upon "suitable cases": "The usual assumption is that an easily analyzable case (usually a case of hysteria) is ideal, but this may not be a tenable assumption." Knapp et al. (17) reported a bimodal distribution of hysterical cases which indicates that as a group they resemble the little girl with the curl in the middle of her forehead, "When they are good they are very, very good; and when they are bad, they are horrid." These authors also raise the question of the meaning of "suitable." There are "two distinctly different goals involved in the selection of cases for supervised analysis. . . . First, cases are selected with respect to the procedure in question, i.e. supervised analysis . . . on the other hand, we wish to provide the learning analyst with an optimal opportunity to have a learning experience. It is not probable that the same case will satisfy both requirements to the same degree." These authors also suggest that obsessional patients might be a better choice than hysterical patients, because of their "somewhat more consistent favorable response to supervised analysis." Also

DeBell remarks the perenial problem of "the dearth of suitable patients for supervised analysis."

Reviewing "special difficulties" involved in the supervisory situation, DeBell alludes to the series of articles devoted to the dangers of the misuse of the supervisory position for narcissistic purposes (18, 19, 20, 21, 22, 23, 24, 25). Among the difficulties listed are "disciple hunting" (26); conflict among supervisors' theoretical positions (27). He also reiterates the disagreement between those who would perceive supervision as primarily an interactional task between supervisor and supervisee (Ekstein) and those who perceive it as more of a learning experience with the patient primarily the focus, so that utilization of mechanical aids is particularly appropriate.

"Research and study" of the supervisory process, according to DeBell, has been almost absent from the literature. He reports on the results of the responses of education committees of various Institutes to questions from the Committee on Faculty (of which Kubie was chairman) in the Rainbow Report (4), and noted that only three education committees replied to Kubie's suggestion regarding recording of analytic sessions and the relevant supervisory hours. "From Los Angeles came the statement about the technique of supervision: 'We have no experience with recording devices and most of our members are against it.' And regarding research: 'The supervisory session is essentially a teaching experience and should not be a research experience. Some students and teachers would not object to being audited or recorded, others do object.' Of the other respondents, one (Southern California) indicated only that a study group on the problem of supervision had been started, and Western New England responded with 'a note of caution: here (when dealing with supervised work), as in other cases, research to develop standards (with the unfortunate connotation of uniformity) is urged along with a tendency to ignore the complex variability and the many intangibles of the supervisory situation. The supervision of a controlled case might be described as the psychoanalysis of a psychoanalysis. It presents ever changing and changeable factors: the supervisor, the candidate, their interrelationship, the patient, and the interrelationship of the patient and candidate. This is a complex context within which to conduct a study of supervision. . . . The danger confronting such studies lies in an *a priori* emphasis on the ideal of literal and therefore static concordance.'"

Concerning the training and selection of supervisory analysts, DeBell states that there is no published work dealing exclusively with this subject, and only a few references to it (3, 4). Lewin and Ross had reported some efforts to instruct the supervisor, noting Fleming as "presenting tape recordings of supervisory hours to a group of training analysts for study and discussion. They also report sporadic attempts to have new supervisors audit the supervisory sessions of experienced supervisors, but they indicate that there is not much enthusiasm for this procedure. A modification of this has been tried by Mahler, with much success. As they describe it, she sits in on supervisory sessons conducted by a junior colleague. Evidently the position of the junior supervisor is more satisfying when he is active than when he is merely a passive auditor." DeBell also recognized that most of the "training of supervisors" has been conducted by means of seminar discussions of supervision by groups of supervisors, pointing out that "such discussions provide a useful learning experience for all participants, but there must be a differential advantage to the junior members."

B. *Studies*

1. *Ekstein-Wallerstein* (12)

In 1958 Ekstein and Wallerstein (12) published a pioneer monograph on supervision which "grew out of a ten-year collaborative experience" within the Menninger School of Psychiatry. The original purposes of their work were to provide "a vehicle for the teaching of psychotherapy to students in the clinical psychology training program; for the teaching of the skills of supervision to a supervisory group of staff psychiatrists . . . and for the systematic study, by a workshop method, of the theory and technique of supervision itself." The settings in which their tasks placed them were the postgraduate training of psychology trainees and of residents in psychiatry at the Winter VA Hospital, and the Topeka State Hospital. In their preface, they point out that their report of supervision of psychotherapy is to be perceived not as a textbook of psychotherapy, nor as a sociological text, though they consider the "administrative" context in which

supervision takes place. Their discussion is successively focused upon:
(1) the training setting, (2) beginning phase, (3) learning process,
and (4) end phase.

The authors schematize their view of supervision according to a
model which they call "the clinical rhombus," a four sided geometric
figure whose points are labeled therapist, patient, administrator,
supervisor; the interactional lines between these four points are perceived as the total "psychological situation with its inferred human
relationships. . . . The personal aspects of this clinical rhombus will
be experienced by each of the participants in a different way, since
each of them—student, supervisor, patient and administrator—has a
different place in the hierarchy of interrelationships. We are talking
not simply about the variety of human relationships which exist
among four people, but about those stratifications of the relationships
which reflect the different functions that the participants carry. . . .
As the student in his corner faces the other three corners of his clinical
world, he confronts three kinds of problems which, we hope to
demonstrate, are but external representations of typical internal
situations."

In their discussion of the administrator or administration, Ekstein and Wallerstein emphasize their importance in setting a context
and an ideology, which may at times conflict with the purposes and
goals of supervisor, patient and therapist. Their concept of the ideal
administrator is a person who would provide an ideal balance between
total separation and extremely close contact with those in his administrative setting. Brief mention is made of the fact that the administrator himself is by necessity functioning within an institutional
context, which itself may be at odds with the four major actors in the
supervisory situation.

In their discussion "Training for Research," the authors construct
"a hypothetical, ideal professional community," pointing out that
training and research functions may appear as dichotomized. In the
ideal system, the type of professional training which permits its students a range of choice is perceived as ideal, though basic to that
ideal is the concept that total freedom of choice would be the absence of any inherent value system. "To be a researcher is not necessarily better than to be a clinician nor the reverse. . . . The supervisor's goal should be to help each student explore and define the
degree of choice available to him." Difficulties are sometimes encoun-

tered in students' reactions to research: "There may indeed be some students for whom research constitutes a slogan under whose banner they can legitimately defy established methods. . . . There is another group of students . . . who can not allow themselves to become committed to a therapeutic method; they can not trust it nor can they really trust themselves or their teachers. Such students, the Don Juans of psychotherapy, try one method after the other . . . enthusiastic at first and then abandon the method in disgust."

To Ekstein and Wallerstein, the supervisory process itself "ideally utilized, will constitute for the student a form of self discovery, a constantly critical evaluation of what he is doing, of what he is taught, and will move him toward those internal commitments he needs in order to learn the use of psychotherapeutic techniques." As he develops the capacity for independent psychotherapeutic work, "he should be ready for serious research work if he so desires." The authors urge that supervisors, during the process of supervision, encourage their supervisees to develop any special capacities or interests in research they may have. They are concerned about the timing of such work, noting that the first criterion is "a sufficient level of technical skill so that he knows well the problems of the area of research, and the methods that he is experimentally deviating from." A further issue in the development of research interests is the administrative structure, which should not "stifle research creativity." The authors feel that certain training centers, as opposed to "the more usual academic setting in which a variety of theoretical schools of thought can well be represented," ought not attempt to be eclectic: "Imagine the kind of problems that would arise if patients in the same clinical setting were in fact treated partly by psychoanalytically trained therapists and partly by Rogerian nondirective therapists. Competing schools of thought in our field must therefore develop their individual clinical settings." Though it appears to be an ideal training program which proposes to teach the young therapist a variety of methods, it is "actually unfeasible and nihilistic in its effect. It stems we believe from ignorance about the nature of training for psychotherapeutic work."

In "The Professional Identity of the Psychotherapist," the authors draw attention to what has become an increasingly debated issue. Discussing Kubie's paper (28) they agree that there is some value in defining psychotherapy as a profession, but do not perceive that it is "likely to be soon achieved." (However, the movement persists: A recent addition to the much publicized debate between proponents of the "medical model" and those who feel psychotherapy is primarily a separate enterprise purports to demonstrate that there exists a functional "fifth profession" (i.e. psychotherapy), by means of a series of questionnaires designed to emphasize the commonalities rather than the differences between the various professional disciplines (29) which practice psychotherapy. A questionnaire sample from three major metropolitan areas—New York, Chicago and Los Angeles—showed that 4,300 psychotherapists were "startlingly similar in terms of cultural origin, social class, career mobility, religious background, political affiliations, influences on their choice of profession and influences on their choice of a specialty.")

The next major section is devoted to the "beginning phase" of supervision, and deals with the importance of outlining the "rules of the game" for the supervisory interaction, which is also to be perceived as operating within the structure of the institutional setting. Various issues must be discussed at the outset: the arrangement of the mutually convenient appointment times, the selection of a suitable patient and so forth. In this first confrontation, typically, the supervisee will begin to express his disappointment about "unhappiness over things that are not going quite as well as he had hoped and expected." Early enthusiasm for the therapeutic enterprise is already beginning to wane, as the student is not immediately given the magical gifts he wishes for. The pattern of the first interview of supervision, "not unlike the first dream which the analysand brings to the analyst, and which reveals the core of the neurosis, may reveal the way in which the student will go about learning and at the same time opposing necessary change." The student's behavior is such that it leaves "very few choices to the supervisor," that is, the supervisor must "fit in" with many of the "givens" of his supervisee, certainly at the outset of supervision. (This parallels the challenge facing the therapist with his patient.)

The major section, "The Learning Process," discusses: first, the relationship between supervisor and student under the rubric "problems about learning," and that between therapist and patient under "learning problems," and finally, the relationship between supervisor and student, and therapist and patient, perceived as "the parallel process." Special problems are analyzed, such as "the psychology of emergencies," followed by a discussion of the "supervision versus psychotherapy dilemma."

Ekstein and Wallerstein believe that "the supervisory process embodies two major purposes. One is to maintain the organization standard of clinical performance through the knowledge (and supervision) of the nature and the quality of the professional service. The other is to help the student therapist toward the acquisition of increased professional skill. . . . The major obstacle to the smooth growth of psychotherapeutic sensitivity and competence . . . is the mobilization during the process of learning of idiosyncratic patterns that determine the way in which a given individual learns. . . . These 'learning problems' encompass the whole complex of ways of acting and responding within the psychotherapy situation. . . ." Supervision, then, is necessarily focused on "the nature of the difficulties in the therapy resulting from a therapist-patient interaction. . . . The area and range of change sought . . . is different," in the case of the patient and therapist. In the case of the patient there is an entire range of "personal problems" which may become "grist for the psychotherapeutic mill." For the new therapist, the change which is sought is "limited to one area, that of the manner of the use of one's self in the psychotherapeutic relationship. . . ." However, even in that narrow area the change desired may be "equally farreaching and deep."

Ekstein and Wallerstein distinguish between "problems about learning" and "learning problems." They perceive that learning problems may be "the predisposition to react in a particularly patterned way toward the patient," as opposed to issues in the relationship between supervisor and therapist which are "problems about learning." The authors explicitly state their belief that "in order to do certain types of psychotherapy (not psychoanalysis), personal therapy is not an essential concomitant or prerequisite—except in such cases where an individual has both "learning problems" and "problems about learning." The supervisory process itself undertakes "to offer help with the learning problems and the problems about learning as they unfold, "and is predicated upon the capacity of the individual supervisor to make effective alterations in his professional self, without necessarily significantly changing his personal self. The two are not necessarily parallel." The authors emphasize that "the problem about learning is not only to be seen as an obstacle on the pathway to increased professional skill, it is rather the very road the student and teacher have undertaken to travel together toward their common goal." Among other difficulties encountered in this phase is the classical resistance in the supervisee's claim that he needs "therapy," rather than supervision, since "supervision does not go far enough."

In the chapters regarding learning problems and problems about learning, the authors have described and illustrated what many observers of supervision have labeled "the learning alliance," and the phenomenon of the "parallel process" which takes place between the supervisor and the student and the therapist and the patient. (This experience, which is often quite astonishing to beginning supervisors, has been well described by Searles (30) and Arlow (31), among others.)

Discussing the psychology of emergencies, Ekstein and Wallerstein illustrate the need for the supervisor to "maintain the environment which can provide for open communication" with a vignette from Bernfeld (32). An acquaintance one night urgently phoned Dr. Bernfeld, asking to see him as soon as possible, which he arranged for the next morning during office hours. As the friend arrived, he "sat down in the office, and in a leisurely way began to talk about the weather, a picture on the wall, in every way giving an impression entirely different from that transmitted over the telephone. . . . Dr. Bernfeld was puzzled and did not quite know what to say as he compared the memory of the call with the person chatting with him at the moment. Since there was a little too much draft in the room, he got up and closed the door, which by chance had been left open. . . . As he sat down again, he noticed that the behavior of the other person changed suddenly. He looked with relief at the closed door and with renewed insistence wondered whether he could borrow $50 from his friend." The manner in which the supervisor meets emergencies and crises is particularly important, and encompasses all aspects of the "clinical rhombus." The supervisor is well warned to consider all these aspects in any response to a "crisis."

Analogizing with the game of chess (quoting Freud's reference), the authors note how important the middle game of supervision is in terms of its individualized qualities. They observe that the beginning and end game strategies are somewhat generalizable, but that the middle game of supervision, as in psychotherapy, is almost infinite in its variable complexities. This area constitutes "the major bulk of the actual work" of supervision. Specific examples from their own experience illustrate some of the "turnings" in the ways of supervision.

Regarding the classic dichotomy "supervision versus psychotherapy," Ekstein and Wallerstein delineate "essential differences" between these processes. Preliminarily, they cite Bertram Lewin's (33) discussion of the various uses to which the method of free association can be put: "There are doubtless many other purposes that free association might be made to serve." Among those mentioned are: "1. literary creation; 2. psychological science; 3. mystical experience; 4. ethical and philosophical guidance or inspiration; 5. therapy. As a drug is only *materia medica* in itself, and variously utilizable for experiment or therapy or pleasure, so are free associations capable of varied employment. They can be elaborated, superseded, used analogically for moral illumination, or permitted to lead to buried memories, according to the interests and intentions, conscious or unconscious, of the self observer." This same kind of distinction holds true, as well, for the essential difference between supervision and psychotherapy. Ekstein and Wallerstein recognize clearly that the *contract* is the fundamental basis for the distinction. The uses to which any skill and knowledge may be put are varied. The issue essentially is whether the parties to the contract have agreed upon the use to which any expertise is to be put. (In the social life of psychiatrists, the universal experience, on being introduced, is to hear the partially serious question "Are you going to analyze me?" from those who are, as the supervisee is, concerned about the non-explicit levels of the relationship.)

Concerning the "definitiveness" of both supervision and psychotherapy, the authors note "we are no longer surprised that a psychotherapeutic experience cannot be considered final and that frequently out patients and also we as therapists need to go back into further treatment. The same may be true for the learner. He may need to go back into supervision again for a new experience of growth." One of the interferences with the post graduate psychiatrist's utilization of further "help" is his apprehension or prejudice regarding "the nature of helping. . . . The teachers of psychotherapy should preferably be people who are identified with a philosophy in which the true helper has humility rather than power motives toward the helping process. Such humility is a part of genuine self-acceptance, the basic ingredient without which the best of techniques will not bear fruit."

In "The End Phase," Ekstein and Wallerstein review the utilization of recordings, and the problem of evaluation and selection. They believe (with Fleming and Benedek) that mechanical devices may well be of use, but that they are not "the whole truth," nor is the goal of a totally accurate recreation of the therapy hour the primary baseline for supervision.

With respect to the evaluation of therapists, "it is not possible . . . to develop a structured learning situation in which many people are trained that is so flexible that it can adjust to every given individual need, or to any given wish expressed by the student or the supervisor. Any structural arrangement will impose certain limits which will perhaps preclude training certain individuals who might be successfully trained elsewhere. Any clinical organization will have to stand for certain regulations which might make it impossible to use certain teachers who cannot fit into its basic structure and philosophy . . . the task of the supervisor then is to work through a given structure, rather than in spite of it or against it. This too is the task of the student."

The authors describe the technique of evaluation and selection at the Menninger center which involved the writing of "process notes" independently, following the supervisory hour, by both therapist and supervisor. They conducted an experimental test of their evaluation procedure in which the students selected two supervisory sessions from their process records for comparative study. Both the supervisor and student independently studied the material selected, and, once again independently, wrote an evaluation of the supervised work as reflected in the interview. These evaluations were then studied and discussed in a joint evaluation conference, "the result of which would be a final summary, prepared by both together, in which an attempt would be made to integrate the two evaluations and to formulate recommendations to the administration on the future training status of the students." The result was, as might be predicted, an exhibition of parallel processes which had already taken place in the supervisory sessions. Both negative and positive findings were in evidence, but one of the most rewarding was the experience in the final conference "of togetherness, of having said the same thing . . . which was often surprising to both the supervisor and the student." This method of evaluation presented in microcosm one of the avowed goals of supervision, which is integration of various aspects of the learning experience.

The evaluation process also served as a selection vehicle, in which the issue of "suitability for psychotherapy" is raised. The correlation of supervision with process notes, and the administrative function of the "psychotherapy supervision committee" avoids many of the pitfalls possible to training centers where these supervisory functions are either fragmented or not in existence. In addition, Ekstein and Wallerstein perceived that there is a natural development from "supervision to consultation . . . the latter is a form of advanced training and practice which can be introduced at a time when the practitioner of psychotherapy knows his basic job, when he can do independent work, but needs occasional help. Much later, perhaps, even consultation may cease, to be replaced by the occasional sharing of clinical experiences with other experienced colleagues who are partners in clarification, rather than supervisors or consultants." (Compare this with the feelings expressed in the papers by Kolb (34) and by Regan and Small (35).)

Following "graduation," Ekstein and Wallerstein envisage the development of the psychiatrist as moving toward that of a staff member, in which the cycle is repeated, as "he will then suddenly find himself in a position where he repeats the total training process in reverse order. He will be confronted with the anxieties of the young teacher, and will have to learn to identify himself in a new way with his profession, for which he has selected himself and for which he was selected to the evaluative training process we have been discussing."

2. Fleming and Benedek (14)

Fleming and Benedek have compiled an impressive distillation of their years of study and research in the work of psychoanalytic supervision. Following an historical review of supervision, they explain their view of psychoanalytic learning as "experiential," and describe their supervisory project, with specific attention to selected details from many hours of supervision of two psychoanalytic candidates as they treated four cases. They divide the supervisory process (as did Ekstein and Wallerstein) into initial, middle, and end phases, and then discuss the evaluation of the supervisee.

The authors begin with an analysis of the classic "dilemma of the supervisor . . . the double function which faces all clinical teachers," and for which each supervisor is forced to find some solution. They note that supervisors may stress the instructional aspect of teaching, or become so patient-oriented as to "become the analyst of the patient," or role-limited, in that he continually focuses upon the student's "blind spots for countertransference," and confuses "therapeutic with teaching objectives." Fleming and Benedek studied recordings of the supervisory interactions which they had with two of their students at different stages of professional development, and were both surprised and reassured at their considerable consensual validation in many fundamental areas, and were impressed also with "their empathic communications" as they read the transcripts of their material.

Historically, formal psychoanalytic supervision began with its "invention" by Eitingon in the early 1920s at the Berlin Institute. Benedek records her own memories of the early days of that Institute, and its training methods. The early concept of supervision was one in which the supervisor as a clinician focused primarily on the treatment of the patient and on his student only as an intermediary. Later (after 1925), supervision depended "on the student's positive transference to his teacher, on his devotion to psychoanalysis and obligation to his patients." Balint (36) termed this kind of teaching "super ego training." Following various debates about the function of the "Analysen-Kontrolle" and its variations, the conference on education in 1946 began a continuing study of the issue of training in psychoanalysis. In 1957, the "Revised Minimal Standards" stated didactic goals for supervision, including the aims of the supervisor: "1. To instruct the student in the use of the psychoanalytic method; 2. to aid him in the acquisition of therapeutic skill based upon an understanding of the analytic material; 3. to observe his work and determine how fully his personal analysis has achieved its aim; 4. to determine his maturity and stability over an extended period of time." Reviewing the panel discussions of the American Psychoanalytic Association of 1955 and 1956 on the subject of supervision, and their attempt to formulate a general goal of supervision, Fleming and Benedek point out that "such a task is an interminable process," though a necessary one.

Psychoanalytic learning is described as "experiential," and primarily dependent upon the therapist's experience of his own therapy, following which, his phases of development include "identification (didactic learning); theoretical knowledge (usually by means of clinical conferences) and on-the-job training (the practice of analysis under supervision).

Recalling the classical injunction for continued self analysis by the postgraduate analyst (citing a paper by Maria Kramer (37)) Fleming and Benedek observe that the primary obstacle to continued learning is "the inevitable resistance," and emphasize that the self analytic processes which proceed "more automatically" in an experienced analyst require the assistance of the supervisor in the trainee's early experience, so that the supervisor serves as a catalyst for the never ending process of self analysis.

Describing the methods of their study of supervision, Fleming and Benedek point out that "the investigator is called upon to empathize with the patient, the therapist, and the total supervisory process." For this task, they developed a method which allowed them to keep in focus the goal of their project, which was to identify and understand the process of communication rather than evaluate the content in microscopic fashion. Although their psychoanalytic training tended to keep them focused on the individuality of experience, they were able to borrow conceptual models from others for a larger view of their study: particularly they acknowledge the assistance of the work of Lennard (38) and of Bales (39) which added "a framework of social interaction theory and problem solving concepts," and assisted in ordering their data "in a way so that they could isolate episodes and trace them according to the educational experience of the student."

Fleming and Benedek diagram a model of supervisory activity (charted on p. 68 of their book) by means of three columns of parallel supervisory processes: 1. "Overall Aims; 2. Pedagogical Diagnoses; 3. Teaching Targets," each of which is perceived as an aspect of the continuous functioning of the supervisor, moving toward specific tasks of each aspect and in which "overall aims moves toward assisting pedagogical diagnosis, and then toward evaluating and teaching targets, and finally towards decisions to orient the supervisee toward theory and correct technique." The authors place a horizontal line separating the first three from the second three sets of activity in order to "call attention to the fact that the content of the supervisor-supervisee transaction includes both conscious and preconscious aspects, both interpersonal and intrapsychic processes. Some idea of the methodology is illustrated by the supervisor's "decision making activity" which involves "not only the target, but the pedagogical technique."

These authors have categorized four classes of "supervisory tactics": 1. Clarification, or calling attention to some gap in information or understanding of the patient; 2. confrontation or calling attention to a mistake in technique; 3. demonstrating the supervisor's work habits, and 4. prescribing or telling the supervisee what he should do."

These teaching tactics are "based on a fundamental strategy of teaching which follows three principles: 1. That the teaching-learning process is similar to the psychoanalytic process and takes into account the necessity for diagnosis, interpretation, and the working through of resistances by both student and teacher; 2. that the supervisory process progresses through numerous short-term tasks but in an orderly progression through objectives of increasing complexity to a long range goal, the development of the student analyst as an analytic instrument; 3. that to achieve this long range goal the supervisory experience trains and exercises the self analytic faculties of the student in relation to the patient without attempting to analyze his personal conflicts."

In the initial phase of supervision, the basic objectives include: 1. To learn to listen with free floating attention; 2. to learn to make inferential interpretations of meaning that are beyond the awareness of the patient but explanatory of his behavior; 3. to learn to estimate the patient's level of anxiety and resistance."

The middle phase is more concerned with "learning to judge timing and dosing of responses in tune with the equilibrium in the patient-therapist system, in other words, 'to develop the tact or system responsiveness' required for skillful interpretation. General learning problems of the middle phase are concerned with 1. recognizing the shifting nuances of transference; 2. technique of interpretation; 3. self analysis. Learning problems relevant to transference phenomena include a. failures of recognition and diagnosis (due to inexperience); b. transference-countertransference reactions in the analyst (due to unsolved conflicts in the analyst); c. transference reactions to the supervisor."

Discussing the end phase of the supervisory process, the authors recall Kris' (40) description of "regressive reliving" in the transference. It is their opinion that "what can be learned by careful supervision of the terminating phase of an analysis is of the utmost value for the student analyst," since it is the consolidation of previous work. The end phase covers three steps: "1. Recognizing changes in the patient which indicate that termination should be thought about; 2. deciding on a date; 3. terminating." The task for the student at this phase is primarily one of integrating what had initially appeared as isolated events, and resolution of the transference.

Regarding the "evaluation of progress as an intrinsic part of teaching," Fleming and Benedek emphasize that the evaluative function of the supervisor is in constant operation, and have analyzed this function in terms of "an educational diagnosis of learning difficulties," and a "prognosis for professional development." The educational prognosis contains two kinds of evaluations: 1. Severity of the learning difficulties observed, and 2. an estimation of the student's basic aptitudes. In making the educational diagnosis, criteria include "aptitude, knowledge, experience and character problems." The same categories are used in the "prognosis for professional development," but this judgment begins with "an assessment of basic aptitude."

Additionally, the supervisor serves an administrative function which the authors feel adds to the clinical teaching-learning situation in a specific manner. Fleming and Benedek agree theoretically with Ekstein and Wallerstein's clinical rhombus, though their own study concentrated primarily on conceptualizing the supervisory process in terms of supervisory activity. Reviewing their own material, the authors questioned themselves regarding the information that an education committee would find useful, and offered the following outline: "1. A good report gives more than the dynamics of the patient and the state of the transference or the process of countertransference. 2. It should evaluate the therapeutic alliance and the learning alliance by describing the skill of the student in communicating with the patient and with the supervisor. The student's capacity for communication is revealed in his pattern of recording. 3. The supervisor's report should also include the persisting areas of learning needs, with the diagnosis of probable causes, an estimation of the student's awareness of these needs, and what the supervisor has tried to do about them. 4. In subsequent reports there should be a follow up statement of outcome. 5. The most valuable supervisory report will include evidence of critical incidents that correlate learning difficulties with learning objectives. . . . 6. An evaluation of the student's self analytic functioning is a most important point. . . . 7. Any information concerning a student's ability to apply theoretical concepts. . . ." In addition, periodic evaluations are of use in the learning of both the student and the teacher. Finally, the authors feel that the Menninger method which utilizes process reports and explicit meetings regarding evaluation "deserves serious consideration," despite the many objections to these procedures.

Fleming and Benedek review the history of one of the debatable issues in supervision, emphasizing the necessity to separate "the supervisory situation" from the "supervisory process," feeling that the teaching situation provides the setting, whereas the teaching activity provides the conditions which facilitate learning; therefore, the theory of supervision should be primarily a theory of teaching rather than a theory of learning. (It is difficult to understand how a teacher, however, could operate successfully without a theory of learning, just as a therapist requires a theory of therapy.) The authors note the scarcity of studies in the teaching and learning processes, and cite several "beginnings" made in this direction (41, 42, 43).

Fleming and Benedek contrast their theory of supervision with some others previously proposed, and insist that their own needs to be distinguished from one which "assumes that the clinical teaching of psychoanalysis is largely a matter of demonstrating technique." They feel that the latter formulation is primarily a patient-centered, rather than a student-centered pedagogic approach, and is based on a theory that learning occurs primarily by imitation. A second rejected theory is one "largely based upon the instructional and demonstrational tactics of the first, making the supervisor responsible for formulating the dynamics of the patient, and prescribing what should be interpreted." They feel that, although this theory is more student-centered, the "correctional" approach depends upon the student's ability to "handle his neurotic limitations," and may work very effectively, but may also avoid giving important assistance to the student. (The authors disagree with Tarachow, observing that this type of supervisor "has not developed a teaching philosophy to handle the supervisor's dilemma over his double role as therapist and teacher.") The authors are in agreement explicitly with Arlow

(44) and with Ekstein and Wallerstein's understanding of the supervisory process as a "new experience of growth with the stress on the concept of supervision as an experience involving the whole personality of student and teacher."

Fleming and Benedek base their theory of supervision on three broad assumptions derived from the nature of analytic work: "1. An analyst's education is necessarily more experiential than cognitive. 2. The basic objective of his educative experience is the development of himself as an analytic instrument. 3. Each phase of his training contributes in different ways to this basic objective."

In conclusion, the authors remark upon the process of "working through" their material during the task of writing up their investigation for a report to others. (An elaboration of the process of "writing up," as well as setting up such a study, and its relationship to the "supervisory process," would be a major contribution to the literature on the subject. One would also like to hear about the impact of this kind of research upon the actual processes of supervision, in terms of the effect upon various participants, as well as upon the system within which it is conducted.)

3. *Tarachow* (13)

Tarachow has written a seminar-based introduction to psychotherapy, its conversational style reflecting his interchange with residents and supervisors at Hillside Hospital (and reflecting the emphasis upon hospital supervision).

In "Problems Relating to Administration," Tarachow espouses the viewpoint that administrative and therapeutic functions ascribed to first year residents who are conducting therapy with hospitalized patients ought not to be "split" into separate compartments, since this is unrealistic in terms of the actual function of these residents. He distinguishes this function from that of the out-patient psychotherapeutic situation in which the therapist need not "side against" any hospital administration.

Three chapters of his book are specifically devoted to supervision, and are concerned with: 1. Outline of supervision; 2. the teacher-critic dilemma; and 3. the transference. Tarachow emphasizes his "basic rule of supervision: the teaching of the resident should be instruction in terms of the problem and needs of the patient, as expressed in the specific clinical phenomena of the patient. The supervisor is an instructor and not a psychotherapist." The "legitimate areas" which comprise the supervisor's function include "educational and didactic functions, then moving in the direction of the resident toward 'special measures which concern primarily the resident.'" Tarachow describes then a continuum of supervisory activity from a patient-centered focus to a resident-centered focus, and does not adhere as rigidly to his "basic rule" as many reviewers have described.

In outline, Tarachow's areas of supervisory interest include, under "educational-didactic": 1. Problems of the specific clinical phenomena; 2. general problems of patients, subdivided into theory of therapeutic relationship, theory of hospital treatment (which includes focus on various in-patient problems as well as relationships with the family). Moving in the direction of interest in the resident, the supervisor is concerned with: 1. Problems of residents in general, including (a) countertransference as a theoretical problem, and (b) lines of authority and complication of administration in hospital treatment; 2. problems of the specific resident, in terms of clinical results, and/or behavior of his patients, or problems of the resident's relations to other services or personnel in the hospital. Finally, functions which concern 'special measures' (in the direction of the resident): 1. Personality profile of the resident; 2. utilization of the transference possibilities to the supervisor."

Tarachow reiterates his supervisory model in terms of "being an ideal *Erzieher* and stimulating the resident in that indirect way. There are two large avenues of approach, either via an empathic seduction or via an intellectual seduction, depending on the needs of the resident and the route via which the resident can be most effectively reached."

Addressing himself to the classical dichotomy "teacher or critic" (Chapter 21), Tarachow recommends: first, the "evaluation of the resident by means of a personality profile" in order to deal with "especially difficult residents." He disagrees with the methodology of Ekstein and Wallerstein, wherein the supervisor and supervisee share frequent "process reports" involving the evaluation of the resident. Also, "one is to stay away from the psychotherapeutic position and to stay away from infantilizing and to keep the position of the teacher and not the psychotherapist. . . . This is why you should do even a confronting kind of supervision only as a last resort. You should teach every resident from the beginning as though he had no problems in learning and as though he had no problems in his seeing the material of his patients. . . . You go to the side of *his* problems last."

Discussing "The Transference," Tarachow distinguishes between transference relationships with residents in supervision, and "actual transference," on the basis that the supervisory situation is "not a *treatment* relationship," and recommends what he calls "utilizing the transference by displaying himself as a model," with the hope that the resident will identify with his response to the patient. With respect to supervisory training, the most important element is "going through a personal analysis." In offering one's self in as real a way as possible, without interpretation, the supervisor does not "interpret the transference, but uses it."

In response to his seminarists' questions, Tarachow points out that, in his conduct of the seminar, he adheres to his own "basic rule": "You may have noticed that in our meetings, we have stayed away entirely from converting this into a group therapy session of ourselves. We have been talking about our students all the time, our residents. If there are any differences among us, it is all to the advantage of the resident. We have kept even our discussion of the problems of supervision focused on the resident and away from ourselves. We are assuming we have no problems, an ideal assumption, I must admit."

Tarachow emphasizes particularly the "supervisor's responsibility to the patient: I would differ with the official policy of the hospital which makes the supervisor responsible for the treatment. The resident will learn more when he is responsible."

Questioned further by the members of his supervisory conference regarding his differences with Ekstein and Wallerstein's approach, Tarachow replies: "I am not insisting my approach is the only one: it is simply one orderly way of thinking based on a conception of the factors increasing the difficulties in teaching. In fact, the use of transference, though it is last in my outline, is at work in the first moment of contact with the resident. It belongs at the end of the outline in terms of the progressive context. This is not an outline of behavior: it is an outline of conception. . . . The resident can be inspired even by the hospital, by identification with the spirit of the hospital. I am inclined to feel that Ekstein and Wallerstein get too close to psychotherapy with their residents. I would be inclined to think that the learning block depends more on the character of the resident's own problems than on his repetition of the patient's problems. . . . Ekstein and Wallerstein use the resident's behavior with the supervisor as a model for the understanding of the patient's posture to the resident. I would not regard such an approach as patient oriented. . . . In effect then they plunge at once into analysis of the transference of the resident to the supervisor. I would rather 'use' this transference than 'analyze' it . . . however, one might differ with their method, but it does have the advantage of a systematic approach. However it is too close to psychotherapy to suit me. They start with the resident. I start with the patient."

4. *Semrad* (45)

In Chapter 5 "The Work of Supervision," Maltsberger and Buie (46) make a specific effort to formulate a supervisory model for the beginning phase of learning psychotherapy. "Successful supervision demands the establishment of a *supervisory alliance* . . . the essence of the supervisor's work is to diagnose what the resident needs in order to treat his patient and to supply what is needed by the resident. Diagnosis of the need requires as a first step gaining an understanding of *areas of interference* which are preventing a resident from doing his therapy. Second, the supervisor must discover what *defense mechanisms* are used by the resident in connection with such an area. Finally he must determine the *supervisory maneuver* appropriate to the distress of the resident in the light of the interference and the defense."

The authors delineate six broad areas of interference with the resident's functioning as a therapist: 1. Personal emotional burdens; 2. ignorance and inexperience; 3. need for omnipotence and omniscience; 4. distress with instinct; 5. countertransference; 6. relative inability to understand empathically. The "next task" for the supervisor is that of determining "defense mechanisms and interferences with learning" in the resident's struggle with therapy. In addition to "the normal defensive patterns of everyday life" (repression, isolation, displacement, rationalization, and so forth), there may be others which will present more difficulty, particularly denial and projection.

The major discussion centers upon "supervisory maneuvers, i.e., the activity required to supply the therapist's needs." The need for a specific maneuver is "dictated by assessing the quality and intensity of the painful affect which threatens the resident." The maneuvers are classified as: 1. Sustaining; 2. supporting, and 3. gratification.

A. Sustaining maneuvers:

 1. Showing a resident how to proceed
 2. Telling a resident how to proceed
 3. Providing an opportunity for the ventilation of feelings about a patient
 4. Allying one's self with the resident's competence

B. Supporting maneuvers aim at the development of the resident's potential for helping patients. These include:

 1. Confrontation, which ought not to be tactless. Indirect confrontation is advocated, often by means of an exemplification and illustration.
 2. "Sharing some of one's own experience"
 3. Making clarifications
 4. "Interpretation." Interpretation is distinguished from clarification in that it refers to comments directed at "deeper psychic structures." "This device is used sparingly and interpretations are not made about the resident's life outside the therapy he is conducting. There is some risk of the same shock effect that may occur in confrontation, and effective interpretation in the supervisory situation requires a strong alliance."
 5. Setting limits, which often comes about when the supervisory session itself is particularly threatening to the resident. Ultimately "in some instances it may be necessary to suggest that personal psychotherapy or psychoanalysis for the resident is in order. After extensive supervision and psychotherapy, some beginners will discover that they are most effective in areas of psychiatry other than psychotherapy."

C. Gratification maneuvers

In this area, the authors feel that perhaps the term "maneuver" is least appropriate, because the activity of the supervisor is minimal. The two modes of gratification are: 1. Validation, and 2. catalysis.

In conclusion, the authors emphasize that though they have defined these categories as if they were encapsulated, in actual practice the experienced supervisor utilizes these maneuvers in combination. They reiterate the progressive and developmental process that is supervision, noting that it moves from a supervisory alliance to a collaborative effort. The entire process is described as "difficult but valuable—as Spinoza remarked 'all things excellent are as difficult as they are rare.' "

II. STUDIES FOCUSED ON THE RESIDENT

A. *Background*

1. *M.D.*

Grete Bibring's (47) long standing interest in the teaching of psychiatry to medical students led her to plan the symposium held in 1964 in Cambridge, Massachusetts, studying the goals and techniques of the teaching of psychoanalytic psychiatry. She recalls that "one question is asked persistently: 'Can a physician adhere to the strict rigor of cause and effect that is medical science, while still maintaining the open spirit of explanation needed in understanding and appreciating a life?' . . . A second question (Whitehorn, 1963) (48) is of even greater importance: where clarity is the ideal, can the physician embrace a profession that must live consistently with ambiguity? He has learned to pursue action vigorously in diagnosis as well as in therapy, because more often than not the well being of his patient depends on quick and determined procedures. . . . (Erik Erikson called this the convergence of data) (49) . . . Can the doctor be professional toward his patient and at the same time care in a personal and responsible way that signals his concern to a human being who is troubled? Can he be dispassionate in comprehending and explaining a patient's emotional problem while at the same time the patient is attempting to involve him personally in a transference relationship? These are some of the contradictory patterns which create problems and difficulties for any student of psychiatry."

Bibring then addresses herself to the "methods" by which their teachers attempt the education of students of psychiatry: "the primary means by which we convey these messages are provided by personal contact between the student and an experienced instructor . . . supervision must never be applied as Sherlock Holmes applied it to Watson, that is, by answering Watson's stumbling attempts to offer his opinion with a barrage of brilliant, although in his case even correct, solutions. Conan Doyle took care of this. He made it easy for Sherlock Holmes to be infallible, much easier than life makes it for us, the supervisors."

Dr. Bibring also feels that the supervisee should be invited to become a collaborator, and an investigator in his own right with the function of expressing his reaction to the instructive viewpoint and checking it against further material of the patient. An essential principle of supervision is that the search for the total presentation of data from the supervisee is an impossible expectation (in this she agrees with Fleming and Ekstein and Wallerstein). The responsibility of the experienced psychiatrist is "to wait and observe the further development of the case . . . [with] a certain tolerance for the opinion of others, an attitude which the student has to acquire or maintain, as the case may be, vis-à-vis his patient, in the same manner in which he experiences it in the instructor's attitude toward himself; it introduces a safeguard against the inclination of some students to accept finally the teacher's point of view, a tendency which often leads to an equally blind effort to prove him right by collecting confirmatory data for the next supervisory meeting . . . the student can learn from this principle that errors are not a disgraceful sign of incompetence—neither for the teacher nor for the student—but rather they offer a most valuable opportunity to broaden our understanding . . . all in all I do believe that supervision is of more importance in the education of the student, for whom it provides the opportunity to learn, not through memorizing but through identification with an accomplished teacher, than it is a direct contribution to the treatment of any one individual patient under discussion."

In the discussion following the presentation of papers at the conference mentioned above, Erik Erikson stated: "The important factor . . . is the relationship of . . . underlying values to the need of each trainee both for competency in method and for identity of personal style. If the trainee wants to be honest, systematic, and helpful in his diagnostic capacity and in his choice of treatment methods, he will have to know something about the method and the findings of psychoanalysis . . . yet whenever we try to teach something about these values to students, for whom such values have not yet become part of a professional identity—and this concerns undergraduates as well as medical students, we come up against a resistance which has not been fully dealt with in this conference. Basic resistance is often hidden behind the specific resistances against insight into sexual or aggressive wishes or thoughts. In fact, many people today accept such wishes or thoughts far too easily, while retaining the basic resistance to which I am referring. This is the recognition that, in vital matters of decision, we are not functioning according to the dictates of "free will" or according to the logic of the secondary process. The first shock in any confrontation with psychoanalytic thought concerns not its content but the fact that there is that much we do not know about ourselves. Furthermore, whenever we speak about psychoanalytic method, we (both teachers and students) are always emotionally involved; and it is important to realize that what we call transference and countertransference in therapy is also an inescapable part of teaching, not only as between teacher and student, but also as between teacher and teacher, and student and student. The fact that this is not systematically acknowledged often causes that ambivalent and ambiguous atmosphere which expresses itself in strange tensions, not to speak of gossip and professional antagonisms.

". . . Now to come to the question of identity; you are probably as tired of this word as I am. It has already become what some people call an 'ashcan concept,' hospitable to all manner of trash, as well as to some valuable insights which should not be thrown away so carelessly. In particular, one aspect of identity—the negative identity—needs to be considered much more carefully.

"One is always nostalgic for one's earlier identity, even if one must repudiate parts of it constantly or reconvert it to make it a part, the more inclusive identity, of one's later development. I do not mean to single out doctors in this respect (some of my best friends are doctors), and to use myself as an example. I am sure my writings show only too clearly how my earlier role of artist struggles for recombination with my later experiences as an analyst. But we're speaking here of medical school, and I wonder whether a certain nostalgia for a certain earlier, more strictly medical identity may at times make it difficult to avoid identifying with the demands of the student's resistance by representing the mind too mechanically and too practically, or on the other hand, to identify with their all too frenetic conversion to psychoanalytic thinking. Students, regardless of their level, must gain from us some kind of shock experience. Dr. Kubie has called it a therapeutic experience, but I'm not sure that this is the right expression. . . . The student should learn to experience the possibility that, in his functioning identity, he may combine traditional medical concern with a totally new kind of insight, not only one needed for the understanding of certain symptoms, but also one that cannot help revolutionizing one's views of man—including one's self."

Dr. Milton Rosenbaum, during the same discussion, alluded to his own "nostalgia for our old identities . . . perhaps this nostalgia explains my fantasy of what I want to do on my sabbatical—be an intern in the emergency room. It is interesting to note that whenever psychoanalysts get together in a conference on how to train psychiatric residents, we emphasize that we do not teach residents enough clinical psychiatry. Why do we emphasize this? Because this is what the residents yearn for. Why did we go into medicine? The reasons that made us go into medicine have nothing to do with understanding people. They have to do with mastering anxieties on the deepest level, through action. It is our effort to beat the game of life, our effort to prevent our own death. That's why we go into medicine. Then we have to master something else: passivity versus activity."

Castelnuevo Tedesco (50), in a questionnaire distributed to 218 Los Angeles area psychiatric residents and fellows, reviewed 112 responses in which the residents ranked in order of subspecialty their feelings regarding the "best taught and best learned" subjects versus the "poorest taught and poorest learned" subjects in clinical and preclinical undergraduate education. Thirteen percent felt that psychiatry was the best taught, 20% thought it was the best learned; however 16% stated it was the poorest taught and 4% the least learned. In contrast, medicine was perceived by 41% to be the best taught and 24% the best learned, in both cases the highest ranking of any specialty. The findings also recorded that about one third of the residents had decided before medical school in favor of specializing in psychiatry, one third during, and one third after medical school. Also "the decision to become a psychiatrist was ascribed to personal factors and to contact with psychiatric patients, more than to the effect that the teaching received . . . the features of their training most prized by those who reported a positive experience, and most missed by those whose experience had been disappointing, were contact with dedicated teachers, and generous opportunity for clinical experience."

The use of psychiatric supervision among medical students, as a recruiting as well as facilitating enterprise, was reported by Karl Lewin (51) at the University of Pittsburgh. He feels that "psychiatric supervision by direct observation provides the student with opportunities not readily afforded by demonstration interviews or by classical supervision. A patient confronted by two interviewers shows a variety of expressions of affect and ego defenses. Nonverbal communication can be more accurately examined. Comparing his own approach to the patient with that of the preceptor gives the student some insight into countertransference and into his own relationship with others."

Hilliard Jason et al. (52) reach a similar conclusion regarding the use of videotape in assisting their medical students to "acquire the skills necessary for professional relationships with patients, overcome anxieties in confronting patients, adopt a comfortable self image, and begin involvement in clinical medicine. . . ."

For the past several years, the views of Dr. Thomas Szasz regarding the appropriateness of the "medical model" in the work of psychiatry have become a source of polemic polarization. One of Szasz's (53) students, Leifer (54), has discussed "The Medical Model as Ideology," (arguing along lines similar to Szasz, and further presented in his own book *In the Name of Mental Health: The Social Functions of Psychiatry*). A rejoinder by Brown and Ochberg (55), "The Medical Muddle," claims that Leifer has not understood "the theory and practice of psychiatry," which includes many models, not merely the medical. Discussions of these presentations by Nemiah, and Albee, with a final rebutal by Leifer makes for a fair sampling of the spectrum of opinions on these issues.

The psychiatric educator, faced with the multiple role conflicts, dichotomies, and conflict-of-interest controversies of our time in his attempt to provide a synthetic model for his residents, is led to formulate a point of view which perceives psychiatry (and medicine itself) as a compromise and transitional social force which serves as a pragmatic buffer between conflicting polarizations between society and individuals. As medicine historically has often served as a social compromise, it has not perceived itself as vacuumatic and neutral. Illness as a social role has never been assumed or perceived neutrally —psychiatry has served as the Alsace-Lorraine of mind-body dualism; of determinism versus voluntarism. Particularly, with its "psychosomatic" viewpoint, it functions to mollify the antinomies of a democracy which depends on an "as if" version of total responsibility for its citizenship, while acknowledging the medical or psychological ambiguities of self determination. Behavior is seen in psychiatry as "overdetermined," but the idea of multiple or conflicted motivations is still antithetical to the fundamental legalities of a democracy. Therefore, psychiatry often is utilized as a kind of social pragmatism, between the "stigmatization of mental illness" and the educational effort toward understanding the bases for behavior. By remaining within the medical field, psychiatry is in a stronger position to legitimize the social compromise it formulates, whenever behavior unacceptable to society conflicts with the issue of responsibility. The fundamental difficulty with the Szaszian viewpoint is that it promotes a socially tendentious, literal acceptance of the legal concept of responsibility for behavior, disregarding its as-if basis. To say that psychiatry should be aware of those aspects of itself which are "socially abused" is undebatable; but to demand a simplistic Cartesian split of psychiatric function in the service of bringing theory up to date with behavior, is to misapprehend the nature and functions of institutions, the manner and methods of their change, and to obscure the possibility for constructive analysis in a cloud of revolutionary rhetoric.

2. Personality

In "The Development of the Psychiatric Resident as a Therapist" Brody (56) states "as a general proposition, I would say that the nature of the psychotherapy practiced by any individual will be a function of his identification with his profession, as well as his teachers and supervisors in therapy." Emphasizing the distinction which his studies had revealed between psychology trainees and residents in psychiatry, Brody reports: "The resident tended to meet crises more with authority and directive action, while psychology trainees tended to meet them more with withdrawal and detachment. The residents identify with doctors who direct the treatment of patients and act as strong advisors. The clinical trainees identified with psychologists who in the field of disturbed human behavior were scientists and observers, rather than responsible participants . . . another element possibly contributing to differences between trainees in psychology and psychiatric residents was the fact that in contrast to residents, the young psychologists limited therapeutic activities to one or two patients at a time. All their countertransference eggs were in one basket, and consequently, the supervisory situation became a more loaded one. (Compare this situation with the similar investment of the analytic candidate in his supervised analysis.) The remainder of their clinical work, mostly psychodiagnostic in character, casts them into the role of a sampler of behavior who is not a constant part of the patient's life. The residents' energies, on the other hand, were dispersed among a large number of patients, some of whom were seen briefly; some carried in intensive, prolonged psychotherapy; some treated mainly with physical-chemical techniques; and some through social manipulation methods. This means of course that much of the resident's therapy did not involve an intensively concerned supervisor."

Brody remarked the degree of freedom which the psychiatric resident requires to develop capacity for independent judgment in clinical situations. He recalls that this question was raised in Bertram Lewin's survey of psychoanalytic training in America, wherein he noted there was a "persisting almost compulsive need for supervision" which analytic training apparently fostered. Brody felt that "such a need does not seem to be engendered by psychiatric residency training of itself, but grows during the superordinate training in psychoanalysis during which the doctor begins to look upon himself less as a physician practicing as a subspecialty of medicine, than as a particular kind of psychotherapist."

Riess (9) in "Selection and Supervision of Psychotherapists" has reviewed some of the studies related to therapist selection. He reports on the book by Holt and Luborsky (57), who studied the Menninger residents in some detail, attempting to discover specific indicators for future competence in psychiatry. Among their conclusions was the finding that batteries of tests were no better indicators of the future performance than individual clinicians' interviews. They also concluded that "we have considered the possible consequences of concentrating on selection, recruitment, or training as approaches to the basic problem of satisfying mental health needs. The experience of carrying out our research, as well as some of its findings, convinces us that it is education that will in the long run repay increased cultivation with the richest yield . . . we like particularly the new kind of selection research closely geared in with an experimental approach to education."

Riess also reports on the selection process at the Postgraduate Center in New York for their candidates, which includes a Rorschach test, among others, as well as interviews. These methods were "not totally unsatisfactory and are being continually revised, currently in terms of matching initial test scores against supervisory judgments at one year intervals during the course of the training." The research Riess has reviewed "points to the need, in such investigations, of a group of continuing supervisors who remain in contact with the student for a relatively long time."

Plutchik and his colleagues (58) found that of 90 physicians applying for psychiatric residencies at Albert Einstein College of Medicine, who were "studied on a 32 item scale," a common personality characteristic was "a greater than average tendency to compartmentalize their thinking and to intellectualize their relationships with people; they also showed a high need for achievement and low impulsivity."

Studies of the differences between psychiatric residents and those in other professional training programs (internal medicine and Ph.D. programs in biochemistry) were evaluated in comparison with two residency programs in psychiatry in Chicago and showed that primarily psychiatric residents were particularly vague about the career identity and task confronting them, compared with residents and graduate students in other disciplines. This was reflected in the staff response during the residency, according to Bucher and his colleagues (59): "It is clear that the staffs of these psychiatric residencies do not believe that a beginning resident in psychiatry can take major responsibilities for patient care—even though staff may treat the resident *as if* they respected his professional autonomy. Nor do they assume that the resident has much of any idea as how to proceed when confronted with a patient. Therefore they set up a system that assumes that entering residents know little or nothing. The whole framework of curriculum supervision proceeds on the assumption that the trouble which residents will encounter is due to: first, lack of substantive knowledge, and second, the resident's own intrapsychic responses."

Frayn (60) reviewed the literature on personality studies of psychiatrists, including the Whitehorn and Betz 1962 study which distinguished types A and B in the treatment of schizophrenic patients; Loweringer and Dobie's study in 1964, which found that the competent therapist is "one who is aggressive, ambitious, and outgoing," and reviewed the studies of Truax, Epstein, and others who have attempted to find "the qualities of the good therapist."

Frayn reported that, of the 25 residents he studied with personality questionnaires (MMPI and other tests) and rating by 10 psychotherapy supervisors, there was high agreement among experienced supervisors regarding the psychotherapeutic ability of these residents. The highest agreement "occurred in rating those residents who were regarded as good psychotherapists" (coinciding with the findings of Holt and Luborsky). "The psychotherapists rated by their supervisors as having the greatest ability were described as being assertive, flexible, and less concerned about social conformity, while those with less ability were compulsively rigid with a need to conform. . . ."

B. *Beginning and Early Problems of the Resident.*

Kahana (61) has observed that "the main stress of psychiatric training is a concentrated exposure to the emotionally disturbed behavior of patients, especially states of extreme anxiety, despondency, helpless appeal, bizarreness or withdrawal, and attitudes of aggressive demandingness, provocativeness or seductiveness." Other sources of pressure lie in the technical task of observing each patient carefully, understanding and evaluating the patient, remembering interviews, and guiding reactions according to therapeutic aims, at the same time responding with spontaneity. Further tasks are schedules, responsibilities of administration, the necessity to adapt to competitive peer groups and confront the injunctions and judgments of supervisors, and the "almost limitless body of knowledge to be gained." Some of the strain may be "ameliorated, and the resident's learning enhanced, by appropriate dosage and timing of clinical experience and responsibilities, by the support of peer group and supervisors, by institutional arrangements, procedures, traditions and morale, through personal psychotherapy or psychoanalysis, and by the cumulative assimilation of information and technique, organized and vitalized by theory."

Among the difficulties facing the beginning psychiatric resident, some are related to the problem of input overload. Bond (62) recalls among his early experiences a story of Ernst Kris which amusingly highlights this issue: Kris told him, "Look, there are two things that you have to remember. There are only two ways, two features of the human mind, that you can use to overcome resistance; one is intellect and the other is positive transference. If you insult the intellect and get a negative transference, it is not going to be a big surprise if people do not learn from you. I think that many people who start to teach think that it will be easy, particularly because they think they know what they want to say. Once they become actively involved, they are not so sure what it is they want to say, and usually they pay not the slightest attention to what the student wants to hear. This is rather important because if the student doesn't want to hear it, he is not going to learn it. This is a little reminiscent of the Thurber story of a third grade girl who was given a book on seals by her teacher and went off and read it. The teacher asked her if it was a good book. She said "Yes it is a good book." The teacher asked her if she liked the book. The child said "No, I hated the book." "Why?" said the teacher. "Because it told me more about seals than I wanted to know."

Semrad (45) emphasizes the importance of the beginning stage in psychiatric training. "The beginning student of psychodynamic psychiatry requires his own opportunity to research, to hypothesize, and to reformulate our discipline. His treatment of patients becomes his classroom—laboratories for the investigation of psychodynamic principles. . . . Supervision begins with the structuring of selected data into a significant framework. The paucity of information will lead to questions of how to collect data in order to obtain a broader base for diagnostic hypothesis. . . . The beginning resident . . . sees his supervisor as one who can catalyze the learning process, provide necessary guidelines and reference points, and help him validate his researches. By mixing, fusing, and crystalizing observed facts with knowledge, theories, and experiences, the supervisor helps the therapist become available to the patient even as learning commences. . . . The skills needed to become a seasoned therapist are slowly developed through errors and disappointments, and most psychiatrists require around ten years to grow into maturity."

Merklin and Little (63) have observed that the psychological response of the resident to his first year of training is characterized by many emotional disturbances. They perceive these as "transient and adaptational which will lessen in intensity." They review the work of Sharaf and Levinson (64), and Halleck and Woods (65). They feel that the residency is "a time of extraordinary stress . . . when many residents develop into mediocre or inadequate psychiatrists partly as the result of a failure to work through the anxieties attendant upon being a resident." The impact of the first year on the resident involves a difficulty with identity, and results in a tendency to become "obsessively preoccupied with conventional medical details, as a reaction to the impact of the first encounter with psychiatric patients." The authors agree with Halleck and Woods that "the most brilliant and perceptive supervisors, judging by our experience, are much less interested in and therefore less willing to become involved in *in-patient* supervision." Further difficulties involve the alienation from previous colleagues in surgery or medicine, "intensifying the resident's sense of estrangement from his former sources of status and feelings of adequacy."

Worby (66) described among the difficulties of the first year resident in establishing a professional identity: "ambiguity about role choice; intimacy with patients; relationships with peers, authority figures, and members of allied disciplines; definition of therapeutic goals; and acceptance of the public nature of the work." Other difficulties include the probability that there will be a resulting period of therapeutic nihilism, as residents find that they are not effective in their ventures. Worby emphasizes the importance of the supervisor's support in these problems, advocating "a developmental perspective of the residency . . . which may clarify how these phase-specific needs of the resident and the increasingly complex requirements of clinical work may be more realistically integrated." (Kubie has also emphasized the importance of timing in education and in psychotherapy (66a).)

Weber (67) points up the difficulties of supervision which he has observed over several years at the Columbia University Psychoanalytic Clinic. He advocates the useful effect of "the language and focus of adatpational theory" in conferences supervising residents.

With this framework in mind, he feels that a general outline and goal of treatment may be reached compatible with the limitations of time, personality and life experience of the patient, and experience of the therapist. Weber believes that the adaptational model avoids complex theoretical discussions, thereby preventing "the therapeutic pessimism common to many beginning residents." Also, this viewpoint tends to diminish the apparently ubiquitous trend among residents which "scorns anything but psychoanalysis as superficial and supportive."

C. General and Developmental Issues

Tichener (68) and Ornstein (5) utilize two classic stories to illustrate the difficulties of the beginning resident. Tichener observed that the tendency to mimic the supervisor is a not uncommon phenomenon in the supervisory situation; while Ornstein points out that the present situation in psychiatric education has strong potential for recapitulating the difficulties illustrated in the tale of the Sorcerer's Apprentice in which "the apprentice attempted to acquire the magical power of the sorcerer by imitation, and failed to control the process he could initiate, because he could only repeat the words of the sorcerer without first-hand knowledge of the nature and processes of sorcery." Ornstein pictures the consequences for the resident-apprentice in which "he might have become completely disillusioned and forever convinced that magic is a tricky business . . . that it should not be undertaken unless one is born a sorcerer, since these tricks cannot be learned."

In "The Beginning Resident and Supervision" Tischler (69) has recorded the reactions of 12 psychiatric residents at the Yale University Department of Psychiatry during their initial year of training. The characteristic prelude to each resident's report was the statement "I for one felt very insecure in psychiatry not knowing what I was doing." Discussing the painful aspects of the resident's confrontation with the supervisor, Tischler states, "in singling out teaching, modeling, support, and judgment as the critical dimensions of the initial supervisory experience, the resident reflects his intent on utilizing the process to facilitate role transition." Focusing upon the issues of "role development," Tischler analyzes the resident's concerns in terms of "the noncomplementarity of the contract between supervisor and resident: the resident comes to expect his supervisor to be interested not only in his patients, but in his reaction to the first year, to his being a psychiatrist. The supervisor is seen solely as an agent of the resident responsive to the multiple needs generated by the transitional and intraceptive demands that characterize the initial year of training . . . there is an obvious discrepancy between the role partners' conceptualization of the appropriate range of activities for the supervisor. . . ." It is Tischler's view that the supervisor is "primarily the agent of the training program," and that the supervisory experience in the beginning of residency training is particularly self contradictory. "They have taken a programmatic given, supervision, and transformed it into a vehicle for facilitating role transition." Tischler's suggestion to correct this difficulty is "introducing a role system into the training constellation more congruent to the resident's expectations." Tischler proposes a preceptorial system, splitting the supervisor from a "preceptor who acts solely" as the resident's agent. "The preceptor will then be prepared to talk with the student about experiences in adapting to a new role and in working with patients . . . the preceptorship should not be thought of as a substitute for supervision, but as a supplemental relationship that enables the resident to direct his expectations surrounding the act of becoming onto someone other than the supervisor. While this does not resolve the question of agency as it applies to the supervisory process, it does allow the student to relate to the supervisor less equivocally as a teacher—an outcome that can only enhance the value of supervision as a learning experience." The issue of agency, with which Tischler reports particular difficulty, is also discussed by Wagner (70), in terms of the fact that the supervisor is a representative of the training organization, as well as an agent of the institution responsible for the setting. There is no mention by Tischler that the supervisor is also, in some sense, an agent of the patient.

D. General Developmental Problems

Kogan (71) and his colleagues, in their study "Personality Changes in Psychiatric Residents During Training," recalled that Holt and Luborsky had previously described qualitative personality changes in the psychiatric residents which he had studied. Kogan's group attempted to quantify changes over the course of residency training in 19 trainees in the Department of Psychiatry at the University of Washington School of Medicine. Among a series of 18 factors, 3 were perceived as significantly changing over the course of the residency program: residents' perceptions of themselves and others changed toward "(a) less resentment of supervision, (b) less self-sacrificing and supporting of others and (c) more self-aggrandizing during the training program." Of their other findings, some were perceived as suggesting "that the residents see themselves as lacking in self-reliance and being too indulgent in contrast with what they considered desirable." Their study, they felt, points up the need for more sophisticated investigation of psychiatric development in the planning of psychiatric training programs.

Grotjahn (72) analyzed "The Role of Identification in Psychiatric and Psychoanalytic Training" and emphasized the importance of "the ability to identify as one prerequisite for psychoanalytic work." He also recognized the existence of "a counteridentification" in the supervisor with his supervisee, as well as difficulties in responding to resentment and hostility from the supervisee.

"Emotional Problems of Psychiatric Residents" by Halleck and Woods (65) reviews the various difficulties encountered by the resident when first exposed in his training to the conduct of out-patient psychotherapy. Among the problems he faces are the situation and climate in which he must work. First, he generally begins with patients who cannot pay for treatment, and therefore his sources are limited to "Veterans' Administration Mental Hygiene Clinics, in-patient services, community clinics, or university student health services. (Also) the patients are likely to come from a socio-economic background markedly different from his own." (Halleck and Woods' discussion of the climate of psychotherapy for the psychiatric resident is one of the few specific allusions to the problems of the residency context; Hollingshead and Redlich (73) have emphasized the difficulties of attempting to work with patients from different backgrounds, a task often impossible even for experienced psychiatrists.) Other problems are the fact that patients are sometimes treated by the resident on a "non-fee basis," and often in this group are many who are "economically unproductive by virtue of severe deficit of ego strength." Thus the resident may well begin with a group of patients less motivated, with less ego strength, than would be optimally desirable. Further difficulty arises from the limited time scale available for out-patient psychotherapy: "it is unlikely that very many of his patients in intensive therapy will respond with major achievements during the 1½ years of out-patient experience provided by most residency programs."

The resident also suffers from psychotherapy supervision itself, since this relationship is perceived as "almost inherently conflictual and ambiguous . . . if (the resident's) needs are met, the supervisor becomes an important ego ideal, and powerful identifications ensue. If his needs are not met, his initial insecurities are magnified by his frustration and anger, and his anxiety mounts still higher. Unfortunately, not all good psychiatrists are good supervisors, and the resident usually has little choice in their selection. Most residencies provide for more than one supervisor on a rotational basis, and while this helps minimize the possibility of poor supervision it sets up additional factors of conflict." The resident is also exposed to a conflicting variety of viewpoints from his mentors, and in his inexperience, is unable to judge for himself, particularly when he respects equally the proponents of various viewpoints. Additionally, the supervisor often assumes the role of a "quasi-therapist," during the examination of the resident's countertransferences. "As anxiety increases the resident-supervisor relationship may move in the direction of a therapeutic one, often covertly. Szasz and Thompson, in discussing the ambiguities of the training analyst-analysand relationship, have pointed out the difficulties inherent in therapeutic intervention by a person who at the same time exercises the realistic role of an evaluator." (Tischler (69) and Escoll and Wood (112) have addressed themselves to this inherent "role conflict"; Dorn (74) and the discussants of his paper have also focused upon the perennial problem of the supervisor as pedagogue-critic. It is noteworthy that although the supervisory process itself is similar in analytic and psychiatric education, the special situation in the psychoanalytic institute's training analysis is not comparable on the basis of the multiplicity of supervisors as well as the variety and number of cases in supervision in psychiatric residency training, allowing the resident some relief from the exaggerated anxieties of the uniqueness of the analytic training case.) Further emotional problems of the psychiatric resident include the effects of emotional stress of therapy itself, which may lead to "a therapeutic nihilism which may never remit. . . . Residents who react in this manner often become cynical, unbelieving and chronically dissatisfied . . . just as serious a problem as the nihilistic resident is what might be called the 'band-wagon resident,' who latches onto whatever philosophy is prevailing at the time and endows it with the status of fact." Other sources of stress include the effect upon the resident's family resulting from his displacement away from his previous medical context, the threat of psychiatric and psychological discussions, for which most residents' wives are ill prepared, and often conflicted reports of the resident himself regarding his psychological efforts with his patients. The authors conclude that though residency programs are aware of their residents' stress, "provision for psychiatric treatment or counseling for disturbed residents . . . are usually inadequate . . . inquiries to other psychiatrists and residents in training throughout the country indicate that many programs are minimally concerned with these problems. It is our belief that lack of attention to the emotional problems of residents leads to psychiatric casualties and the development of too many mediocre psychiatrists."

Emphasis upon the "educational" aspects of psychiatric education, as distinguished from "therapy models for teaching of residents," is the thrust of "Professional Development in Psychiatric Residents: Assessment and Facilitation," by Miller and Burstein (75). "It is the educator's duty to exhaust proximate measures . . . residents should be protected from taking inappropriate refuge in the 'therapy model' as illustrated by the attitude 'I don't need to read that book, what I really need is an analysis' . . . With due recognition of the relationship between character difficulties and learning problems, we wish to highlight that source of difficulties in professional development which is intrinsically educational. . . ." The educational goals of the residency are primarily the acquisition of the basic skills of observation, understanding, and purposeful action. Outside of "neurotic interferences," the causes of variation in residents, according to Miller and Burstein, are "(1) constitution, (2) education, (3) psychopathology, and (4) stylistic variations." In order to improve their assessment procedure, they designed a method utilizing a one-way mirror through which two supervisors observed the resident conducting a diagnostic interview. Afterward, the resident and two observers wrote their impressions about the interview, then met to discuss these impressions. Finally, the supervisors wrote their evaluation of the resident's work, sending it to the "Director of the Residency Training Program."

DeWald (76), in his discussion of psychoanalytic supervision, also labeled the major difficulties as "learning problems." Among the supervisee's difficulties are some involved with "conflicting motivations between his wish favorably to impress the supervisor in order that he will receive the proper credit . . . and the need to expose his areas of weakness, uncertainty, and lack of skills, in order that he may receive the instruction, guidance, and help that he needs to correct insufficiencies and improve his overall performance."

DeWald categorizes the learning problems of the supervisee in seven major groups: "(1) cognitive knowledge, (2) clinical experience, (3) countertransference, (4) the student's relationship to the supervisor, (5) the supervisor's relation to the student, (6) the supervisor's relationship to the patient, (7) the student's basic aptitude for analytic work." DeWald is one of the few discussants of supervision who gives explicit attention to the supervisor's relationship to the patient: "The supervisor may sometimes face something of a syncretistic conflict between the learning needs of the student and the therapeutic and clinical needs of the patient. Usually this is not a major problem, but there may well be instances when the two demands placed on the supervisor become irreconcilable and one must be temporarily sacrificed in favor of the other." Tarachow has also explicitly pointed out the importance of clarification in the contract between supervisor and supervisee regarding the issue of the fundamental responsibility for the patient; Schuster and Freeman (77) in their discussion of supervision of the diagnostic interview, have pointed out the need on occasion for the supervisor to intervene on behalf of the patient during the process of supervision.

Sharaf and Levinson (65, 78, 79) have reviewed extensively the issue of "the quest for omnipotence" as it appears in the professional development of the psychiatrist. The authors consider the "context of the resident" including the setting (i.e. Massachusetts Mental Health Center, over a seven year period, 1953-1959), in which a total of 95 psychiatrists were studied. They state pointedly that "since the literature on psychiatric education is very meager, we have no rigorous empirical basis for comparing the situation described here with those at other places and times." They review specifically the historical changes in "the relative emphasis and prestige" given to various psychiatric subspecialties. For example, they observed that the prestige of "research and administration" grew sharply during the period studied. Adopting a term from Henry A. Murray (80), "intraception," the authors define the task of learning psychotherapy as an "intraceptive task." By intraception they mean "a syndrome of psychological qualities such as psychological-mindedness, empathy with others, self-awareness—a proclivity to seek out and to enjoy the subjective and personal in human affairs." Intraception, then, is a "required personality characteristic in modern dynamic psychiatry." Sharaf and Levinson recall the difficulties the resident faces in dealing with the intense emotions of his patients, as well as his own, in addition to the lack of previous experience, on the basis of his prior medical training, in psychological work. Paradoxically he is, despite his "limited competence, given high professional status in the hospital, both officially and unofficially."

The resident attempts to deal with the insufficiency of his professional competence at this stage by attempting to gain reassurance from "membership in an elite professional group. . . . The sense of professionality provides much needed psychological support. . . . Psychoanalysis, with its long term, subtle, and intensive exploration of the patient's inner life, represents for many residents the elite group within the profession." In addition the supervisor is often used at an unconscious level as a magical figure in a fantasy of future omnipotence. The authors had previously classified "two modal patterns of professional ideology and role definition among residents: the analytic and the eclectic." These two types of residents pursued their "quests for omnipotence" in contrasting ways. The "analytic" resident focused particularly upon psychodynamics, and hierarchized patients and staff figures and therapeutic modalities along a continuum of analytic versus management. Vicissitudes of this quest occurred with shifts in emphasis from the learning of special techniques to the learning of general emotional attitudes, and upon experiential aspects of the psychiatrist's role, such as emotional empathy, rather than intellectual insight. In this early phase there develops also a "quest for omnisentience." This is paralleled by a shift from a medical background toward a more abstract, less active model of medical specialization. (The final phase of the quest for the analytically oriented resident is described in tones reminiscent of the emotions of the protagonist in Kafka's *The Trial,* as the resident becomes an applicant to the Psychoanalytic Institute.) On the other hand, the "eclectic residents" are committed to other aspects of clinical psychiatry, administration, or research. In their quest, the shift toward omniscience is modeled upon the "renaissance man," in which the eclectic residents perceive their guides to be not only within but outside the analytic profession. Though they may indeed apply to the analytic institute, they do so in the tone of incorporating "the totality" of psychiatric experience. Elaborating upon their observation of the historical shifts in the "quest for omnipotence," the authors trace the movement from the earlier identificatory figures as analysts, toward the "new hero" who is described as "the ideal role model: a triple threat—therapist, administrator, and research professor . . . possessing the combined powers of omniscience, (and omniscience about more than psychodynamics), omnisentience, and omnifacience. The particular emphasis will vary in any given role model, but all three have been embraced in the myth of the new eclectic hero." (The triple threat here described, is reminiscent of Funkenstein's three styles of "new physicians": the quest for omnipotence is a fundamental medical dream, reflected partially in the insistence upon the "undifferentiated" medical student or physician.)

Finally, Sharaf and Levinson assert that the quest for omnipotence is advantageous toward the development of competence in one's profession, by means of: (1) facilitating a re-examination and perhaps a change in the self; (2) the usefulness of identity models as transitional bulwarks against anxiety; (3) an assistance in being able to tolerate one's early ineptitudes and failures, which could be attributable to one's supervisors; (4) a support in being able to tolerate criticism and opposition from significant teachers; (5) assisting in promoting a 'youthful enthusiasm,' as a facilitative factor in growth and development."

Ornstein's paper "Sorcerer's Apprentice . . ." (5) reviews the major tidal movements in psychiatric education over the past several years, as he surveys various difficulties developing under the impact of psychiatry "riding madly in all directions" (81), and perceives many problems attendant upon the struggle for eclecticism. Ornstein is particularly concerned with the lack of a "pedagogic solution to the impact of the information explosion and of the emergence of new areas of study and new forms of treatment," and observes that the conference on psychiatric education of 1952 and the second conference in 1962 had recommended broadening the curriculum without attention to educational methods. Re-examining the educational and training philosophy of psychiatric education, Ornstein is particularly concerned not only about this lack of methodology, but about what he perceives as the dilutional overemphasis upon content in the residency experience. "The emphasis on what to learn and how much to learn has to shift to an emphasis on how to think, a shift which has recently revolutionized pedagogy from grade school to higher education. Curiously enough, it has thus far failed to have sufficient impact upon training and education in psychiatry." Emphasizing the importance of the clinical experience of the psychiatric resident, Ornstein reasserts the statement of the 1962 report: "the principal element of the core curriculum is the patient-physician relationship, and the psychiatrist's other diverse activities must evolve from this foundation." In corroboration of this viewpoint, he cites Gaskill and Norton (82): "Our objective is the training of psychiatrists in the fundamentals of diagnostic evaluation and dynamic psychotherapy . . . fundamental to this is an increasing awareness and understanding of the dynamic unconscious and intrapsychic conflict as it relates to the patient and the therapist. The dyadic therapeutic relationship is conceived of as the primary model of the clinical psychiatrist. Knowledge of the intricacies and complexities of this relationship with all of its theoretical and therapeutic implications and unknowns is the unique tool of the psychiatrist of both today and the future."

Ornstein lists the "basic skills" of the psychiatrist as "observation, evocative listening, empathy, intuition and introspection." In view of what he perceives as "the absence of a satisfactory learning theory," Ornstein suggests analogizing from the psychotherapeutic situation itself, in which the first order of business is "to utilize the patient's experiences systematically, so that he may develop the skill necessary for his participation in his analytic task. The list of these necessary skills is identical with the basic skills of the psychiatrist." Warning against a confusion of the "therapeutic and the pedagogic methods," Ornstein stresses the importance of the creation of an emotional climate and methods of teaching that will allow reliance upon one's own experiences with patients as a source of learning for the resident. "The idea is not to exclude the reasonable authority of the supervisor or the textbook or reference to someone else's previous experience, but the proper timing and manner of their introduction into the training and educational curriculum." Ornstein is particularly concerned to avoid the "apprentice complex" resulting from premature identification with the supervisor; also, the supervisor's supportive approach, by leading to anxiety diminution, will not enhance the trainee's trust in himself. Excessive support, according to Ornstein, is conducive to "the shift towards eclecticism and the disappointment in psychodynamics and psychoanalysis. . . ."

These concepts are summarized in a pedagogic emphasis upon the resident's creative and self-reliant impulses, and toward the focus on the doctor-patient relationship and the processes of their interaction. Ornstein perceives a close parallel between the "working alliance" (by which Fleming and Benedek have described the supervisor-supervisee relationship) with what Fliess has pointed out as the primary vehicle of analysis, the "work ego" of the patient. These general principles are actualized in Ornstein's practice of supervision by means of early focus upon "the patient's present illness, the precipitating circumstances, and the specific details of the first encounter between patient and doctor." These are "the essential data" and this encounter is the nucleus upon which are based the multiple complexities of psychotherapeutic transactions. Ornstein advocates the model of T. M. French (83), especially his concept of "focal conflict." Fundamentally, Ornstein perceives the elemental task in the process of becoming a psychiatrist is "to discover his own mode of thinking and feeling in his professional experiences."

Chessick (84) in "How the Resident and the Supervisor Disappoint Each Other" (and expanded in *Why Psychotherapists Fail* (6)) has reviewed the difficulties described in most of the literature on supervision, and notes at the outset that "it is surprising that with the exception of one paper by Emch, almost no authors have defined the term supervisor." Undeterred, Chessick defines the supervisor as "a person assigned by the training committee to work with the novice psychotherapist in order to somehow facilitate the transition from novice to trained therapist. This can include the individual supervisor or the group seminar leader." Chessick discusses his theme in terms of "a clarification of this definition," and lists the questions at hand: (1) "What are the problems the resident is facing?" These constitute a "crucial triad: (a) development of his *identity* as a psychotherapist (85); (b) the *anxiety* attendant upon the development of psychological-mindedness; (c) developing a *conviction* about the meaningfulness of psychodynamics and long term intensive psychotherapy." Chessick agrees with Ornstein that "the shift toward eclecticism and the disappointment in psychodynamics and psychotherapy are *symptoms that the training program is defective*" (84).

Chessick's second question "How can the supervisor help the resident?" is self answered by reviewing a variety of techniques including the importance of the therapist's personal life as a "training unit" (this concept is based upon Spiegel, J. "Factors in the Growth and Development of the Psychotherapist") (86). "The relationship with one's own wife and children is emphasized as a 'laboratory' in which the therapist can apply what he has learned from books and from his own treatment." Other means by which "the supervisor can help the resident" include identification as a means of assisting the growth of the "work ego," and enhancing the development of a "supervisory alliance" as a parallel to the "therapeutic alliance" of psychotherapy.

Chessick's model of supervision is "a hierarchy of tasks over an extended time, and . . . the supervisor as the person in whom both the qualities of teacher and psychotherapist are fused, and used according to the specifics of the situation." (This position is closest to that in our own out-patient department, with the exception that it does not consider to any great extent the total context [institutional] nor the patient [in terms of characteristics] as mentioned by Sharaf and Levinson.) Chessick feels that "the anxiety level is the crucial factor in determining to what extent the supervisor should be purely didactic and to what extent he should begin to approach unconscious processes in the resident that are interfering with his work with patients. Thus, the anxiety level of the resident becomes a crucial factor in determining the supervisory maneuvers." This viewpoint, Chessick states, is "completely analogous" to that he utilizes as the approach to psychotherapy in *How Psychotherapy Heals* (87), in which the therapist is urged to take the patient as far toward uncovering and self understanding as the patient is able to go, using the anxiety level as a gauge of what the patient can tolerate.

Having raised the above issues, Chessick asks "certain prior questions": (1) "What does the resident yearn for?" In reply, he lists realistic and magical "remedies," such as are involved in the acquisition of "power and competence." Also, "The resident hopes to please his supervisor, to make an impressive presentation in seminars, and to have his work accredited. . . . Additionally there are "severe personal pressures" resulting in what Sharaf and Levinson discussed as quests for omnipotence, omniscience and omnisentience.

A second question asked by Chessick is "What does the supervisor expect and why does he supervise?", and he notes that there is a "remarkable paucity" in the literature regarding this question. (Dr. Richard Lower, of the University of Pennsylvania, addressed himself to this issue, among the topics reviewed in a panel discussion at the APA meeting, May, 1971: "Psychotherapy Supervision: Role of the Supervisor" (100), and included among the secondary gains of the supervisor: the supervisor's needs to be "respected, loved, and defended;" and in order to achieve these, he utilizes many "seductive and rivalrous maneuvers.") Chessick feels that the primary gains of the supervisor, "laudatory" as they are stated to be, are not sufficient to motivate most supervisors, and that some of the secondary gains involve "the relief of professional loneliness for the psychotherapist who is isolated in an office, a chance to discuss his ideas and to expose himself to the criticism of intelligent residents, an opportunity to rethink his basic assumptions and to review the literature, the maintenance of a teaching appointment which has competitive value, and whatever narcissistic gratification is involved in being a member of a faculty alongside one's former teachers, and in having a voice in the accreditation of future colleagues." Lazerson has further elaborated upon the teacher's roles and needs in "The Learning Alliance and Its Relation to Psychiatric Teaching" (87a).

"How do the resident and the supervisor disappoint each other?" Some of the ways in which disappointments occur include particularly the disillusion which follows "the faith of the counsellors" (88), who often place their reliance on "short cuts and expediencies." Chessick also reviews Tischler's "rather amusing reports of the resident's perception of his initial supervisory experience," paralleling Grotjahn's, as well as Chessick's own original experiences with supervision. (Other difficulties are cited, as illustrated in Allen (89).) Further sources of disappointment in supervision include the assumption that residents have technical knowledge beyond their actual attainment. This is often based upon the resident's need to save face, particularly since for the resident, supervision is "a narcissistic injury" in which the "supervisor becomes an ambivalent object of painful growth" (45).

Chessick is unique in the commentators on supervision in explicitly considering whether "the prolonged bombardment of the supervisor by the ambivalent emotions of residents over the years, will not, unless special precautions are taken, lead to first a feeling of boredom (which masks anxiety, of course) and eventually to a loss of the desire to teach. Just as the resident may lose his desire to learn, due to a failure in the supervisory alliance, and manifest this by coming late to sessions or forgetting sessions, and so on, so the supervisor may act out in the same way."

Chessick recommends ten methods for avoiding disappointments in supervisory relationships: (1) resolving the conflict between service and teaching demands; (2) more seminars, emphasizing study of the humanities, literature, philosophy, drama, and other aspects of human experience; seminars constantly evaluated by residents and the training committee; (3) a regular seminar for supervisors; (4) a clear definition of an "outside supervisor" (citing Escoll and Wood's (112) attempt to foster cohesion among their private practice supervisors by scheduling monthly dinner meetings, and noting their regret that "it must be admitted that the outside supervisors do not come regularly," Chessick feels "either it must be made clear what the demands of the program are upon this outside supervisor and just what his role will be, or the program should abandon the use of outside supervisors altogether"); (5) the use of the "preceptor system"; also a resident organization allowing the residents to speak to the training committee as a group; (6) careful assignment of supervisor, in terms of his willingness and ability to perform the task (Chessick recalls Rosenbaum's attention to this issue, urging the matching of supervisors with residents in terms of personality and developmental stage); also supervisors should be involved in the selection and evaluation of residents; (7) developing *esprit de corps* in the institution, which also serves as a recruitment device; (8) periodic evaluation of the supervisor by the resident, along with residents' evaluation by the supervisor; also, the length of supervision of each resident by an individual supervisor should be variable; (9) the need for personal psychotherapy should be emphasized as an absolute necessity for training in psychotherapy. "If the resident by the second year of his training does not strongly feel the need for personal psychotherapy there has been either a mistake in selection or a pedagogic failure . . . it almost goes without saying that no supervisor, preceptor or administrator in the program with contact with residents should simultaneously be giving psychotherapy to these residents, since this obviously sets up a malignant peer competition." (10) The need for supervisory rewards, including "remuneration, meetings, flexibility about seminar and supervisory time, status, title, university appointments, and regular promotions."

Chessick expands the paper outlined above in a chapter from his book *Why Psychotherapists Fail* (6), adding an outline of education for psychotherapy which is based upon a fundamental effort to bridge C. P. Snow's "Two Cultures," by means of a synthetic "Kultur." "Of the various factors that cause failure in psychotherapy, the one that can be remedied most easily is the psychic field of the psychotherapist . . . [which optimally consists of] a humane attitude on the part of the therapist."

Outlining a four year program for psychotherapists, Chessick emphasizes a philosophy of education similar to that of "St. John's College, Annapolis, Maryland." The use of the seminar as a major vehicle for the teaching of psychotherapy has not been reported in the literature as "particularly helpful" (as noted by Guiora (90)), however Chessick recommends the use of a type of seminar he had conducted over the past ten years at "Northwestern, Illinois State Psychiatric Institute, and the U.S. Public Health Service," in which the residents were given an opportunity to present a case, following which the group made "predictions" regarding the course of the therapy. Questionnaire replies from the residents who had attended this seminar gave Chessick the impression "that they profited considerably from it."

III.   STUDIES FOCUSED ON THE CONTEXT OF SUPERVISION

As many students of supervision have pointed out, perhaps the only discussion primarily directed toward the context of supervision is a pioneer paper by Emch (23), which focuses upon the complexities of the psychoanalytic supervisory situation, particularly the mathematical combinations of its "seven basic elements," wherein the permutations reach "the tremendous total of 5,040." Emch includes in the basic elements of the psychoanalytic supervisory situation: (1) supervisor; (2) student; (3) patient under discussion; (4) student's analyst (training analyst); (5) another past or present supervisor; (6) institute committee on education; (7) clinical conference instructor.

The presentation of conflicting points of view simultaneously, particularly at conferences, is perceived as paralleling transference issues between supervisors and supervisees. Emch recommends various solutions, including "direct communication between at least two authority entities in the supervisory setting," as well as "setting up informal groups of training analysts, where in seminar fashion any topic may be discussed . . . , providing for regular additions to the group of supervisors, arranging for meetings of supervisors with student groups, and an increased awareness on the part of supervisors of the tremendous complexities in which the supervision takes place."

Among the few papers concerned with the impact of context of residency programs upon the resident's development, Sharaf and Levinson's pointed out the importance of the ideology of the training center, as well as extramural shifts in psychiatric emphasis, which have influenced the evaluative hierarchy of psychiatric enterprises. An informative follow up study, which extended the original observations they made at the Massachusetts Mental Health Center, is that by Ching-Piao Chien and Appleton (91) "The Need for Extensive Reform in Psychiatry Teaching: An Investigation in Treatment Ideology and Learning," in which the attitudes of residents and of the training center toward the use of drug treatment in psychiatry were investigated. Of particular concern to the authors was the finding that, as Klerman (92) stated, "psychopharmacology is regarded by many residents as of low priority, and by some residents as extraneous to the main goals of their training." Also, as Freyhan (93) emphasized, "first year residents are often given what amounts to a free hand when it comes to drug treatment, while systematic supervision is—rightfully—considered an absolute necessity for psychotherapy." Piao-Chien and Appleton studied 24 beginning psychiatric residents by means of a questionnaire regarding chemotherapy attitudes during the first week of their residency, and again six months later, following their completion of a systematic course in psychopharmacology: The residents were previously divided into "psychotherapeutic" and "eclectic" groups. At the outset, there were "16 residents in the psychotherapeutic category and 8 classified eclectic . . . 25% of each of these groups changed their ideology within the six month period of study." The finding that "psychotherapeutic residents administer drugs as frequently as the eclectic in the treatment of in-patients" was attributed to "pressure from ward staff operative on all residents to effect immediate alleviation of psychotic behavior; also the administration of drugs to establish a rapport for psychotherapy." (That the hospital milieu itself places contextual pressure upon the resident toward the use of medication seems not to have been considered by the investigators as a factor in their study.)

O'Connor (94) studied the influence of the peer group upon the resident's viewpoints, and noted that most of the literature has stressed the importance of the mechanism of identification with the supervisor as the most important factor in the choice of psychiatric viewpoint (citing Fleming, Ford, and Grotjahn; as well as Coker (95)). According to O'Connor, little attention has been paid to the influence of peer opinion, which "may in part offset more influential status of the teachers." In support, he cites Kalis (96) who found that the attitudes of first year residents "more closely agree with those of fellow residents and ward personnel at the end of the first year than at its beginning." However, as O'Connor recalls his own residency experience, he recognized the importance in retrospect of his teachers' personalities as outweighing the content and ideological propositions of any specific psychiatric philosophy. Also operative in influencing the resident's point of view is the timing at which he is exposed to various individuals and their theories, considering the emotional cycles through which he passes (as noted by Halleck and Woods), including periods of "therapeutic nihilism" and rampant eclecticism. As the residency nears its end, "the resident feels particular pressure for adopting a specific philosophy, since there is less room for experimentation with various approaches." Finally, O'Connor concludes that the two factors which are most important in the decision to adopt a particular school of psychiatric thought in the residency are "group support and the protective devices inherent in the theory."

At the University of Cincinnati, Kurtz and Kaplan (97) studied "the social system of the training center as a contributing factor in the developing attitudes and value system of psychiatric residents," and compared the residents at two psychiatric training institutions, one characterized by strong ideological commitments, the other by low ideological commitments. Hypothesizing that "attitude congruence toward treatment concepts would be greater between resident and staff in the center with the strong ideological commitment rather than in the one where the staff was less committed," they studied 32 psychiatric residents and 20 faculty psychiatrists for congruence of attitude (by Osgood's Somantic Differential) and ideological commitment (by Strauss' Ideology Scale). The results did not support their hypothesis, but they did feel there was evidence for a relationship between the ideology of a training center and the manner in which residents develop attitudes toward types of treatment. In their discussion, Kurtz and Kaplan speculated that "a resident's resistance to attitude assimilation is lower in a social setting with less ideological structure, because his developing professional identity and sense of competence are not focused upon his acceptance or rejection of any strongly held point of view. Perhaps in such a social setting he feels less threatened and thereby remains more open to attitudinal influence."

Colman (98), following his first year in-patient experience at Langley-Porter Psychiatric Institute, reported his response to the specific treatment philosophy and methods of the ward program in which he had worked. Pointing out that the first year resident spends a great deal more of his time in group meetings and in group therapy than he does in individual psychotherapy, Colman reports that his supervision experience was "richer in the group modality," because of staff attitudes as well as the necessity for multiple group meetings. "Prior training experience had been as a physician, with a well delineated role and function; psychiatric residents however find no clearly defined role or function." Although the individual psychotherapist's role might have assisted in allaying the anxiety of the beginning psychiatric resident, "the resident on the ward cannot identify himself as an individual psychotherapist. He can only seek security in the role of group and family therapist, or more broadly, he may see himself as leader of the various therapeutic groups into which his main energies are funneled." In this situation, further problems beset the resident: "(1) his experience and training with group and group functions is negligible; (2) privacy of the medical interview and privileged communications is a sacred cow in medical tradition, and its violation by the necessity of exchanging common experiences in the group situation can be disconcerting, particularly when combined with the presence of a co-therapist." An additional difficulty in this setting is the resident's feeling that he may be "marking time while learning group and family techniques, since he may still envision his future professional role as individual psychotherapist or even analyst." Further role diffusion results from the necessity to "change roles radically in various meetings," but Colman perceived some supportive aspects of the resident's first year situation, including "his administration of drugs and ECT, as well as his identification with the supervisor and other residents."

Decision making responsibility is also influenced by the first year resident's group role, and Colman feels that the ward personnel value the resident in the role of group therapist, while his patients at times experience difficulty in integrating "different faces of the resident in various group settings." In summary, Colman concludes "on a ward in which relatively short hospitalization is an important goal . . . the resident's broad grasp of the patient's life situation and reaction patterns provides the basis for a strong voice in all decisions made."

It is noteworthy that in the literature on supervision, very little attention has been paid to the situation of the patient in the tetradic relationship between supervisor and supervisee, patient and context. Tarachow and Schuster have commented, *en passant,* regarding the issue of responsibility for the patient on the part of the supervisor. Brody mentions, incidentally, the issue of the selection of patient types as a relevant concern of the supervisor. General mention is made of the fact that first-year residents are primarily assigned to hospital in-patient care and, therefore, primarily deal with patients in severe states of decompensation, usually schizophrenic or depressive. However, in out-patient psychotherapy, although some mention has been made of the disparity in the Hollingshead-Redlich Index between therapist and patient in clinic populations, there has been very little discussion of patient selection as a supervisory responsibility, except in terms of "intensive versus supportive" issues. In most residencies, there seems to be an implicit rule that one or two "intensive cases" are all that the resident will have either time or capability to handle. The process of selection of these patients from an out-patient clinic population, as a preliminary contractual element between supervisor and supervisee, is rarely mentioned, nor is the "fit" between the personality as well as the skills of the resident to the specific personality style, psychopathology, and life situation of the patient. Again, many residencies perceive the one or two psychotherapy cases usually treated by the resident during his training as "paradigmatic," which in most residencies has meant the treatment of one hysterical female patient and one obsessive-compulsive male patient. The timing of the introduction of these patients, in terms of the residency program, is another supervisory concern not much discussed in the literature. Certainly it would seem that one of the primary tasks of the supervisor in out-patient psychotherapy would be a preliminary discussion with the supervisee regarding the relevant factors in choice of appropriate therapy patients, whereby the basic elements of the supervisory situation may be brought into explicit focus: the context of the residency training program (ideology, clinic population, service commitments, models of psychiatric treatment); issues of the supervisor-supervisee relationship (explicitude of the supervisor's psychiatric point of view, the "ground rules" of the supervisory situation); the resident's own situation (developmental stage, personality, career ambitions, and directions, and previous experience in psychotherapy).

IV.   STUDIES FOCUSED ON THE SUPERVISORY PROCESS

A. *General Comments*

Gardner (99), in a round table discussion on the training of clinical psychologists, described "the development of the clinical attitude . . . though our present day teaching methods do not enable us to create the artist, they definitely do enable us to recognize and eliminate the 'hacker.' The only teaching method we have at the present time is prolonged individual supervision of the psychotherapist. This is true and will continue to be true, I feel, for the majority of our workers in the several mental health disciplines; and to the supervisor-teacher in our midst, falls the task of imparting to the trainee as much as he can concerning the student's assets and liabilities as a potential therapist, and of equipping him with specific skills and techniques that he will use with the patient. I need not add that we need more and better supervisors in all our fields if we hope to train the therapists that we need, and therapists who are imbued with the clinical—or better, therapeutic—attitude."

Ekstein (100) in a panel discussion at the American Psychiatric Association's meeting in May of 1971, "Psychotherapy Supervision: The Role of the Supervisor," explicated his basic model of the supervisory situation, the "clinical rhombus" at each point of which the respective participants in the process were located (resident, patient, supervisor and administration); the task of the supervisor was described as oscillatory, moving across the various participant elements of the supervisory situation. Hollender (100) stressed the importance of the contract between supervisor and supervisee, emphasizing the importance of the third through the sixth hours as crucial for the "contract." He also emphasized the impact of the preliminary meeting between supervisor and supervisee, prior to the start of therapy, in which the discussion should touch upon issues such as data gathering, the goal of the therapy, what will be offered and what the patient can use.

Lower (100) then discussed the importance of countertransferential feelings in the supervisor, and the need to recognize the multiple gratifications (secondary gains) of the supervisor: recognition, narcissistic gratification, and proselytization. At the same panel, Kaplan (100) elaborated upon the anxiety attendant upon beginning supervision and the necessity to "fit in" with a series of supervisory styles. I presented a modified Eriksonian schema of developmental tasks, in which the residency challenges the trainee to recapitulate and/or attain the stages of identity, intimacy, and generativity. These developmental tasks could also be perceived as applying equally to the supervisor himself. Audience discussion following the formal presentations at this panel was primarily concerned with requests for specific recmendations on the formation of a training program for supervisors. Dr. Ekstein, attempting to describe an ideal program, mentioned that "work in progress" is still going on at Reiss-Davis Clinic in Los Angeles, and that the San Francisco Psychoanalytic Society had just embarked upon a study of psychoanalytic supervision.

The developmental tasks noted above may be perceived as a continuum: the beginning resident's identity crisis; the formation of the ability to tolerate intimacy; and, in the practice of psychotherapy, the necessity for the therapist to proceed to a level of generativity, to be able to conduct and conclude the experience of psychotherapy. Ultimately, the resident is faced with the task of integrating the previous phases of development. Hopefully, the supervisor has been able to achieve his own "identity," capacity for intimacy, generativity, and finally "integrity," in order to be usefully adopted as a role model, the primary and essential ingredient of supervision.

Riess (9), in his excellent chapter, "Selection and Supervision of Psychotherapists," has elaborated upon the role of the supervisor in some detail. He states, "The role of the supervisor is . . . compounded of a need to help integrate theory and practice to deepen the understanding by the therapist of human behavior as it is reflected *in vivo* and to help develop skills and techniques for bringing about change." In this activity, character problems of the supervisee intrude themselves in the therapist-patient interaction as well as in the trainee-supervisor interchange. Thus the first function of the supervisor, his educative role, has "a triple structure," in which the trainee is assisted to develop skills, recognize the areas and ways in which his character problems enter into the therapeutic relationship and overcome resistances to learning. Other functions of the supervisor include his evaluative role, which involves decisions about phase-specific questions in the resident's program. Additionally, the supervisor must evaluate judgments of the resident's progress and perform his institutional role as well. In effect, also, the supervisor "has to be the middle man between the routine demands of the clinic and the resistances of the trainee. . . ." Riess describes the way the Postgraduate Center has dealt with problems of ideological misfits between supervisors and trainees, where a careful study was made of the effect of theoretical allegiance and the supervisor process. "In most instances it was found that the blocks to learning were caused by transference and countertransference resistances." Riess recalls an experimental experience of Max Markowitz in which "a relatively sophisticated therapist's supervisor subjected himself to supervision by a group of his colleagues of varying persuasions. To his surprise he found that his own reactions were determined by his intrapersonal needs and not by the spurious rationalization of differential schooling."

The scarcity of evaluation of the effectiveness of supervision is also cited by Riess, and partially explained upon the basis of the difficulty inherent in the interaction of "two factors, the stage of learning of the therapist and the stages of therapy during which the supervision is done. These two factors can best be described in question form as 'what should a therapist be expected to know and do at the beginning, middle and end of therapy, and what should be expected of a therapist after his first, second or third year of training'?"

The supervisor should be prepared to teach: "At initiation of treatment, introduction of the patient to treatment procedure, handling of inadequate motivations, establishment of an initial rapport, definition of goals, structuring of sessions, establishing of a tentative diagnosis, and dynamics and plan of treatment." In the middle phase the major issues are resistance, transference and countertransference issues, diagnostic hypotheses and plans of treatment modifications as a result of new data and attitudes; and finally, as termination nears, "the translation of knowledge into action is to be handled, together with the reduction of dependency, resistance to normality, and the summarization of progress to date."

"At the Postgraduate Center an attempt has been made to derive a more objective rating scale from the experience of a group of supervisors who met regularly once a week to assess candidates and problems in supervision. As a result a five point scale was established as an experimental supplement to the more open-ended evaluation of each trainee."

"The Function of Individual Supervision" by D'Zmura (101) narrows the issues to the primary function of individual supervision perceived as the promotion of the personal growth of the therapist. In agreement with this position is Kaplowitz (102), who points out that there are several "maneuvers" particularly important for supervisors to be able to utilize; one of these is the questioning of the supervisee for a "relevant personal life experience so that he can make contact with his patient." Additionally, Kaplowitz aligns himself with "the principles of those teachers who focus on the student-therapist in the supervision, with the added dimension of probing the supervisee's intrapsychic processes only as they relate to his therapeutic work . . . my chief aim has been to give the supervisee the ability to be aware of himself on a feeling level, as he relates to his patient and to his supervisor. In this way he can be helped to use his native endowments and sensitivities, in order to develop his capacity for empathic responsiveness." (In this emphasis Kaplowitz agrees with Ornstein and Fleming and Benedek.) He lists several techniques he considers important for the supervisor: "(1) asking the supervisee for relevant life experiences; (2) investigating the supervisee's dominant emotional quality in supervision as it relates to his patient; (3) examining the supervisee's countertransference problem by probing his intrapsychic processes in relation to the supervisor; (4) utilizing the supervisor-supervisee relationship as a living emotional experience so that the therapist student can truly sense himself in relationship to his patient. Emphasis is placed on the parallelism between supervisory and therapeutic relationships; (5) utilizing the supervisor's personality as a model for the supervisee, not hesitating to expose his own transference problems if they appear."

The supervisory task and the therapeutic relationship are perceived as "battlegrounds" by Schwartz (103). Since this battle is perceived as "inevitable," the task of the supervisor is "not to help the therapist to achieve self-limiting abrogation of affect. Rather it is to help him to utilize his state of unsettlement to promote his own professional learning. . . ."

Arlow (44, 2, 31) has written extensively on the supervisory situation, analogizing it with artistic creation as well as analytic therapy. His opinions parallel Searles' regarding the importance of the counter-transferential responses of the supervisor to the therapist as an emotional indicator regarding the situation between therapist and patient. Nonetheless, "in the supervisory situation only the surface of the therapist's reaction to his patient is laid bare. Because it lacks depth and genetic dimension, supervision does not lend itself to be used for real structural change in the therapist. Supervision is a part of reality, and it cannot accomplish *per se* that which the personal analysis may set in force by way of broadening insight and stimulating receptivity to new self-understanding."

In 1955, Searles (30) established the point of view that the specific responses of the supervisor during supervision often provide 'valuable clarification of processes currently characterizing the relationship between the supervisee and the patient." Hora (25) is equally convinced that in the supervisory process many of the therapist's presentations are parallel and unconscious representations of his patient's material. He labeled this phenomenon the "patient within the therapist."

An extreme position regarding the therapy-pedagogy controversy is advocated by Woodmansey (104) who explicitly urges that the supervisor be quite explicit in his viewpoint that "the teacher must give not only formal instruction, but also what may be regarded as actual psychotherapy to the trainee, directed specifically towards helping the latter with the inner conflicts that interfere with his clinical casework—and are re-experienced in the supervision." Since "the same ultimate basis" exists for difficulties encountered in treating individual patients as in supervision, the training method should primarily be "regarded as actual psychotherapy."

A shift in focus to include the patient in the supervisory process is advocated by Wagner (70) who recognizes that the supervisor is indirectly responsible for the treatment of the patient. "From the viewpoint of training, the therapist must be given the opportunity of learning . . . but it must not take place at the expense of the patient's welfare. The judgment as to when intervention becomes necessary may be difficult, but the risk of this kind of teaching does not seem great. Supervision is not a chaotic phenomenon, but a highly differentiated process, where the main controls are internalized through the therapist's loyalty to the structure of therapy, and realization of his personal responsibility toward the patient as well as to himself."

B. *Specific Issues and Problems*

Ackerman (18), in 1953, recognizing that there was yet to be established a "program of supervision," emphasized that the role of the supervisor was particularly important in the area in which the supervisee must deal with "unresolved conflicts in theory . . . while the supervisor may try to protect the student from conceptual confusion, he must not try to conceal these theoretical conflicts from the student or try to get him to accept uncritically some fixed ideological system. An important part of every student's education should be that he acquire a critical appreciation of these unresolved controversies." Recalling his experiences with transferential and countertransferential problems in supervision, Ackerman urges that the supervisor "try to view the phenomena . . . within the broad frame of several overlapping interpersonal relationships." And also in 1953, Rosenbaum (105) recognized the importance of the selection of a specific kind of supervisor, in the effort to "match" the personality and level of training of the resident.

One of the few supervisors who reports more than one experience in supervision, Grotjahn (106) recalled that "in my work in recent years, I have found supervision becoming more and more of a problem, a challenge, and a reason for dissatisfaction to me . . . when I asked others what they remembered about their own experience of being supervised, several of my senior colleagues . . . said in effect 'I always saw to it that I went to a supervisor who would interfere with me as little as possible.' " Grotjahn decided "to return to the role of the supervisee . . . this experience was so educational that I can recommend it to other psychoanalysts, no matter how late they may be in their careers: in my own case I underwent the experience of being supervised again after almost 25 years." In his practice of supervision, Grotjahn did not hesitate to visit in person the offices of his supervisees, and observe them in the actual conduct of their psychotherapy. (This is akin to the method utilized at our center wherein the supervisor sits with the patient and therapist during his initial out-patient diagnostic interview.)

Grotjahn divided the phases of supervision into " (1) the period of preparation; (2) growing insight into the psychodynamics of the patient's personality and his sickness, and (3) working through."

There have been very few extensive reports by supervisees of recollections of their own supervision. However, several reminiscences were included in a section of the Journal of the William Alanson White Psychoanalytic Institute entitled "Views on the Supervisory Situation," edited by Ruth Moulton (107). She reports that in 1959 the Institute initiated regular meetings of supervisors to discuss "general problems in supervision; the result of the discussion between students and supervisors proved so much more useful in promoting good teaching alliances than written explanations of training processes and goals, that arrangements were made to hold such discussions at least once a year." Further developments included a monthly study group meeting on supervision with the plan of the formation of parallel committees with a student group which would meet three or four times a year jointly. In "Multiple Dimensions of Supervision," Moulton advocates that the supervisor focus upon the student's anxiety in the supervisory sessions. Reporting on her own experience under three supervisors, Moulton ("My Memories of Being Supervised") reminisces about Erich Fromm, Harry Stack Sullivan, and Frieda Fromm-Reichman. Describing Harry Stack Sullivan's point of view regarding supervision, she recalls that "he certainly did not favor orthodox pomposity or unnatural neutrality, but he did not believe in foisting on a patient data about one's self that could only make him anxious and serve no purpose. Thus he advocated that political views, private matters of taste, details of family life and the like should be kept out of the way of the patient, who had enough to deal with from within himself without having to contend with extra burdens." (Contrast this point of view with that of Halleck in *The Politics of Therapy*.) Other anecdotal papers are included by Bush (108) and Paidoussi (109); Paidoussi recalls one of his supervisor's questions reminiscent of the supervisory style recommended by Kaplowitz, "Can you think of an analogous situation from your own life experience?" Beckett (110) records his conclusions about supervision: "1. Becoming a psychoanalyst is a process of self-appointment; each candidate must assess where he is in his development and what he needs to work on to further that development. 2. The effectiveness of supervision depends upon the working alliance between candidate and supervisor and upon the way each participant handles his own transference reaction to the situation. 3. Factors which hinder the development of a working alliance in the supervisory situation may arise from sources in the supervisor or the candidate."

Fleming (111) analyzes various models of the teaching process in supervision: first, the "jug-mug model," in which a supply of information is poured into the student's mind; second, on the analogy of the "potter" who turns unformed clay into a shape which has utility and beauty; and third, on the analogy of the "gardener who prepares the soil, plants the seed, nurtures the seedling and encourages growth to maturity by all possible means." The third style of supervision "exercises the student's mind" rather than demonstrates "the supervisor's viewpoint. . . . Our own viewpoint regarding the fundamental task of teaching psychotherapy is the situation of watching and being watched, being informed and being corrected, are partial learning experiences. They prepare the ground but they do not cultivate the growth potential as it is possible to do in a supervisory situation." Fleming takes issue with Kubie and others who advocate the use of technical strategies of teaching (such as one-way screens, T.V., case conference presentations etc.) since she feels that these are "passive methods of teaching in which the situation is reversed, so that the student becomes the performer and the teacher becomes the observer" along the lines of the "potter-pot strategy," and does not reach the third model of supervision which she espouses, the "nurturing gardener."

C. Methodological Studies

Among the residency programs which have described their methods (most of them consisting of direct or indirect observation of resident interviews), Miller and Burstein (75) described the methodology of their program which involves observation and subsequent discussion by two supervisors of the resident's diagnostic interview. They feel that "the discussion phase of our format not only provides an opportunity to explore the resident's thinking in the light of his observed behavior, but also presses him in the direction of an active involvement in the assessment process. Sequential assessments at successive stages of the residency . . . offer several advantages." One of these is that these assessments become "in effect a potential evaluation of the educational program when consistently repeated over time and with many residents." Also the objective view obtained within this systematic framework provides "a valuable contrast with informal and anecdotal evaluations."

Schuster and Freeman (77) describe their experience in the supervision of psychiatric residents during their second year assignment of six months to the out-patient clinic at the University of Rochester. Their format involves the actual presence of the supervisor with the resident during the initial diagnostic interview, with these advantages: 1. Immediacy of data for the supervisor, by virtue of direct observation; 2. opportunity for the supervisor to intervene or elaborate upon the interview; 3. realistic impact of the supervisor's presence, as contrasted with imaginings by resident and patient of a viewer behind a one-way screen, with consensual validation of access to first-hand material; 4. opportunity for the resident to observe the supervisor's interview technique, and not with a patient in whom the resident has no investment but one which will be his own case in all likelihood.

Escoll and Wood (112) described a similar procedure at the University of Pennsylvania recommending that the preceptor join the resident in the interview since "in watching alone behind the screen . . . the observer feels isolated, and effective supervisor-resident interaction is inhibited." (They also cite Zinberg (113) as recommending the same practice.) Escoll and Wood also mention their reservations concerning the use of tape recordings, in psychotherapy supervision: "Tape recordings have a definite place, but can be used by the resident to avoid formulating a case, or confronting the preceptor directly, and as with the use of the one-way screen, interaction may be slowed." They also recommend, with the hope of solving the peda-gogue-critic dichotomy, an "inside preceptor and an outside precep-tor" for the beginning resident. However, this approach contains problems of its own, as they observed "the tendency of the inside preceptor to abandon his administrative role, and a tendency of the outside preceptor to become isolated from the administrative and the resident group . . . he may even be seduced into joining the resident's manipulations against the administration." The length of the preceptorial assignment, according to Escoll and Wood, should be optimally one year. Occasionally, residents request specific precep-tors; here the authors' response is "individualized," since "the resi-dent may utilize a variety of preceptors to fractionate his professional life, being the analyst, the social psychiatrist, the behavioral therapist, as he mimics each preceptor in turn. He thus may not only shun controversy with the preceptor, but also avoid evaluating and in-tegrating these approaches. . . . (Additionally) we find it very helpful to have female members of the department as preceptors; they are of particular help to female residents, and may work particularly well with certain male residents who for competitive or other reasons resist learning from men."

A "fieldwork" program at the University of Virginia is described by Volkan and Hawkins (114, 115, 116) which was inaugurated for first year residents. Six first year residents were assigned to a tutor who shared five hours per week with the group. The tutor became "an auxiliary therapist" forming a learning alliance with the therapist resident and other group members. The residents treated in-patients in rotation, while the group observed the actual treatment through a one-way screen, and discussion of the treatment followed these observations. The tutor's chief aim was to "open a way for a learning group to evolve rather than a therapy group." One of the basic assumptions of the program was that "psychiatric practice includes an element of art which can be passed on to beginners only through preceptorship." Agreeing with Ornstein that the funda-mental experience of working in depth on a one-to-one basis is the essential task of the psychiatrist, they analogize between "psychoanalytic treatment aimed at ego building and the teaching techniques applicable to the first year resident, whose ego is deficient in therapeutic experience."

Guiora et al. (90), describe their program at the University of Michigan, in which, recognizing that supervision is a cornerstone of training, yet is subject to great variation, they cite several modifications such as "role reversal" (advocated by Jose Barchilon (117)): "While the reversal of role technique may present agonizing difficulties and self supervision may clearly be inadequate, their very advocacy points to some dissatisfactions both latent and not so latent with the traditional system. The continuous case presentation is an established adjunct to individual supervision, and . . . its efficacy is taken for granted and rarely if ever questioned" (118).

The authors examined the continuous case seminar and found it to be of limited value, but "that the problems faced by a group discussing at an intellectual level a process that is only in part intellectual, are very serious. We have at this time, however, no final answer to the question as to whether group supervision of this kind must inevitably entail . . . contradictions."

Muslin and Carmichael (119) describe a method of teaching at the University of Illinois based on the filming of the teacher-student dyad, the showing of the film followed by "group supervision of the instructor by a workshop group." The members of the "group workshop" who discuss the observed interview consisted of "the coordinators of the psychiatry clerkship in the third and fourth years, with the addition of invited members of the faculty, plus the coordinator of the undergraduate program, and the head of the department of psychiatry." (A similar method of teaching clinical psychiatry to medical students was utilized at State University of New York Upstate Medical Center, Syracuse, by Hollender (120), wherein he and medical student clerks observed and commented upon the continuous therapy of an out-patient by a senior staff member.)

Further experiences in observed psychotherapy and experimental methods in role reversal are described by Titchener et al. (121) at the University of Cincinnati. This group reported on their teaching of "conjoint marital therapy," by means of a format whereby the teacher conducted the treatment, while residents observed by closed circuit T.V., and supervised the treatment in 40-minute discussions after the 50-minute treatment session. The authors recall Barchilon's developmental sequence in this type of teaching situation, and were able to define phases in such a development, which were "1. pseudo-didactic; 2. investigative; 3. participatory." The development of the group discussion progressed through these phases until "the supervisory sessions assumed a real rather than a play-acting-for-learning quality" in the final phase of participation. This method of teaching, they concluded, "should perhaps be offered more often and earlier in the psychiatric educational experience." A modification of the classical supervisory arrangement was described by Rosen and Bartemeier (122) who report on their experience with psychotherapy sessions "conducted jointly by psychiatric residents and their supervisors" in Baltimore, Maryland. Fourteen hospitalized patients were treated by ten psychiatric residents and a single supervisor over an 18 month period. Despite the relative "anxiety provoking situation," the authors observed a shift in the resident from "participant observer to active therapist."

Among the investigators focusing on the supervision of the first year resident, Bonn and Schiff (123) examined the supervisory situation with particular emphasis on the training of residents as ward physicians, on an in-patient service of the VA Hospital at Topeka, Kansas. "Although we . . . are ultimately responsible to the hospital administrators for the welfare of the patients, the residents are primarily responsible for the day to day care of the patients. . . . As much as we can, we avoid interjecting ourselves into the doctor-patient relationships the residents establish . . . our role with the residents is largely consultative." The authors feel they are in a superior position as supervisors because of their ability to amass a great deal of data "from other sources than the residents, so that as supervisors of both the treatment program and the training program on our service, we have the opportunity to observe the interactions of all concerned . . . rarely have we had to explicitly interfere with and negate a resident's own planning." In their supervision of the first year residents, these supervisors advocate the use of "all three methods of supervision" (patient, process, and resident- or supervisor-centered). The use of resident- or supervisor-centered supervision was reserved for "a persistent learning problem that failed to respond to other methods." They report upon their use of the Menninger process notes evaluation of the resident, recognizing that "reactions varied with individual resident and with the resident-supervisory relationship. When the resident reads the report, we discuss it with him. Generally, reading the report seems to enhance the resident's capacity for accurate self appraisal. This is particularly helpful to the resident who denies his ability in his self evaluation of his functions as a resident. Writing the report also enhances our own supervisory acumen."

D. *Technical Procedures*

Several authors have devoted themselves to the technical aspects of the supervisory situation (124, 125, 126, 127). Including discussions of the use of tape recording, one-way screens, and most recently, video-tapes, Berger (128) has compiled a series of papers on this subject, and in his introduction to a section on training, reviewed the uses of television in the teaching of psychotherapy. He explicitly recalls Barchilon's methodology, believing it to be "the ideal medium for teaching technique, know-how, and practical considerations almost impossible to learn elsewhere." He also records Barchilon's finding that "students ordinarily most refractory or insensitive or not psychologically minded in their previous residency experiences have surprisingly come forward in this type of exercise and demonstrated profound awareness, sensitivity and competency. His creative and courageous technique was successful in undermining passivity and reducing resistance or antagonism to learning."

Gruenberg et al. (129) emphasized the importance of the "therapist's lack of awareness of his own nonverbal communications to the patient" in his reports to the supervisor in the classic supervisory method. Reviewing the literature related to "the problems inherent in psychiatric supervision," Gruenberg et al. cite Grotjahn's dissatisfaction with the methods of supervision available in 1955, and report on the work of many pioneers in the use of video-tape both as a therapeutic and a teaching device. Some of the advantages reported by the advocates of video-tape include: the attention to kinesics, the accuracy of the data, and the increased emphasis upon the "presentation itself" which is supposedly more evident on video-tape. One advantage which Gruenberg cites is that "too often the patient can become the forgotten man as a result of our concern with and focus upon the teaching-learning experience. We may lose sight of the patient's need for help. With the greater sense of engagement with the patient provided by video tape, the experienced supervisor can protect him against possible antitherapeutic maneuvers by the resident." The residents who have been taught by this method, according to Gruenberg et al., report that "while they may not have learned faster how to do psychotherapy, they have learned it better."

Froelich (130) describes his use of video-tape simulation, "which is the use of a combination of role playing and video-tape in which the teacher selects a common clinical situation appropriate to his teaching goals, which has as part of it role conflict and interpersonal disagreement, yet one which has no clearcut management procedure." Froelich concludes that on occasion "the level of frankness and the honesty of comments approaches that in a T-group," and enthusiastically reports "we have not found any teaching method that creates as much student participation or involvement as does video-tape simulation."

Other chapters devoted to the subject of teaching of psychotherapy by closed circuit T.V. include Trethowan (131) who describes the use of closed circuit T.V. in the United Kingdom, and lists various useful applications; and Gladfelter (132), who describes the use of video-tape in the supervision of group psychotherapy conducted by co-therapists. (He urges that the supervisor have personal experience in viewing himself on video-tape as a group therapist.)

In a detailed description of his use of video-tape in a training program, Kagan (133) emphasizes a "*caveat* for the social sciences" in the use of video-tape. He feels that it is of specific rather than general utility, and most particularly helpful in the development of a technique which he and his colleagues termed "Interpersonal Process Recall," in which a subject of the video-tape was given control of the replay, or stopped at various points and asked questions regarding his feelings at these times. Kagan's use of video-tape in his training program was perceived as composed of three phases. In the first phase, the supervisee was acquainted with the concepts of his supervisor, shown video-tape models of "good therapy," and was asked to rate each video-tape along the dimensions of "affect, understanding, and specific versus explanatory." In the second phase of this supervisory system, the supervisor dealt particularly with two inhibitory dynamics of beginning counselors. "1. Feigning clinical naivete, and 2. tuning out" (by which Kagan and his colleagues mean "ignoring the other, usually by focusing on one's self"). In the second phase, the task was "to set up a counselling session and do little or no recall with the client, but rather to conduct a recall and interrogation session of the counselor." The third phase places the counselor in the position of performing the function of interrogation with another student client. Thus the counselor has an opportunity "to try out confrontive behavior with the support of the video tape to fall back on, and the realization that he is working with his peer's client, not his own. When he and his colleague switch roles, the counsellor's partner then does recall and interrogation with one of the counsellor's clients. The counsellor is permitted to observe the session through a one-way mirror and so learns about his client's recalled reaction to the session which they have just concluded together. Both counsellors' supervisor is available to be of assistance with any technical problem and to discuss with both students their reaction to the aggressive role of interrogator, and to the feedback they got from their clients." Kagan feels that he has evidence that this system is effective, since it has shown significantly "better ratings of a group of counsellors given interpersonal process recall experience as opposed to those who did not receive such training." Additionally, Kagan describes the use of his method in medical education, utilizing simulation technique, in a project at Michigan State University, where the system was found "to have worked well, and statistically significant gains were found in student interview skills." Kagan also advocates the addition, for research purposes, of "physiological measurement devices to the interpersonal process recall system" in order to get further parameters of "feelings that are very basic determinants of human interaction."

Miller and Tupin, at U. of California (Davis) have described their methods for second-year medical student teaching of psychiatry as "multimedia teaching," utilizing a "diagnostic inventory." They are explicitly concerned with "style" as well as "content" in teaching (133a).

The term "cyberneticide" has been coined to describe the replacement of human workers by technological advances. The supervisory process, and its relationship to the teaching and learning of psychotherapy, are in the central path of the march of technology and must adapt, or become obsolete (134). Nonetheless, Fleming's cautionary response to the use of mechanical devices in supervision might well be reiterated (135). The essential task of supervision is not the insistence upon the accuracy of detail, nor the mutual observations of what is inevitably a displacement from a dyadic transaction. This is not to minimize the value of video-tape for many educational enterprises, nor to insist on a "generation gap" between supervisors and supervisees, which would emphasize their differences in terms of classic issues of confidentiality, the special qualities of the dyadic relationship, and a not so subtle shift in the "tempo" of the milieu in which residents now grow and learn to do psychotherapy, i.e., a world in which McLuhan may have more theoretical impact than Freud.

E. Training Studies and Models

Despite the explicit recommendations of the GAP Report of 1955 emphasizing the need for educating clinical supervisors ("Adequate training of supervisors has been neglected in medical education, particularly outside full-time medical school faculties. In psychiatry supervisors presumably have administrative and clinical duties or research interests in addition to their teaching responsibilities. More often than not, the staff physician is appointed not primarily because of his proved expertness as an educator and rather, finds the role of instructor thrust upon him. Although the effective teacher must be a competent clinician, not all competent clinicians can teach. A minimal amount of systematic training and supervision given junior staff psychiatrists by experienced and gifted teachers improves a residency program tremendously."), there have been few reported efforts toward extensive analysis of the rationale, methodology, or effectiveness of the teaching of psychotherapy to residents. The classical model of seminars for supervisory discussion, which has been in existence at several training centers (Chicago, Cincinnati, Topeka, Boston, New York), has not been modified to any great degree as the major vehicle for training of supervisors. Nor has there been reported any research upon the effectiveness of this method of training. (In fact, the only research reported on the evaluation of supervisory training methodology was that described by Kagan in the training of counselors.)

Kubie (28) and others have noted similarities in the processes of consultation and supervision. A report on consultation research by Mannino and Shore (136) discussed the possibility of formulating an empirical classification of consultation. They particularly were impressed with the research of McClung (137) which derived an empiric schema containing descriptions of several types of consultation, and fixing upon four definitive parameters: "Contact with clients, degree of consultant's responsibility for case disposition, direction of the consultant's responsibility, and degree to which the consultant was willing to participate in the personal processes of the consultee." (These categorizations have parallel implications in the supervisor-supervisee relationship.)

As Mannino and Shore emphasized, the attempt to derive an empirically based classification is a fundamental step in research. Semrad (45) described an attempt to discover the commonalities among various supervisors of psychotherapy, based upon 100 responses to a questionnaire sent in 1962 to 150 Harvard Medical School supervisors. It was felt that the questionnaire succeded in outlining the "general assumptions of our own academic community . . . some of the generally recognized practical problem areas, and (noted) that the questionnaire technique samples only the surface derivatives of inner feelings and deeper motivations, which themselves do not yield except to a more personal and painstaking investigation." Some of the factors singled out as particularly significant of ways in which teachers might contribute to residents' learning difficulties were revealing: "1. The teacher not understanding or disregarding the learning processes of the resident; 2. the teacher's overloaded schedule not permitting fulfillment of his desire to teach." Other common causes of difficulties in learning were felt to be primarily "the resident's neurosis," followed in decreasing order of importance by "inadequate preparation and time for reflection, overloaded schedules, neurotic choice of vocation, and the temptation to slight one's training to make money." The somewhat disappointing result of this questionnaire, may be more attributable to the small size of the sample, the explicitly discussed difficulty of the data itself as not available by means of a questionnaire format, the problem of questionnaire design, and finally insufficient variety of sampled centers of training (45).

Riess (9) has described at some length the methodology utilized at the Postgraduate Center in the training of supervisors. One of the important features of that program is the development of a specific evaluative questionnaire for supervisors, which focuses on many discrete areas involved in the supervisory process, and in so doing "trains the supervisor" to focus on specific aspects of his task. (This method recalls Weed's series of papers in the New England Journal, "Medical Records that Guide and Teach" (138).) Also, there is a course for supervisors at the Center which utilizes techniques such as role playing. Riess cites Kubie's pioneer description of the method of comparison of taped interviews of patient-therapist sessions and supervisory sessions with the therapist: this technique "can easily be modified for teaching supervision where the emphasis is on what the supervisor said and why, rather than on the training and performance of the supervisee." (This method is also utilized at our own out-patient department.) Beyond the specific issues of training, Riess asks, "For what are we training psychotherapists? Almost all students will admit under pressure that one reason is basically economic. On the other hand, very few training institutions will grant that they are training practitioners for private practice. There is in general little stated concern with the improvement of public welfare and preventive mental health. . . . This should be, in my opinion, a most important direction in the future of educational institutions. Adequate preparation for a consultant or participant role in community projects and agencies requires specialized technique and skills. . . . One essential element in such a course is an attempt to arrive at the value system with which our therapy operates. Implicit social and economic biases must become explicit in order to evaluate their effect on both hypothetical assumptions and practical interventions. [This point of view is carried to its extreme in Seymour Halleck, *The Politics of Therapy* (139).] Practitioners have only recently come out of the analytic deep freeze to admit that we do make judgments, and that part of our task is to help patients examine their values, the stereotypes which disguise values, and warp their observations of reality. A philosophy of life and some basic education in ethics should be fundamental in training. So too, attention should be paid in a systematic manner to the codes of ethical practice evolved by the participating professions."

Some research into the process by which students learn psychiatric interviewing has been carried on by Muslin et al. (119). They utilized "an experiential model" in the teaching of two groups of senior medical students during their University of Illinois psychiatric clerkship. The skills they focused upon included: 1. Observational; 2. collating; 3. data gathering and therapy. They compared the members of the two groups in terms of clinical diagnostic interviews and psychological testing. The hypothesis which emerged from their data was "changes noted in interview behavior demonstrated the impact of the teaching program, and more specifically the impact of the teacher on the student." However they also found that "thus far none of the specific data on psychological examination seems to indicate ways in which to analyze and assist those students who do improve or do not improve in their interviewing techniques." They concluded that "the teaching-learning situation seems to involve a unique and separate relationship on the basis of the student's needs of the teacher and the teacher's needs of the student. Thus, study of the teaching learning situation may not be predictive of performance by the student in the clinical interview."

Further investigation of instruction by means of video tape is reported by Schlessinger, Muslin and Battle (140) in their study of the effect of an orientation course for beginning residents which was also designed "to evaluate the use of video tape as a method of instruction and developing a hierarchy of observational learning tasks, to study the process of teaching and learning observations, and devising better means of testing for learning." The authors concluded that the video tapes were a means of providing more accurate data, and the active participation of the residents appeared to facilitate learning. However "there are distortions" introduced by video taping . . . "the limitations of the method must also be stressed. Teaching observational skills in this way constitutes an activist approach to the problem, directed toward bringing to the attention of the group the rudiments of observation. It is a useful adjunct to the traditional supervisory experience which has a more powerful potential in the exploration of individual problems in and about learning." The same authors reported a previous investigation of the teaching of psychotherapy (141) in which they felt that their data, relating to the very earliest phase of supervision, could be viewed as either "learning, therapy, or more pertinently, as a relationship which is a precursor to both. If the supervisory relationship remains at this initial level, the result can only be an unconscious analytic relationship from which the apparent data of therapy are used as currency for the unverbalized and unrecognized needs of both therapist and supervisor. At any phase other than the very outset of supervision, such a relationship can be viewed only as a contamination of the learning situation."

Whitman et al. (142) at Cincinnati studied the patient-therapist-supervisor triad in order to investigate particularly some of the ideas espoused by Searles, Arlow, and others about the parallelisms in the relationships between the members of this triad. They studied the dreams of resident therapists, patients, and supervisors, utilizing ten patient-therapist-supervisor triads, collecting dreams on nights preceding or following conferences regarding supervision. In their commentary, they note that their original hope was that the resident therapist and the patient would all dream of each other, but this hope was not realized. Rather "each of the groups studied dreamed of the next 'higher' observing group, i.e., the patient about the therapist, the therapist about the supervisor or experiment, and the supervisor about the experiment." (In their discussion, the authors do not mention the possible effect of the experimental situation itself upon the content of the dreams of the participants.) Among their findings, they noted "there is also some suggestion . . . that the group process of supervision is significantly different from the individual process of supervision. Manifestations of this appear in dream allusions to mobs or gangs wherein the intimidating effect of numbers appears in the form of both threatening and controlling crowds . . . in this regard a presentor had a dream in which . . . he associated to Shirley Jackson's well-known short story 'The Lottery,' wherein a victim is chosen each year, by an otherwise pleasant little hamlet, to be stoned to death." They suggest that a supervisory technique which might be facilitative, given these findings, would be "asking for the therapist's dreams when they deal with either the patient or the supervisor . . . in these instances the dream should be dealt with in terms of its ego defensive and synthetic adaptation to the therapeutic and supervisory task, rather than deeper personal problems of the therapist. For this purpose we have found the careful use of the manifest content to be sufficient. . . ."

Ornstein (5, 143) has made several contributions to the study of supervision; in "Selected Problems in Learning How to Analyze" he conceptualizes learning in the supervisory situation in terms of a shift in the identification process. Citing Sandler and Rosenblatt's (144) distinction concerning the mechanism of identification, in which, though it is a continuous lifelong process, the content and end results differ depending upon the "developmental stage at which the mechanism is used," he observes that in the supervisor-supervisee relationship "the supervisee's representational world contains . . . a distinct self representation and a distinct object representation of the supervisor. As to the supervisee's professional self, there is confusion between his own professional self-representation and the supervisor's professional object representation." Ornstein feels that if this relationship is a productive one, the process of separation of the supervisee's professional self from the supervisor's professional object representation will be accomplished. There are stages in this development, in which first, the supervisee is in "confusion," as he unconsciously imitates the supervisor; this is replaced by "conscious awareness of attempting to conduct the therapy deliberately the way the supervisee thinks the supervisor would. In the advanced stages of the separation from the supervisor, there is "a decathexis of the supervisory object . . . and a use of the energy in cathecting the professional self, thus making it a stable professionally permanent autonomous ego structure."

Ornstein and Kalthoff (143) propose a schema for the teaching of clinical psychiatric evaluation, delineating the methods used and distinguishing these from the processes of evaluation within the doctor both during and after the clinical interview, as well as organizing the descriptive data along the lines of clinically important psychic functions. They also attempt to separate clearly the observational from the interpretive process, as well as "to integrate the former with the latter." First, they analyze the clinical psychiatric interview in terms of (a) psychology of participants, and (b) methods of the clinician, as they become important in connection with the purpose of the interview. Reiterating Ornstein's fundamental concept that "meeting another human being in our professional role as physician differs very little, basically, from meeting him man to man," the authors emphasize their belief that the psychiatric trainee will enhance his professional development "if he can accept himself as the instrument of clinical psychiatric evaluation." The clinician's basic skills include " (1) evocative listening; (2) empathic-intuitive-introspective capacity" (by which they mean something akin to "intraception," as cited by Sharaf and Levinson).

The authors then discuss the essential elements of the patient to be noted in the psychiatric interview: " (a) Behavior, (b) experiences which become known to us from the verbal expression of his views of his inner and outer world and (c) somatic phenomena he may present." Next they describe the "communicative process between patient and doctor as a two-way system" with the physician methodically evaluating the following functions of the patient: "1. Cognitive-intellectual; 2. affective-emotional; 3. adaptive-defensive." A model of the clinical psychiatric evaluation is presented in terms of a "condensation of the two-pronged process of descriptive and interpretive synthesis." "Descriptive synthesis" involves a consideration of the phenomena under scrutiny according to "1. Registering both the how (form) and the what (content) of the patient's behavior; 2. describing his characteristic ways of thinking, feeling and behaving; 3. delineating, selecting and grouping those aspects of his thinking, feeling and behavior that are adaptive, deviant, or maladaptive; 4. comparing our findings with our own past clinical experiences and with textbook pictures of psychiatric illness, using them as 'templates' to arrive at a clinical diagnosis."

A hierarchy of functions and their mutual influence upon each other is perceived as useful for the clinician to consciously consider during his examination. However, "it should not dictate to him the procedure to be used." The authors also describe the necessity for the clinician to make "an interpretive synthesis." In this "the diagnostician cannot tune in on the many levels of meaning all at once. Yet, . . . his interpretive activity in the form of evocative listening and some tentative interventions goes hand in hand with his fact gathering."

Observing that it is difficult to determine exactly how we arrive at diagnostic or therapeutic interpretations, the authors feel that among the "variety of diagnostic interpretations there are many that cannot be turned directly into therapeutic interpretations. However, these can be used as guides in finding appropriate derivative therapeutic interpretations which can bring us closer to the patient's immediate experience and can be couched in his own language. The manner, timing, dosing, and the specific intent for which an interpretation is to be communicated to the patient comprised the *process of interpreting.*" The authors emphasize that "interpretive synthesis" is the fundamental factor in the transaction between therapist and patient, and propose several models for this activity. The best suited models for "the purpose of interpretive condensation" they feel are those of French (83) called: "1. Focal conflict, and 2. nuclear conflict." The elements in these conflict models consist of: "1. Disturbing motive in conflict with 2. reactive motive resulting in 3. solution(s); 4. precipitating events or circumstances that brought the problem into "dynamic focus" and sparked the solutional attempts."

F. *Postresidency Supervision*

There are very few specific programs for continuing education in psychotherapy, although (as noted above) (35) there has been considerable recent interest in the educational status of the postgraduate psychiatrist.

Several years ago, it was not an uncommon practice in many residency training programs for supervisors (faculty members) to "buy supervision" from senior, experienced clinicians. This self-generated form of continuing education appears to be no longer very much in evidence—perhaps its last residue is reflected as a partial motivation for entering psychoanalytic training.

Grotjahn (145), who had previously described his own experiences in returning to supervision after many years of practice, suggests that the "psychiatrist, working usually in isolation, has more difficulties in communication about his patients than do other specialists. A more frequent use of consultation from psychiatric colleagues is advanced as a means of overcoming this problem, and as an important step in the training and maturation of any psychotherapist." Reviewing the literature about psychiatric consultation from colleagues, Grotjahn cites Lawrence Kolb (34) and perceives the postgraduate consultation as a rather short term relationship between the psychiatrist and his senior and more experienced colleague. Although this is not a continuing supervisory relationship, it has a parallel with certain kinds of supervision available to the resident during his training, particularly that concerned primarily with his diagnostic interview. Grotjahn recalls Sigmund Freud's practice as a consultant, mentioning his own paper (146) on this subject and his belief that psychiatric consultation will be "much more utilized by the younger psychiatrists" particularly because of their enthusiasm about "using the new technologies of auditory or visual taping."

This discussion is primarily focused upon the supervision of individual out-patient psychotherapy, and has not attempted to review the supervision of variations of individual psychotherapy, including group and family treatment. However, as an example of the ubiquity of most of the issues in supervision, attention is called to a paper by McGee (147) who outlines four models of supervision: 1. The dyad, based on the relationship in individual psychotherapy; 2. the triad, in which two co-therapists are supervised by a third person; 3. group supervision, wherein a supervisor meets regularly with a group of supervisees in group psychotherapy; 4. co-therapy supervision, wherein two individuals conduct a therapy group, the senior co-therapist also assuming the role of supervisor. McGee feels that recommendations can be made regarding supervision in group psychotherapy so that an appropriate decision regarding each model might be made, by considering the varieties of approach in terms of contextual and individual needs and convenience.

Though many express concern for the necessity for continuing education in psychiatry, there appears to be no widely accepted method for pursuing this goal. It would seem that unless certain external incentives are introduced (such as recertification or peer review), psychiatrists will, along with their other medical colleagues, be "too busy" to continue their training beyond the years of residency. (Perhaps, during the five days of the annual APA meeting, a seminar or pilot effort might be launched in which supervision, at least of preliminary diagnostic and evaluative processes, might be initiated.) Certainly, the classically informal "corridor consultation" is no substitute for supervisory training of postresidency education. It is unlikely that the maximal two years of residency experience in out-patient psychotherapy qualifies the graduate resident as a seasoned psychotherapist (Semrad has mentioned a ten year estimate for the development of a psychotherapist). The incentive which appears to have been most productive, at least in activity, has been the conduct of research and/or investigative program into supervisory processes. There is no experimental evidence that this activity results in "better supervisors" or "better therapists"; however it at least has the advantages of drawing attention to the issue, and providing some element of sophistication for the investigators. Another side effect of research or at least focus upon the supervisory situation, which has come as a personal observation, has been the increasing sense of "an alliance" on the part of the supervisee who perceives himself as a colleague in the investigation of the transaction, as opposed to the passive recipient of a "didactic" endeavor.

TRENDS AND ISSUES IN SUPERVISION

Throughout the literature dealing with psychotherapy supervision, two commonly held principles have been evident: 1. That the core of the psychiatrist's identity is his role as a psychotherapist; and 2. that individual supervision of psychotherapy is the most important single educational method in the training of psychotherapists. The "varieties of supervisory experience" in which these principles are put into practice range along a continuum from "intrapsychically focused" to "interpsychically focused." Ekstein and Wallerstein's work is representative of a primary emphasis upon the therapist's personality, while Tarachow and Semrad's group tends to deal primarily with the therapist's behavior and technique. Fleming and Benedek's supervisory approach is representative of a compromise between these emphases, and a refusal to be trapped in the quibble of "therapy versus pedagogy."

The modes of supervision which devolve from the two basic principles are reflections of the trends toward increased social involvement now seen in all professions, as well as the assimilative effort by which psychiatry is now attempting to deal with burgeoining technologies involving computers, videotapes and closed-circuit T.V. These social and technological forces are reflected in theoretical divergences from the traditional assumptions: 1. That one-to-one psychotherapy is the ideal form of psychiatric treatment; 2. that "modeling" is the optimal educational methodology for training clinicians; 3. the "restrained" view of the clinician's function (that is, whereby he waits for "pathology" to be brought to him for "cure," as opposed to prevention of illness, or "health care.") These newer values are analogically reflected in the supervisory methods utilized by their adherents. The differences in the supervisory techniques now proliferating represent common trends which, first, tend to devalue one-to-one interactions (and correspondingly elevate the importance of "milieu," group, or community interaction); second, tend to devalue expertise and authoritative hierarchization, in favor of an egalitarian blurring of role definition; and third, tend to scrutinize the styles and values of one-to-one interaction by means of technical procedures, inherently undermining the givens of traditional supervision, while demonstrating how much has been neglected in the established models of teaching psychotherapy.

One of the major results of these trends has been the creation of multiple modes of supervision so that the historically narrow range of difference between theorists of psychotherapy supervision (for example, Ekstein-Wallerstein versus Tarachow), has been widened and fragmented, paralleling the multidimensional functions of psychiatric activity. In addition, individual supervision, which has not by any means achieved a satisfactory level of theory or practice, is being displaced from its central position, under the pressure of demand for "delivery of services" which in turn requires suitable models of supervision not based on one-to-one contact.

The supervisory literature reveals this fragmented, *ad hoc* concern with special tasks, and the need for synthesizing theory becomes increasingly evident. Nor, unfortunately, is there much evidence of a concerted effort towards the education of supervisors for the needs of the future. At our own center, tentative efforts have been made toward this goal; however the "supervisor's conference" remains a relatively casual and haphazard means of educating supervisors, either for classical or newer modes of supervision. What is most needed is a formal educational enterprise in the training of psychotherapy supervisors which would address itself toward sophistication in issues of cultural context, organizational theory, psychiatric role models and the specific expertise relevant to these models, and explicit hypotheses of educational theory which would facilitate evaluative studies of the theories.

In the following section, some of the trends in the education of the psychiatric clinician will be reviewed and will illustrate the increasingly imperative need for improved supervisory training.

V. THE FUTURE

A. *Context: The New Society and Its Quest for Health*

Criticisms of the health care system, as well as of the education of the physician, have become increasingly widespread, frequently labeling the problem as a "crisis" (148, 149). Among others, Millis (150, 151) has specifically addressed himself to analysis of the situation, and made recommendations for solutions. Social pressures, including "consumerism" and the "right to health," have raised problems for the medical profession, demanding that it bring medical care to relatively deprived segments of the population, and demanding immediate and accelerated or improved health care. Educationally, pressures mount for increased involvement and training of paraprofessionals, concomitantly with the general tendency toward egalitarianism and disapprobation of expertise. Although Millis' survey is overtly directed toward "financing" of medical education, it provides a paradigmatic summary of the issues confronting modern medicine. Millis observes that there is an insistent public demand for more service, but a lack of recognition of "the growing basic inefficiency in medical education," as society demands at the same time more service and enlargement of medical schools. "Millions of people, believing they had been given a right to health, demanded the promised medical care whether there were funds provided or not . . . (the result is that) . . . we as a nation are a faced with a crisis in medical education." Tracing the origins of this attitude toward health service shows a change from the fundamental concept that the role of the physician in the past was "the cure" of illness (a view which has come to be called "secondary prevention") to the expanded concept in the public perception of the role of the physician as including the concept of health "care," (now labeled "primary and tertiary prevention").

The resulting effect upon the world of the physician is a change in his role vis-à-vis other professionals. In the world of medical cure, the physician was the central factor; in the world of health care, the physician "very frequently is in the position of having to share responsibility, decision, and action with others as associates, that is, as peers and sometimes as superiors." A further important change in the physician's role resulting from the shift from cure to care is the inherent restraint in the physician-patient relationship previously obtaining in the world of medical cure, as opposed to the current consideration of larger and larger segments of the population, as well as the appropriate units to which "health care can be rendered." These include enlarging concepts of "health units" such as family, industrial plants, neighborhoods, organizations, and finally, cities, regions, states, nations, and ultimately to the cosmic area of "space medicine."

Describing the kind of "output" (a revealing term) which is needed from the system of medical education, Millis includes, first, a diversity of physicians, both in ability and in terms of social responsibility; "physicians are needed for both one-to-one relationships and one-to-group relationships." Also, physicians are needed who are capable of "rapid adaptation to change, that is, who are both doers and learners." Finally physicians are needed for "biomedical research, as well as for delivery to the entire population." Among the problems of medical education, Millis lists various anachronisms including "traditionalism, discontinuities, fragmentations of accreditation," and suggests the creation of a "rational public policy" for medical education based upon "relating medical education to medical service." Among the recommendations are "the need to produce a diversity of physicians in place of physicians of a uniform pattern . . . in order to accept students of heterogeneous background, the system of education must become a substantially individualized experience," and the curriculum must be modified along vertical lines in contrast to its classical horizontal scheme. The goal of the undifferentiated medical school graduate is no longer reasonable, and should be altered to the "multiple track concept." In order to increase the numbers of graduate physicians, medical education should be shortened by means of an analysis of the entire medical educational process, and at the same time "improved." This may well be achieved, according to Millis, by means of earlier admission and elimination of the internship. "It is possible to omit the internship only if medical schools provide much improved clinical training," and accordingly Millis opposes the suggestion to cut medical schools from four to three years "for all students."

Because of the "discontinuities" in postgraduate training, Millis recommends strongly that residencies be based "at a university," and finally urges continuing education and peer review as a necessary means of improving medical education.

B. *The New Physician: Role and Methodology*

Funkenstein (152) has reviewed the historical changes in medical education since the Flexner report of 1910. Labeling "three eras" of medical school training (1. general practice, 2. scientific, 3. community), he perceives this shift as reflected in changes in medical students' premedical education, which is currently toward "a more sociological viewpoint." Funkenstein reported on his survey of Harvard medical students: the class of 1971 when "undergraduate fields of concentration showed 70% devoted to humanities and only 8% to social sciences, as opposed to 1973 (class of 1973) with 36% concentrated in the social sciences and 48% in the humanities." (He also felt that many students who might have chosen psychiatry as a specialty, on the basis of their wish to "work directly with people," "now that family medicine is again becoming a respectable career, and the function of the internist is being redefined to include the art of medicine and the community aspects of illness," are turning from the original goal of psychiatry.)

Funkenstein predicts that medical students of the future will have a series of characteristics which include: greater diversity, increased sociological and behavioral science backgrounds; increased involvement in the work of faculty and administration; intellectually, less interested in scientific method, more interested in trial by error; more interested in the pragmatic use of science rather than the activities of the scientist; increased interest in mechanical aides, (computers, T.V., etc.); in terms of career plans: increased interest in community aspects of medicine; increased political interests; decreased interest in the private practice and economics of medicine; in interpersonal relationships; increasingly interested in family medicine, increased acceptance of changes in sexual mores, and of drug use; increased interest in social responsibilities, and in the art of medicine as opposed to its science, and attention to personal and emotional aspects of individual patients.

Edelson (153) reviews the development of the program adopted at Yale, illustrating the directions of change according to the "track system." Similarly, in *Psychosocial Aspects of Medical Training* (154), the extent to which the "sociosphere" has become the primary interest for medical students is exemplified in the series of papers presented at a conference at Bowman-Gray School of Medicine held in June, 1969. At this conference, Lief (15) reported on an empirical investigation of medical students at Tulane, stimulated by studies of Merton and his colleagues (156, 157, 158, 159), utilizing the method of serial interviews of medical students (60 students from four classes graduated in '59, '60, '61, and '62). These students were interviewed by two of three psychiatrists an average of 20 times throughout the four years of medical school. Additionally, they were given psychological tests (including Rorschach, Miller Analogies test, and Strong vocational aptitude tests), which were scored on a personality rating scale including "ego strength." The purpose of their study, explicitly, was to determine the changes of personality by which medical students adopt a professional identity, as well as the capacity for dealing with the emotional intensities of the practice of medicine. In other words, the investigation was an attempt to find the personality factors contributing to the development of good doctors. Having reviewed the various parameters of their survey, their conclusions led the investigators to "some implications for medical education: 1. The lock step curriculum is wasteful and may keep the medical student from realizing his full potential; 2. an attempt should be made to insure that the student's personality is fitted for the professional role he will strive to achieve; 3. medical educators should be as much concerned with the development of attitudes as with the acquisition of information and skill; 4. medical students who need psychotherapy should be encouraged to obtain it without feeling that any stigma is attached; 5. the social and psychological factors in medical education need continued study." In comparison with Funkenstein's observations, the Tulane survey shows many correlations, particularly in the area of "cognitive types" with 75% of the sample classified as "doers" as opposed to "thinkers and mixed." In terms of students' primary interest in the practice of medicine, five categories were labeled: scientist-teacher, healer, entrepreneur, security seeker, and disorganized. In the final survey, 65% of the total study population were classified as healers, and 15% as scientist-teachers. The others were evenly distributed among the other categories; this finding is also in agreement with Funkenstein's Harvard survey.

The debates regarding the "ideal physician" and his education, reflected in proponents and opponents of track systems, undifferentiated versus differentiated medical students, and other issues of curriculum and delivery, are discussed by Grinker (160), who reiterates the importance of the fundamental nucleus of medical education. "Within the medical specialties compartmentalized in departments, there are 'core areas" which need to be taught, and within which experience by practice is necessary for adequate mastery . . . there is, however, another core area, which is *basic* for the education of all graduate students, no matter what the specialty or what apparent career goals may be favored at the moment. This is a knowledge of the health-illness system, which cannot be fractured since it denotes a process in continuity over time, i.e. life."

Rudy (161) suggested that a continuum of medical school and residency requires new track systems simulating early residencies, in order to allow students to select special interests in medical school. With the abandonment of the internship, the diminution of undergraduate medical educational time, and the multiplicity of subspecialties, the burden of medical and psychiatric education increases. "Role functions of psychiatrists and clinical psychologists should also continue to overlap. With many departments of psychiatry now referred to as divisions of behavioral science, the psychiatrist is in some ways becoming more like a psychologist. It has been suggested that the resident may qualify for a doctorate in behavioral science upon completion of his training."

Engel (162, 163, 163a, 163b) and Romano (164, 164a) have written of the importance of the clinical experience of the physician and particularly of the psychiatrist. Romano deplores the loss of internship since "the psychiatrist, as physician, brings to the field his ancient heritage of the physician, and broad experience in biology and clinical medicine, as well as in psychology and the social sciences. To reduce the dimensions of the role of the psychiatrist as a physician would seriously impair his contributions as practitioner, teacher, scholar, and investigator." Engel has particularly emphasized the importance of educating the physician in "clinical reasoning." "Clinical reasoning refers to the mental operations whereby the raw clinical data are interpreted in other frames of reference. Clinical examination and clinical reasoning involve an orderly scientific process whereby the clinician successively makes observations, develops hypotheses, and then proceeds to test them with further observations, including the application of appropriate technologies. From such a sequence evolve decisions as to further study, diagnostic formulations and judgments as to the appropriate methods of treatment and care." (Compare Reiser's view of the psychiatrist as the new "synthesizer." (164b))

The issue of "clinical judgment" and its development in the physician have become of increasing interest in medical education. This is reflected in many aspects of curricular reform including the methodology of "independent study," increased use of audio-visual aides, and "learning programs." Lusted (165) cites Osler's dictum that medical practice is "an art which consists largely of balancing probabilities"; Haney (166) has reviewed the "psychosocial factors" in medical decision making, and points up the current diminution of interest in the "biosphere" for contemporary students.

An exemplary opposition to the "new look" and an argument for the necessity for the maintenance of at least a nucleus of "synthetic physicians," is presented by Poser (167) at the University of Vermont Medical School (where Weed promotes the use of "medical records that guide and teach" (138)). Poser is concerned that the preceptorial system, which dominated medical education in the post-1910 era, and was replaced by the basic science system, is now being re-introduced to medical education. "This practice is questionable, since outstanding clinicians do not always make good teachers." In the process of shortening medical education, content has often been "thinned out." Other trends which are also "questionable," include "the demand by many medical students that basic science courses be taught by clinicians." Also questionable are insistences on "self education," audio-visual aides, and bedside teaching. "Students want to know more and more what to do rather than why to do it," therefore, "the intellectual gap between the greater part of our medical school faculties and the student is widening at a frightening rate." The difficulty is compounded by the fact that medical students are less exposed to clinical scholars, who previously had mastered basic medical science as well as clinical expertise, and who could bridge the gap necessary to teach clinical medicine. However, "to be a medical renaissance man today has become impossible, but the properly disciplined human intellect is still capable of exercising critical judgments. If we attempt to reduce this to a numbers game played by a computer, there will be nothing left to the challenge of medicine." To offset this result, Poser recommends that "all medical schools identify the five or ten percent of their entering classes, who are the future clinical academicians." These will be not basic scientists, but clinical scholars with broad background in basic science. Additionally, "the currently popular track or major system forces the student into specific areas of medical practice much too early . . . (and) shortening the medical curriculum will simply reinforce the inadequacy of our physicians' basic intellectual equipment . . . it would be peculiarly shortsighted to turn out large numbers of medical practitioners without thinking of the day when the present generation of teachers will have gone and there will be none to take their places."

C. The New Psychiatrist

"Now let us assume that by some kind of organization we were able to increase our numbers to an extent sufficient for treating large masses of people . . . the conscience of the community will awake and admonish that the poor man has just as much right to help for his mind as he now has to the surgeon's means of saving life . . . it may be a long time before the state regards this as an urgent duty . . . sometime or other, however, it must come."

—*Freud* (168)

The debate about the role of psychiatry and its "proper business" was reviewed by Garber in his 1971 Presidential Address "The Proper Business of Psychiatry" (169). He recalled Alan Gregg's comment of 1944 that "psychiatry will find great extensions of its content and its obligations. There will be applications far beyond your offices and your hospitals of the further knowledge you will gain, applications not only to patients with functional and organic disease, but to the human relations of normal people—in politics, national and international, between races, between capital and labor, in government, in family life, in education, in every form of human relationship, whether between individuals or between groups."

Similarly, Ruesch (170) believes that "what we know for sure is that the technological civilization, and its handmaiden, the large-scale social organization, constitutes the matrix of modern society and that the events of the last few years have forced the psychiatrist into a new role. Willy-nilly he has become a change agent for smaller social systems; and in the process, his focus is moving from individual to group, from psychopathology to social pathology, and from psychodynamics to social dynamics. Consequently, his methods of intervention are shifting from the traditional one-to-one relationship to multi-person interaction, and from treatment to prevention. The psychiatrist of the future will have to shift his thinking from the older person orientation with its focus on human interaction, to the newer system orientation and its emphasis on man-machine interaction. This is the trend of our time."

Miller *et al.* (171) described the "future of psychiatric education" in their summary of the experimental program at the University of Wisconsin, integrating medical school, internship, and psychiatric residency in order to enable some students to complete the total training in six years. Among the advantages of this plan are: younger candidates, since "we feel doctors come to their psychiatric training too late in their learning career," and one group of teachers responsible for integrating training throughout the three phases of training in medicine; the extra time would be available for further training in subspecialties or other areas; economic savings by shortening of educational time; increased manpower output; and finally, "we believe that there is something about the prolonged role of medical student, intern, and resident that has a lifetime dampening effect upon the appetite for further learning . . . going to school becomes the career."

Evidence of the spiraling scope of psychiatric activity is exemplified in Halleck's book *The Politics of Therapy* (139), which advocates that psychiatrists take an active role in the context (specifically political) in which they conduct their treatment. Theoretical parallels to the "sociology" of psychiatric activity are offered by Rabkin (172) who "espouses a new concept of affect in which it is viewed not as a substance or as inner states of one person, but as part of a process in which the tensions and emotions of the family and other natural groups are determined by the configuration and motion of their systems." (And compare Raskin's view of the "public health" trend in psychiatry (172a).)

The new psychiatrist is further described by Funkenstein (173), who observes that the class of students characterized as "student clinicians" who have become interested in psychiatry primarily in order to "practice primarily with patients" may not be "totally acceptable to application committees." In this case "the attempt to discourage these students is a disservice both to the individuals concerned and to psychiatry, since it deprives the specialty of a group different in their makeup from most present-day psychiatrists. The new breed of psychiatrist may well be better suited to work in community psychiatry than most of today's psychiatrists . . . the new psychiatrists may be in fact harbingers of the future, since many of the other type of would-be psychiatrists—those primarily interested in psychological material—are having more and more difficulty in learning the basic medical sciences as these become more complex. A good number in this group may be unable to succeed academically in medical school unless a special curriculum is devised for them."

Bandler (8) has summarized the trends in psychiatric education: "The psychiatrist as an ideal, as an individual model, and as an academic leader, should be able to integrate . . . into his professional self identity" these four models: 1. public health: primary, secondary, tertiary prevention; 2. developmental perspectives; 3. an organizational model; 4. an ecological model. These models should be considered "complementary rather than antithetical, as mutually enriching rather than as polarized opposites. . . . If the psychiatrist has not made this an actuality in himself, how can he be an adequate model for his residents? How can they grow as individuals, or learn as professionals, in order to assume the responsibilities for innovation and creativity which will shortly be theirs?" Bandler has analyzed the issues which confront psychiatric education as comprising three major problems: first "the explosion of knowledge; second, the difficulty of predicting the future; and third, difficulties in manpower and facilities." Returning to the fundamental issue of the psychiatrist's identity, he asks, "What then is the core of our identity as physicians and psychiatrists? . . . The *sine qua non,* I believe, is the capacity to understand one's self and to understand other people. Without this capacity in the human encounter of doctor and patient, doctor and family, doctor and group, doctor and community, I would say the resident lacks the essential tools for becoming a psychiatrist. He needs to know much more, of course, and to develop many skills. But they are all integrated into this central identity. Self-knowledge and knowledge of others naturally go hand in hand. Encounter with the patient and with other people is always also an encounter with one's self . . . our task as educators then is to facilitate the resident's growth and learning and to make available to him the variety, range and depth of experiences, particularly experiences with patients, which will make that learning optimal for him. The crucial teacher is the patient. Our task as teachers and supervisors is to reinforce and to elaborate and to conceptualize what the patient has taught." Bandler sees four major difficulties in the attainment of this ideal: first, the growth of behavioral science; second, the increase in formal curricula which has resulted in what Kubie (174) has called the "retreat from patients"; third, the deemphasis of the importance and contribution of psychoanalytic understanding; fourth, increasing specialization of psychiatry. He well recognizes the importance of the fundamental contact with patients, in terms of the core identity of the psychiatrist: "Before you can be a teacher of psychiatry or an administrative psychiatrist, or a community psychiatrist, you must first be a clinical psychiatrist. . . . I would even argue further the seeming paradox that the practitioner of community psychiatry is the one most in need of clinical and psychoanalytic understanding in depth. The psychiatrist's passport to the community is his core identity, his professional competence and understanding. If he fails to demonstrate his professional role . . . he will have forfeited his credibility in the community and his capacity to serve. If he is anchored in his professional clinical competence, he is unlikely to find himself adrift on the sea of militant social actions."

The impact of the psychiatric resident upon the training program has been facilitated by the increased activity in group and "T-group" training. (A fine summary of some of the issues regarding T-group in residency training is that by Christ (175).) The issue of residency training in community psychiatry is reviewed by Pattison (176). He observes that training in social and community psychiatry in the basic three-year curriculum has been poorly integrated, nor has a consistent methodology been devised. He proposes that community psychiatry training be built upon a preceding solid clinical training experience, prior to enlarging the resident's repertory of skills beyond the clinical arena. (Compare the Philadelphia experience described by Fink and Newman (176a).)

A fitting conclusion to this section is provided by a proposal by Taylor and Torrey (177), who describe a psychiatric educational program in which the residents work together as a "self education corporation." They outline a hypothetical teaching program wherein "faculty members would serve as advisory and teaching consultants to provide individualized education consistent with the emerging track systems of medical education. The residents' involvement in creating and administering their own educational program would provide training in principles of education and administration compatible with the evolving role of the psychiatrist as educator and administrator." (An ironic commentary upon the previous proposal is the result of a questionnaire by Kardener et al. (178), which surveyed 160 psychiatric residents in the Los Angeles area regarding their "need and satisfactions." Kardener remarks that the rhetorical question he heard raised at the conference on psychiatry and medical education in Atlanta in 1967 (179, 180)—"When will we accede to the proposition that students should also have a say about the educational policies that will mold their destinies?"—required empirical data to provide some answer. Among the results—not the least interesting of which was the response rate, which overall was 58% of residents queried in nine institutions—was that foremost on the list of discrepancies between "desirability and availability" to residents were the items dealing with staff contact: "obviously the most important factor is a continued need for role modeling, which should exist throughout one's training and perhaps well into the postresidency years as well. . . .")

D. *Education in Psychotherapy*

Ornstein (5) has reviewed impressively the current status of psychiatric education, and emphasized the difficulties of a fragmented eclecticism. Regan and Small (35) have listed the areas of knowledgeability expected of the psychiatrists of the 1970's, and beyond (which, if presented to Chessick—who required four years of residency for his proposed program—would very likely require not "continuing" but "chronic" education).

It appears that, from one viewpoint, the supervisor's task is the teaching of a methodology of approach, emphasizing various aspects of psychotherapy, according to the resident's personality, phase of development, clinical context, and the supervisor's own biases. Supervision contributes, then, a kind of specificity to the hierarchization of issues based upon an explicit theory of bio-psycho-social functioning. The more comprehensive this model, the more flexible. Supervisory strategies rest upon the fundamental issue of the establishment of a contract, a learning alliance, which in turn derives from the supervisor's operational philosophy, the ethics of his professionalism, his scientific methods (i.e. his overt references to his hypotheses, data gathering, prediction, and evaluation) and explicit discussions of his explanatory models, in which the criteriology of psychotherapy is presented to the resident. This also means facing squarely the issue of multiplicity of agency which confronts the clinician: the shifting alliances with society, patients, therapists, and one's self. Ultimately, the supervisor's "explanatory model" should be presented as criticizable in terms of its "analogic fit," its parsimony, generativity, explanatory scope, internal consistency, and predictive power. The context of supervision becomes, as evidenced in many of the references discussed above, increasingly the major ingredient in the "clinical rhombus." Particularly, the social atmosphere, in which the "quest for intimacy" becomes a kind of universal demand, almost as powerful as "the right to help," has resulted in a kind of pseudomutuality, which could be termed "interpersonal ricochet." The development of sensitivity groups and other "instant intimacy enterprises" are the phenomena of a multiply mobile society, with increasing demands for novel, accelerated, and guaranteed delivery of gratification upon almost every level of experience; social, intellectual, and sexual. Additionally, the demand for instant education of professionals has led to a pseudoegalitarian, anti-work attitude in which expertise is either discounted or easy to come by (or it ought to be), which is far from conducive to long-term strategies, values, or delayed impulse gratification. The widespread adolescent model in which peer group validation, a quasimutual "short cut to identity" (by defining the enemy as the outsider), has led to an emotional "lapel clutching," where the demand for instant delivery of intimacy is antithetical to the traditional belief that close relationships between people are not only slow in their development, but naturally involve a painful growth process which, if hot-housed, results in a spurious hybrid, a facsimile of intimacy. Similarly, self understanding is perceived as available by means of gimmicks, such as drugs,* sensory exercises, and other magical techniques of individual or group enterprise.

As teachers of psychotherapy, itself becoming somewhat anachronistic, we are in the difficult position of both tolerating and appreciating additional complexities of the modern world, in which we are asked to add to our "third ear" a fourth of "kinesics," and a fifth of "cultural context," at the same time inculcating a postponement of gratification in a process of self-understanding which is inherently tortuous, and has few rewards which can compete in a hedonistic marketplace.

---

* Drug use often represents a flight from the threat of intimacy, as well as a pseudomutual avoidance of the hollowness inherent in many group relationships, and echoes the quality of parallel play seen in early childhood.

What place is there for psychotherapy, and for tolerance of ambiguity, for the achievement of long-term goals, and for insight in an accelerating society ruled by demands for multiple and instant gratification? One may be tempted to "meet the demands of the consumer" (as the therapist is asked to "give the patient what he wants"). But it is our belief that it is possible to teach psychotherapy, that is, the process of self-understanding, in a manner that maintains and enhances the values of long-term processes without repudiation of the fundamental style of psychoanalytic psychotherapy. This is achievable, par excellence, by means of the supervisory process: its complexities permit identification, postponement of gratification, partial rewards, and ultimately a sense of competence. In essence, the apprentice moves toward a mastery of his craft, and a skill which, though not overtly in popular demand, still attempts to satisfy a perennial human goal—self understanding, and promotes this by a methodology which is based upon the autonomy inherent in the procedure, as well as the goal.

Future programs will need to take cognizance of the issues mentioned above, as well as the increasing complexity and diversity of the demands upon the new psychiatrist. It would appear that a sequence in developmental terms which would parallel "core" issues of psychiatric training, and then allow some compromise between service needs and individual preferences, could be planned, probably between the first and second years of residency. This undoubtedly will require a shift in supervisory methodology. Even if the currently traditional first year hospital assignment is shortened, the resident will still require supervision focused upon issues of group and system tasks, as well as the primary model of individual therapy. Further refinements of the one-to-one essential activity hopefully would be accomplished by means of appropriate assignment of specific supervisors able to accommodate this phase of the resident's development. In the third year, the "instrumental usage" of the psychiatrist could be consciously synthesized, with the assistance of appropriate supervisory models. Therefore, the future program must consider: 1. the core identity of the psychiatrist; 2. the context of the center; 3. the personality of the resident; 4. the assessment of its faculty; 5. the feasibility of appropriate supervisory fit considering resident, context, and faculty expertise; 6. the education of supervisors and 7. evaluation of the entire educational enterprise.

There are many areas which could be appropriately and routinely emphasized in the training program, which would serve as "synthesizing" influences such as "career supervision"—sequential reviews over the "nodal" points of training. (This concept is consonant with an Eriksonian schema of residency growth, in terms of identity, capacity for intimacy, generativity and integrity.)

Training in supervision, which considers "analogic fit" and the core psychiatric identity, should involve, then, several modalities, not only the classical seminar, but a research program which itself is a training ground for supervisors (as cited in the experience of Fleming and Benedek, Ekstein and Wallerstein, and Semrad). Supervisors will require sub-grouping, according to the focus (bio-psycho-socio) and the methodology of their approach. Their individual representation on a "residency training committee" would insure the continuation of a least common denominator definition of their total psychiatric educational goals.

These elements should result in an increase in morale (Chessick's *esprit de corps*), an important element not only in the quality of the everyday life of the residency training program, but also in recruitment, in experimental data, in evaluation of methods and results, so that teaching and treatment methods are being used and evaluated concomitantly, and also in effectively sharpening the identifying foci for the residents in training, and finally, hopefully, permitting them to feel somewhat less anxious regarding their own "beginning residency crisis." Multiplicity of psychiatric subspecialties could be offset by the reassurance to the resident about the "core of his training," that is to say the development of a clinical attitude, and the process of becoming a psychotherapist. Such a supervisory program would also help sharpen the identity of the training center itself, and provide an important unifying substrate offsetting superstructures of eclecticism.

The model of supervision which is proposed, and partially utilized currently at our own training center, could be schematized according to three axes in which the dimensions represent patient, supervisor, and resident respectively, within a circle representing the context, and the entire system moving across the baseline of time (the developmental continuum of the entire system).

The task of supervision, and the training of supervisors, may well be the most important elements in psychiatric education, considering the dilution factor to which the "core identity" of the psychiatrist is exposed. Despite the "narcissistic blows" of the supervisory process, hopefully both supervisors and residents may reach the point where they can say with Aeneas, "Perhaps one day even these events will be happily remembered."

REFERENCES

1. LEWIN, BERTRAM, D., Education or the Quest for Omniscience, *Journal of the American Psychoanalytic Association*, 6:389-412, 1958.
2. ARLOW, JACOB A., Some Dilemmas in Psychoanalytic Education. Panel discussion at American Psychoanalytic Association Meeting, May, 1971.
3. LEWIN, BERTRAM D., ROSS, HELEN, *Psychoanalytic Education in the United States*, W. W. Norton & Company, Inc. New York, 1960.
4. Rainbow Report. Report of the Survey Steering Committee of the Board on Professional Standards. American Psychoanalytic Association, 1955.
5. ORNSTEIN, PAUL H., Sorcerer's Apprentice: The Initial Phase of Training and Education in Psychiatry. *Comprehensive Psychiatry*, 9:293-315, 1968.
6. CHESSICK, RICHARD D., *Why Psychotherapists Fail*. Science House, New York, 1971.
7. BANDLER, BERNARD. Current Trends in Psychiatric Education, *American Journal of Psychiatry*, 127:585-590, 1970.
8. BANDLER, BERNARD, Current Trends in Psychiatry From the Academic Point of View. Presented to the American College of Psychiatrists, Third Annual Seminar for Continuing Education for Psychiatrists. Atlanta, Georgia, 1970.
9. RIESS, BERNARD F., The Selection and Supervision of Psychotherapists. In *The Training of Psychotherapists: A Multidisciplinary Approach*. Editors: Dellis, Nicholas P.; Stone, Herbert K. L.S.U. Press, Baton Rouge, 1960.
10. Trends and Issues in Psychiatric Residency Programs. Report No. 31. Group for the Advancement of Psychiatry. American Psychiatric Association, 1955.
11. SCHLESSINGER, NATHAN. Supervision of Psychotherapy. *Archives of General Psychiatry*, 15:129-134, 1966.
12. EKSTEIN, R., and WALLERSTEIN, R. S., *The Teaching and Learning of Psychotherapy*, Basic Books. New York, 1963.
13. TARACHOW, S., *An Introduction to Psychotherapy*. International Universities Press, Inc. New York, 1963.
14. FLEMING, J., and BENEDEK, T. *Psychoanalytic Supervision*. Grune & Stratton. New York, 1966.
15. KAPP, R., and ROSS, W. D., A Technique for Self Analysis of Countertransference. *Journal of the American Psychoanalytic Association*, 10: 643-657, 1962.
16. DeBELL, DARYL E., A Critical Digest of the Literature on Psychoanalytic Supervision. *Journal of the American Psychoanalytic Association*, 11:546-575, 1963.
17. KNAPP, P. H., LEVIN, S., McCARTER, R., WERMER, H., and ZETZEL, E., Suitable for Psychoanalysis: A Review of 100 Supervised Analytic Cases. *Psychoanalytic Quarterly*, 29:459-477, 1960.

18. ACKERMAN, N., Selected Problems in Supervised Analysis. *Psychiatry*, 16: 283-290, 1953.

19. BALINT, M., On the Psycho-analytic Training System. *International Journal of Psychoanalysis*, 29:163-173, 1948.

20. BALINT, M., Analytic Training and Training Analysis. *International Journal of Psychoanalysis*, 35:157-162, 1954.

21. BENEDEK, T., Countertransference in the Training Analyst. *Bulletin of the Menninger Clinic*, 18:12-16, 1954.

22. EKSTEIN, R., Panel Report: The Teaching of Psychoanalytic Technique. *Journal of the American Psychoanalytic Association*, 8:167-174, 1960.

23: EMCH, M., The Social Context of Supervision. *International Journal of Psychoanalysis*, 35:298-306, 1955.

24. GROTJAHN, M., Present Trends in Psychoanalytic Training. In *Twenty Years of Psychoanalysis*. Editors: Alexander, F., and Ross, H. Norton, New York, 1953.

25. HORA, T., Contribution to the Phenomenology of the Supervisory Process. *American Journal of Psychotherapy*, 11:769-773, 1957.

26. KEISER, S., Panel Report: The Technique of Supervised Analysis. *Journal of the American Psychoanalytic Association*, 4:539-549, 1956.

27: KOVACS, V., Training and Control Analysis. *International Journal of Psychoanalysis*, 17:346-354, 1936.

28. KUBIE, L., Research Into the Process of Supervision in Psychoanalysis. *Psychoanalytic Quarterly*, 27:226-236, 1958.

29. HENRY, WILLIAM, SIMS, JOHN, and SPRAY, S. L., *The Fifth Profession*. Jossey-Bass, Inc. San Francisco, 1971.

30. SEARLES, HAROLD F., The Informational Value of the Supervisor's Emotional Experiences. *Psychiatry*, 18:135-146, 1955.

31. ARLOW, JACOB A., The Influence of the Psychoanalytic Curriculum on Supervision. Panel of the American Psychoanalytic Association, 1956.

32. BERNFELD, SIEGFRIED. The Fact of Observation in Psychoanalysis. *Journal of Psychology*, 12:289-305, 1941.

33. LEWIN, BERTRAM D., Dream Psychology and the Analytic Situation. *Psychoanalytic Quarterly*, 24:169-199, 1955.

34. KOLB, LAWRENCE C., Consultation and Psychotherapy. *Current Psychiatric Therapies*, 8:1-10, 1968.

35. REGAN, PETER, and SMALL, MOUCHLY, Toward a Continuum of Formal and Continuing Education. *American Journal of Psychiatry*, 128:607-609, 1971.

36. BALINT, M., On the Psychoanalytic Training System. *International Journal of Psychoanalysis*, 29:163-173, 1948.

37. KRAMER, M., On the Continuation of the Analytic Process After Psychoanalysis (a Self Observation). *International Journal of Psychoanalysis*, 40:17-25, 1959.

38. LENNARD, H. L., and BERNSTEIN, A., *The Anatomy of Psychotherapy*. Columbia University Press. New York, 1960.

39. BALES, R. F., *Interaction Process Analysis*. Addison-Wesley Press, Inc. Cambridge, Massachusetts, 1951.

40. KRIS, E., On the Vicissitudes of Insight. *International Journal of Psychoanalysis*, 37:445-455, 1956.

41. MARMOR, J., Psychoanalytic Therapy as an Education Process: Common Denominators in the Therapeutic Approaches of Different Psychoanalytic

Schools. *Science and Psychoanalysis*, Vol. 5. Grune & Stratton, New York, 1962.

42. PIERS, G., and PIERS, M. W., Modes of Learning and the Analytic Process *Sixth International Congress of Psychotherapy*, London, 1964, *Selected Lectures*. S. Karger, Basel, 1965.

43. SZASZ, T., Psychoanalytic Treatment as Education. *Archives of General Psychiatry*, 9:46-52, 1963.

44. ARLOW, J. A., The Supervisory Situation. *Journal of the American Psychoanalytic Association*, 11:576-594, 1963.

45. SEMRAD, E. J. and VAN BUSKIRK, D. (Eds.), *Teaching Psychotherapy of Psychotic Patients*. Grune & Stratton, New York, 1969.

46. MALTSBERGER, J. A., and BUIE, D. H., JR., The Work of Supervision. In Semrad, E. J. and Van Buskirk, D. (Eds.), *Teaching Psychotherapy of Psychotic Patients*. Grune & Stratton, New York, 1969.

47. BIBRING, GRETE, L., The Teaching of Dynamic Psychiatry. A Reappraisal of the Goals and Techniques. In *The Teaching of Psychoanalytic Psychiatry*, Bibring, Grete (Ed.) International Universities Press, New York, 1968.

48. WHITEHORN, J. C., Education for Uncertainty. In *Perspectives in Biology and Medicine*. Vol. 7. Chicago University Press, 1963.

49. ERIKSON, ERIK, The Nature of Clinical Evidence. In *Evidence and Inference*. Editor: D. Lerner. *The Hayden Colloquium on Scientific Concept and Method*. New York, Free Press of Glenco, 1959.

50. TEDESCO, CASTELNUEVO, Psychiatric Residents' Appraisal of Psychiatric Teaching in Medical Schools. *Comprehensive Psychiatry*, 10:475-481, 1969.

51. LEWIN, KARL K., Psychiatric Supervision by Direct Observation. *Journal of Medical Education*, 41:860-864, 1966.

52. JASON, H., KAGAN, N., WERNER, A., ELSTEIN, A., and THOMAS, J., New Approaches to Teaching Basic Interview Skills to Medical Students. *American Journal of Psychiatry*, 127:1404-1407, 1971.

53. SZASZ, THOMAS, *The Myth of Mental Illness*. Hoeber-Harper, New York, 1961.

54. LEIFER, RONALD, The Medical Model as Ideology. *International Journal of Psychiatry*, 9:13-21, 1970-1971.

55. BROWN, B. S., and OCHBERG, F. M., The Medical Muddle. *International Journal of Psychiatry*, 9:22-25, 1970-1971.

56. BRODY, EUGENE B., The Psychiatric Resident as a Therapist. In *The Training of Psychotherapists: A Multidisciplinary Approach*. Editors: Dellis, N. P., Stone, Herbert K. L.S.U. Press, Baton Rouge, 1960.

57. HOLT, ROBERT H., and LUBERSKY, LESTER, *Personality Patterns of Psychiatrists*. Basic Books, Inc., New York, 1958. Menninger Clinic Monograph, Series No. 13.

58. PLUTCHIK, ROBERT, CONTE, HOPE, and KANDLER, HENRY, Variables Related to the Selection of Psychiatric Residents. *American Journal of Psychiatry*, 127:1503-1508, 1971.

59. BUCHER, RUE, ET AL., Implications of Prior Socialization for Residency Programs in Psychiatry. *Archives of General Psychiatry*, 20:395-402, 1969.

60. FRAYN, DOUGLAS H., A Relationship Between Rated Ability and Personality Traits in Psychotherapists. *American Journal of Psychiatry*, 124:1232-1237, 1968.

61. KAHANA, RALPH J., Psychotherapy: Models of the Essential Skill. In *The*

Teaching of Dynamic Psychiatry. A Reappraisal of the Goals and Techniques in the Teaching of Psychoanalytic Psychiatry. Editor: Bibring, Grete L. International Universities Press, 1968.

62. BOND, DOUGLAS, In *The Teaching of Dynamic Psychiatry. A Reappraisal of the Goals and Techniques in the Teaching of Psychoanalytic Psychiatry.* Edited: Bibring, Grete L. International Universities Press, 1968.

63. MERKLIN, LEWIS, LITTLE, RALPH B., Beginning Psychiatry Training Syndrome. *American Journal of Psychiatry,* 124:193-197, 1967.

64. SHARAF, MYRON R., and LEVINSON, DANIEL J., The Quest for Omnipotence in Professional Training. *Psychiatry,* 27:135-149, 1964.

65. HALLECK, S. L., and WOODS, S. M., Emotional Problems of Psychiatric Residents. *Psychiatry,* 25:339-346, 1962.

66. WORBY, CYRIL, First Year Psychiatric Resident and the Professional Identity Crisis. *Mental Hygiene,* 54:374-377, 1970.

66a. KUBIE, L. S., *Evaluation of Psychotherapy and of Education: Influence of Timing.* A.P.A. Meeting, Dallas, Texas, 1972.

67. WEBER, JOHN J., Some Observations on Psychiatric Residency Supervision. *Psychoanalytic Review,* 43:214-219, 1956.

68. TITCHENER, JAMES L., The Epaminondas Phenomenon. *American Journal of Psychiatry,* 122:98-99, 1965.

69. TISCHLER, GEORGE L. The Beginning Resident and Supervisor. *Archives of General Psychiatry,* 19:418-422, 1968.

70. WAGNER, F. F., Supervision of Psychotherapy. *American Journal of Psychotherapy,* 11:759-768, 1957.

71. KOGAN, WILLIAM, S., BOE, ERLING E., GOCKA, EDWARD F., and JOHNSON, MERLIN H., Personality Changes in Psychiatric Residents During Training. *Journal of Psychology,* 62:229-240, 1966.

72. GROTJAHN, MARTIN, The Role of Identification in Psychiatric and Psychoanalytic Training. *Psychiatry,* 12:141-151, 1949.

73. HOLLINGSHEAD, A. B., and REDLICH, F. C., *Social Class and Mental Illness. A Community Study.* John Wiley, New York, 1958.

74. DORN, ROBERT M., Psychoanalysis and Psychoanalytic Education: What Kind of "Journey"? In *The Psychoanalytic Forum.* Editor: Lindon, John A. Science House, New York, 237-254, 1969.

75. MILLER, ARTHUR A., and BURSTEIN, ALVIN G., Professional Development in Psychiatric Residents. Assessment and Facilitation. *Archives of General Psychiatry,* 385-394, 1969.

76. DEWALD, PAUL A., Learning Problems in Psychoanalytic Supervision. Diagnosis and Management. *Comprehensive Psychiatry,* 10:107-121, 1969.

77. SCHUSTER, DANIEL B., and FREEMAN, EDWIN N., Supervision of the Resident's Initial Interview. *Archives of General Psychiatry,* 23:516-523, 1970.

78. MARMOR, JUDD, The Feeling of Superiority: An Occupational Hazard in the Practice of Psychiatry. *American Journal of Psychiatry,* 110:370-376, 1953.

79. SHARAF, MYRON R., and LEVINSON, DANIEL J., Patterns of Ideology and Professional Role Definition Among Psychiatric Residents. In *The Patient and the Mental Hospital.* Editors: Greenblatt, Milton, Levinson, Daniel, and Williams, Richard. Glencoe, Illinois, Free Press, 1957.

80. MURRAY, HENRY A., *Explorations in Personality.* Oxford University Press, New York, 1938.

81. GRINKER, R. R., SR., A Struggle for Eclecticism. *American Journal of Psychiatry*, 121:451-457, 1964.
82. GASKILL, H. S., and NORTON, J. E., Observations on Psychiatric Residency Training. *Archives of General Psychiatry*, 18:7-15, 1968.
83. FRENCH, T. M. *The Integration of Behavior*, Vols. 1, 2, 3. University of Chicago Press, Chicago, 1952.
84. CHESSICK, RICHARD D., How the Resident and the Supervisor Disappoint Each Other. *American Journal of Psychotherapy*, 25:272-283, 1971.
85. BRODY, EUGENE B., Psychiatry's Continuing Identity Crisis: Confusion or Growth? *Psychiatry Digest*, 30:12-17, 1969.
86. SPIEGEL, J., Factors in the Growth and Development of the Psychotherapist. *Journal of the American Psychoanalytic Association*, 4:170-175, 1956.
87. CHESSICK, RICHARD D., *How Psychotherapy Heals*. Science House, New York, 1969.
87a. LAZERSON, ALAN M., The Learning Alliance and Its Relation to Psychiatric Teaching. *Psychiatry in Medicine*, 3:81-91, 1972.
88. HALMOS, P., *The Faith of the Counsellors*. Schocken, New York, 1966.
89. ALLEN, D., ET AL., Resistances to Learning. *Journal of Medical Education*, 33:373-379, 1958.
90. GUIORA, ALEXANDER Z., HAMMANN, ARTHUR, MANN, RICHARD D., and SCHMALE, HERBERT T., The Continuous Case Seminar. *Psychiatry*, 30:44-59, 1967.
91. CHING-PIAO CHIEN, and APPLETON, WILLIAM S., The Need for Extensive Reform in Psychiatry Teaching: An Investigation in Treatment, Ideology and Learning. In *Changing Patterns in Psychiatric Care*. Editor: Rothmen, Theodore Crown Publishers, New York, 1970.
92. KLERMAN, G. L., Teaching of Psychopharmacology in Psychiatric Residency. *Comprehensive Psychiatry*, 6:255-264, 1965.
93. FREYHAN, F. A., On Psychopharmacology of Psychiatric Education. *Comprehensive Psychiatry*, 6:221-226, 1965.
94. O'CONNOR, CHARLES T., Peer Group Influences on the Choice of a Psychiatric Viewpoint. *Archives of General Psychiatry*, 13:429-431, 1965.
95. COKER, R. E., BACK, K. W., DONNELLY, T., and MILLER, N., Patterns of Influence: Medical School Faculty Members and the Values and Specialty Interests of Medical Students. *Journal of Medical Education*, 35:518-527, 1960.
96. KALIS, B. L., The In-Patient Program As Seen by the Staff. Read before the staff of Langley-Porter Neuropsychiatric Institute, January 27, 1965. Unpublished.
97. KURTZ, RICHARD M., and KAPLAN, MARVIN L., Resident Attitude Development and the Ideological Commitment of the Staff of Psychiatric Training Institutions. *Journal of Medical Education*, 43:925-929, 1968.
98. COLMAN, ARTHUR D., The Effect of Group and Family Emphasis on the Role of the Psychiatric Resident of an Acute Treatment Ward. *International Journal of Group Psychotherapy*, 15:516-525, 1965.
99. GARDNER, GEORGE E., The Development of the Clinical Attitude. *American Journal of Orthopsychiatry*, 22:162-169, 1952.
100. EKSTEIN, R., Panel discussion, Psychotherapy Supervision: The Role of the Supervisor. American Psychiatric Association meeting in Washington, D.C., May, 1971. Other panelists were: Hollender, M., Kaplan, E., Lower, R., and Sandt, J. Moderator.

101. D'ZMURA, THOMAS L., *The Function of Individual Supervision in Teaching of Psychotherapy*. International Psychiatry Clinics, Vol. I, No. 1. Editor: Francis H. Hoffman, 1954.
102. KAPLOWITZ, DANIEL. Teaching Emphatic Responsiveness in the Supervisory Process of Psychotherapy. *American Journal of Psychotherapy*, 21:774-781, 1967.
103. SCHWARTZ, D. A., Psychotherapy and Supervisory Focus. *Psychiatric Quarterly*, 40:692-701, 1966.
104. WOODMANSEY, A. C., Science and the Training of Psychiatrists. *British Journal of Psychiatry*, 113:1035-1037, 1967.
105. ROSENBAUM, MILTON, Problems of Supervision of Psychiatric Residents in Psychotherapy. *Archives of Neurology and Psychiatry*, 69:43-48, 1953.
106. GROTJAHN, MARTIN, Problems and Techniques of Supervision. *Psychiatry*, 18:9-15, 1955.
107. MOULTON, RUTH, Views on the Supervisory Situation: Multiple Dimensions in Supervision, 146-150; My Memories of Being Supervised, 151-157, all in *Contemporary Psychiatry*, Vol. 5, 1969.
108. BUSH, GEORGE, Transference, Countertransference and Identification in Supervision. *Contemporary Psychoanalysis*, 5:158-162, 1969.
109. PAIDOUSSI, E. R., Varied Experiences in Supervision. *Contemporary Psychoanalysis*, 5:163-168, 1969.
110. BECKETT, THOMAS, A Candidate's Reflection on the Supervisory Process. *Contemporary Psychoanalysis*, 5:169-179, 1969.
111. FLEMING, JOAN, Teaching the Basic Skills of Psychotherapy. *Archives of General Psychiatry*, 16:416-426, 1967.
112. ESCOLL, PHILIP J., WOOD, HOWARD E., Perception in Residency Training: Methods and Problems. *American Journal of Psychiatry*, 124:187-193, 1967.
113. ZINBERG, N. E., The Psychiatrist as Group Observer: Notes on Training Procedure in Individual and Group Psychotherapy. In *Psychiatry and Medical Practice in the General Hospital*. International Universities Press, 1964.
114. VOLKAN, VAMIK, and HAWKINS, DAVID, The Fieldwork Method of Teaching and Learning Clinical Psychiatry. *Comprehensive Psychiatry*, 12:103-115, 1971.
115. VOLKAN, VAMIK, and HAWKINS, DAVID, A Fieldwork Case in the Teaching of Clinical Psychiatry. *Psychiatry in Medicine*, 2:160-176, 1971.
116. VOLKAN, VAMIK, and HAWKINS, DAVID, The Learning Group. Paper presented at APA Annual Meeting, May 5, 1971. Washington, D.C.
117. BARCHILON, JOSE, Some Conscious and Unconscious Factors in Teaching Psychotherapy with One Way Screens, Closed Circuit T.V., or Movie Films. Unpublished manuscript, 1966.
118. SCHULMAN, JEROME L., KASPER, JOSEPH C., and BARGER, PATRICIA M., The *Therapeutic Dialogue*. C. C. Thomas, Springfield, Illinois, 1964.
119. MUSLIN, HYMAN L., and CARMICHAEL, HUGH T., Exercises in Self Observation: A Workshop for Instructors in Psychiatry. *American Journal of Psychiatry*, 124:198-202, 1967.
120. HOLLENDER, MARC, Personal communication.
121. TITCHENER, JAMES L., ROBINSON, JIM, and WOODS, HARRY B., Observing Psychotherapy: An Experience in Faculty-Resident Relations. *Comprehensive Psychiatry*, 9:392-405, 1968.

122. ROSEN, LEO, and BARTEMEIER, HAROLD, The Psychiatric Resident as Participant Therapist. *American Journal of Psychiatry*, 123:1371-1378, 1967.

123. BONN, ETHEL M., and SCHIFF, SAMUEL B., Clinical Supervision of Psychiatric Residents. *Bulletin of the Menninger Clinic*, 27:15-23, 1963.

124. CHODOFF, PAUL, Supervision of Psychotherapy with Videotape: Pros and Cons. *American Journal of Psychiatry*, 128:819-823, 1972.

125. WILMER, H. A., Practical and Theoretical Aspects of Videotape Supervision in Psychiatry. *Journal of Nervous and Mental Disease*, 145:123-130, 1967.

126. WILMER, H. A. Television as Participant Recorder. *American Journal of Psychiatry*, 124:1157-1163, 1968.

127. SCHIFF, S. B., and REIVICH, R. Use of Television as Aid to Psychotherapy Supervision. *Archives of General Psychiatry*, 10:84-88, 1964.

128. BERGER, MILTON M., *Videotape Techniques in Psychiatric Training and Treatment*. Brunner/Mazel, New York, 1970.

129. GRUENBERG, PETER B., LISTON, EDWARD H., JR., and WAYNE, GEORGE J., Intensive Supervision of Psychotherapy with Videotape Recording; *American Journal of Psychotherapy*, 23: 1969, and Chapter 4 in *Videotape Techniques in Psychiatric Training and Treatment*. Editor: Berger, Milton M., Brunner/Mazel, New York, 1970.

130. FROELICH, ROBERT E., Teaching Psychotherapy to Medical Students Through Videotape Simulation; Chapter 5 of *Videotape Techniques in Psychiatric Training and Treatment*. Editor: Berger, Milton M., Brunner/Mazel, New York, 1970.

131. TRETHOWAN, W. H., Teaching Psychiatry by Closed-Circuit Television. Chapter 6 in *Videotape Techniques in Psychiatric Training and Treatment*. Editor: Berger, Milton M., Brunner/Mazel, New York, 1970.

132. GLADFELTER, JOHN W., Videotape Supervision of Co-therapists. In *Videotape Techniques in Psychiatric Training and Treatment*. Editor: Berger, Milton M., Brunner/Mazel, New York, 1970.

133. KAGAN, NORMAN, Television in Counselor Supervision—Educational Tool or Toy? In *Videotape Techniques in Psychiatric Training and Treatment*. Editor: Berger, Milton M., Brunner/Mazel, New York, 1970.

133a. MILLER, PAUL and TUPIN, J., Multimedia Teaching of Introductory Psychiatry, *American J. of Psychiatry*, 128:1219-1223, 1972.

134. COLBY, K. M., STILLMAN, R., WALTON, R., and ROSENBAUM, C. P., An On-Line Computer System for Initial Psychiatric Inventory. *American Journal of Psychiatry*, 7: Supplement 8-11, 1969.

   B. COLBY, K. M., WATT, J. B., and GILBERT, J. P., A Computer Method of Psychotherapy: Preliminary Communication. *Journal of Nervous and Mental Disease*, 142:148-152, 1967.

   C. COLBY, K. M., Computer Simulation of Change in Personal Belief Systems. *Behavioral Science*, 12:248-253, 1967.

   D. HILLMAN, ROBERT G., The Teaching of Psychotherapy Problems by Computer. *Archives of General Psychiatry*, 25:324-329, 1971.

135. WINDHOLZ, E., The Theory of Supervision in Psychoanalytic Education. *International Journal of Psychoanalysis*, 51:393-406, 1970.

   B. SOLNIT, A. J., Learning from Psychoanalytic Supervision. *Ibid.*

   C. LEBOVICI, S., Technical Remarks on the Supervision of Psychoanalytic Treatment. *Ibid.*

   D. GRINBERG, L., The Problems of Supervision in Psychoanalytic Education. *Ibid.*

136. MANNINO, FORTUNE V., and SHORE, MILTON F., Consultation Research in Mental Health and Related Fields: A Critical Review of the Literature. *Public Health Monograph*, No. 79.

137. McCLUNG, F., STUNDEN, A., and PLOG, S., A Study of the Theory and Practice of Mental Health Consultation as Provided to Child Care Agencies Throughout the United States. Behavior Science Corporation in cooperation with the Center for Studies of Child and Family Mental Health, N.I.M.H., 1-3: 1969.

138. WEED, LAWRENCE, Medical Records that Guide and Teach. *New England Journal of Medicine*, March, 1968; *Medical Records, Medical Education and Patient Care: The Problem-Oriented Record as a Basic Tool*. Cleveland Press of Case Western Reserve, 1969.

139. HALLECK, SEYMOUR L., *The Politics of Therapy*. Science House, New York, 1971.

140. SCHLESSINGER, NATHAN, MUSLIN, HYMAN L., and BATTLE, MARGERY, Teaching and Learning Psychiatric Observational Skills. *Archives of General Psychiatry*, 18:549-552, 1968.

141. SCHLESSINGER, NATHAN, Research on Supervisory Process: One Supervisor's Appraisal of the Interview Data. *Archives of General Psychiatry*, 427-431, 1967.

142. WHITMAN, ROY, KREMER, MULTON, and BALDRIDGE, BILL, Experimental Study of Supervision of Psychotherapy. *Archives of General Psychiatry*, 9:529-535, 1963.

143. ORNSTEIN, PAUL H., and KALTHOFF, ROBERT J., Toward a Conceptual Scheme for Teaching Clinical Psychiatric Evaluation. *Comprehensive Psychiatry*, 8:404-426, 1967.

144. SANDLER, J., and ROSENBLATT, B., The Concept of the Representational World. *Psychoanalytic Study of the Child*, 17: 1962.

145. GROTJAHN, MARTIN, Psychiatric Consultations for Psychiatrists. *American Journal of Psychiatry*, 126:932-937, 1970.

146. GROTJAHN, MARTIN, Sigmund Freud as a Psychoanalytic Consultant. *Psychoanalytic Forum*, 1:932-937, 1966.

147. McGEE, THOMAS F., Supervision in Group Psychotherapy: A Comparison of Four Approaches. *International Journal of Group Psychotherapy*, 17: 165-176, 1967.

148. Carnegie Commission on Higher Education. Higher Education and the Nation's Health; Policies for Medical and Dental Education. McGraw-Hill, New York, 1970.

149. MECHANIC, DAVID, *Medical Sociology: A Selective View*. New York Free Press, New York, 1968; Chapter 18, in *Psychosocial Aspects of Medical Training*. Editors: Coombs, R. H., and Vincent, C. E. C. C. Thomas, Springfield, Illinois, 1971.

150. Citizens Commission on Graduate Medical Education. Commissioned by the American Medical Association, Chicago, 1966.

151. MILLIS, JOHN S., *A Rational Public Policy for Medical Education and Its Financing the National Fund for Medical Education*, New York, 1971.

152. FUNKENSTEIN, DANIEL H., Medical Students, Medical Schools, and Society During Three Eras. In *Psychosocial Aspects of Medical Training*. Editors: Coombs, Robert H., and Vincent, Clark E. C. C. Thomas, Springfield, Illinois, 1971.

153. EDELSON, MARSHALL, The Integration of the Behavioral Sciences and Clinical Experience in Teaching Medical Students. In *Training Tomorrow's Psy-*

chiatrist. *The Crisis in Curriculum.* Yale University Press, New Haven, 1970.

154. *Psychosocial Aspects of Medical Training.* Editors: Coombs, Robert H., and Vincent, Clark E. C. C Thomas, Springfield, Illinois, 1971.

155. LIEF, Personality Characteristics of Medical Students. In *Psychosocial Aspects of Medical Training.* Editors: Coombs, Robert T., and Vincent, Clark E. C. C Thomas, Springfield, Illinois, 1971.

156. MERTAN, H. K., READER, G. C., and KENDALL, P. L., *The Student Physician.* Harvard University Press, Cambridge, 1957.

157. LEVITT, L. P., The Personality of the Medical Student. *Chicago Medical School Quarterly,* 25:201-214, 1966.

158. BLOOM, S. W., The Sociology of Medical Education. *Milbank Memorial Fund Quarterly,* 43:143-184, 1965.

159. ZABRENKO, L., PITTINGER, R. A., and ZABARENKO, R. N., *Primary Medical Practice, A Psychiatric Evaluation.* Warren H. Green, Inc., St. Louis, 1968.

160. GRINKER, ROY R., SR., Biomedical Education as a System. *Archives of General Psychiatry,* 24:291-297, 1971.

161. RUDY, LESTER, Psychiatric Education: New Challenges. *American Journal of Psychiatry,* 128:633-634, 1971.

162. ENGEL, GEORGE L., On the Care and Feeding of the Medical Student: The Foundation for Professional Competence. *Journal of the American Medical Association,* 215:1135-1141, 1971.

163. ENGEL, GEORGE L., On The Care and Feeding of the Faculty: A Responsibility for Students. *New England Journal of Medicine,* 281:351-355, 1969.

163a. ENGEL, G., The Implications of Changes in Medical Education. *Hospital Practice,* 6:109-116, 1971.

163b. ENGEL, G., Must We Precipitate a Crisis in Medical Education to Solve the Crisis in Health Care? *Annals of Internal Medicine,* 76:487-490, 1972.

164. ROMANO, JOHN, The Elimination of the Internship—An Act of Regression. *American Journal of Psychiatry,* 126: 1970.

164a. ROMANO, J., *Teaching of Psychiatry to Medical Students: Past, Present and Future.* A.P.A. Meeting, Dallas, Texas, 1972.

164b. REISER, M. F., *Psychiatry in the Undergraduate Medical Curriculum.* A.P.A. Meeting, Dallas, Texas, 1972.

165. LUSTED, LEE B., *Introduction to Medical Decision Making.* C. C Thomas, Springfield, Illinois, 1968.

166. HANEY, C. ALAN, Psychosocial Factors Involved in Medical Decision Making. In *Psychosocial Aspects of Medical Training.* Editors: Coombs, Robert H., and Vincent, Clark E. C. C Thomas, Springfield, Illinois, 1971.

167. POSER, CHARLES M., Medical Education in the 1970s. *Modern Medicine,* December 13, 1971, 54-64.

168. FREUD, SIGMUND, *Collected Papers,* Vol. II. Editor: Ernest Jones, Hogarth Press, 1956.

169. GARBER, ROBERT S., The Presidential Address: The Proper Business of Psychiatry. *American Journal of Psychiatry,* 128:1-11, 1971.

170. RUESCH, JURGEN, The Old World and the New. Editorial. *American Journal of Psychiatry,* 124:225-226, 1967.

171. MILLER, MILTON H., FEY, WILLIAM F., and GREENFIELD, NORMAN S. The Implications of Changing Medical Education for Psychiatric Training. *American Journal of Psychiatry,* 126:1127-1131, 1970.

172. RABKIN, THEODORE, Affect as a Social Process. *American Journal of Psychiatry*, 125:773-779, 1968.

172a. RASKIN, D. E., Psychiatric Training in the 1970's—Toward a Shift in Emphasis. *American Journal of Psychiatry*, 128:1129-1131, 1972.

173. FUNKENSTEIN, DANIEL H., A New Breed of Psychiatrist? *American Journal of Psychiatry*, 124:226-228, 1967.

174. KUBIE, LAWRENCE S., The Retreat from Patients: An Unanticipated Penalty of the Full-time System. *Archives of General Psychiatry*, 24:98-106, 1971.

175. CHRIST, JACOB, Training Groups for Residents. Presented at APA Meeting. Washington, D.C., May, 1971.

176. PATTISON, E. M., Residency Training Issues in Community Psychiatry. *American Journal of Psychiatry*, 128:1097-1102, 1972.

176a. FINK, P. A. and NEWMAN, R., An Integrated Psychodynamic Community Residency. A.P.A. Meeting, Dallas, Texas, 1972.

177. TAYLOR, ROBERT L., and TORREY, E. FULLER, The Self Education of Psychiatric Residents. Presented at APA Meeting. Washington, D.C., May, 1971.

178. KARDENER, SHELDON H., FULLER, MARIELLE, MENSH, IVAN N., and FORGY, EDWARD W., The Trainees' Viewpoint of Psychiatric Residency. *American Journal of Psychiatry*, 126:1132-1138, 1970.

179. *Psychiatric and Medical Education*, II, 1967 Conference, Garamond/Pridemark Press, Inc. 1969.

180. *Teaching Psychiatry in Medical Schools: The Working Papers of the 1967 Conference*. American Psychiatric Association, 1969.

181. HENDRICK, I., *Psychiatry Education Today*. International Universities Press, New York, 1965.

3

The Ontogeny of the Psychiatric Physician

We wish to approach the clinical supervision of the psychiatric resident from the developmental standpoint, using his three years with us as the span of his professional ontogenesis, which we hope to examine in some detail. We recognize that his development prior to reaching us is of great importance. It would appear that interest in human suffering and in means of alleviating it is one fairly obvious motivation of those entering the field; but the whole complicated matter of who chooses medicine as a career and why is beyond the bounds of this study. During the course of his undergraduate medical school years, the student in recent years has been increasingly and more effectively introduced to social and psychological factors in human health and illness. The quality and scope of this exposure vary from school to school, and regardless of the persistence of ambivalent attitudes toward psychiatry, everyone concerned in medical education has accepted the fact that psychiatric illness must be reckoned with. Even in the face of good teaching, however, some studies indicate a shift in medical students' attitudes as they traverse the first to fourth year in that they tend to become more cynical and less idealistic. Bondy (1) states that students, as they go on in medical school, tend to minimize the importance of psycho-social factors in medical practice which they first became curious about in high school and college. He feels a number of factors in the medical school experience are responsible. He speaks of the need to acquire a "pro-

122

tective carapace": the student must learn to tolerate the suffering of his patient without allowing it to overwhelm him. He must become dispassionate in the face of human pain and tragedy, yet not lose sight of the human qualities of the patient. Attaining this balance is a difficult process, and at first he tends to "overshoot" in the direction of cynicism. The attitudes of his teacher, Bondy points out, are crucial in the attaining of this balance. If the teacher lacks the qualities requisite to this precept, the end result may be minimization of psychosocial factors in human illness. The student may forever turn his back upon certain fundamental aspects of human behavior central to understanding and treating patients.

Relevant to this discussion is the question raised increasingly in recent years: Is it necessary for a psychiatrist to have a medical education? Mariner (2) in a recent paper dismisses the contribution of a medical education when he says: "It seems clear, then, that whatever advantage accrues to the psychiatrist functioning as a psychotherapist stems not from his medical knowledge but from irrational attitudes on the part of his patients, his colleagues, and himself (or, of course, from nonmedical training experiences)." His approach is rather literal and concrete: he lists all the courses he took in his pre-medical and medical education and proceeds to state that most of them did not prepare him for his professional task. Our feeling is that a medical background provides an experience not elsewhere obtainable which uniquely fits a person, affectively as well as cognitively, to understand (and empathize with) human illness and suffering. The medical responsibility for patients' comfort, welfare, and indeed lives develops attitudes of enormous importance in subsequent care of patients. Beyond all this, the medical background broadens and deepens the appreciation of a human being, his development, his health, his illness. A physician cannot view the enormous complexities of human problems in terms of a "client" or the mental operations as an "existential dilemma." He is influenced by what he has learned of evolutionary, genetic, developmental, and biological concepts in his view of disordered behavior. This does not imply that a psychiatrist is a competent internist, who physically examines the patient, but that he views the patient in a medical frame of reference and takes into account factors other than strictly psychological ones.

We do not intend to discuss this issue in detail—the relevance of a medical education to the psychiatrist's task—but the main argument of this study, either directly or indirectly, is concerned with it. Engel (3) has stated it well in saying, "Psychiatrists, who after all are physicians, should be concerning themselves not with dispensing with the medical model, but with updating it to make it more appropriate for the modern understanding of health and disease and the care of the patient . . . the distinctive feature of the M.D. is that his ultimate concern is with the health and illness of each individual. It is this which constitutes the basis for the medical model, not some preoccupation with the body as a machine to the exclusion of psychological or social considerations, as some critics would have us believe."

In addition to the relevance of medical education to the psychiatrist's training is the general state of medicine today. There are at present powerful and conflicting forces being brought to bear on medical education (4) which may appreciably alter, possibly dilute, its quality and standards. We have in mind the simultaneous pressure to eliminate the internship (5) and reduce the time required for undergraduate medical training. Some of this has come about as a consequence of parochial specialty interests, some from certain groups within organized medicine, and some resulting from the impact of the Carnegie Commission's report (6). It is important to note that it has not come, for the most part, from the medical centers and their teachers who educate physicians.

Complex social, economic and political factors have put great pressure on medicine to produce comprehensive care for everyone in accordance with the growing feeling that health care is no longer a privilege but a right. There is in addition a demand for more physicians and for their improved geographic distribution, but without accompanying financial support to accomplish these tasks. A great deal is expected of medicine today, some of it unrealistic and doomed to disappointment.

In the face of all of this, it behooves us to rededicate ourselves to the important task of training the clinician—to maintain high standards of such training amidst the welter of these forces, which at times work at odds with our objective.

We have set the following discussion in the framework of psychoanalytic psychology. Our understanding of both the patient and the process of supervision, as well as of the professional growth of the resident, is unavoidably based on certain basic issues and principles which have been developed by psychoanalysis. We know of no other frame of reference or scheme of thought which offers as comprehensive, economic, or elegant an explanation of human behavior. We will not dwell in the realm of the metapsychological nor entertain theoretical discussion of psychoanalytic concepts. The reader can be referred to excellent discussions of these issues by Brenner (7), Arlow and Brenner (8), Waelder (9) and others. We find the use of such basic concepts as the unconscious mind, psychic determination of behavior, instinctual drive, mental conflict and its production of symptoms and other compromise-formations, primary and secondary process, ontogeny and epigenesis, transference and counter-transference not only helpful but inescapable in discussing behavior.

We sometimes overlook the fact that psychoanalytic psychology has so thoroughly permeated psychiatric thought that residents come to us familiar to a greater or lesser degree with some psychoanalytic theory. At times this amounts to a handful of clichés, or worse, a great deal of misconception. So much of what the resident has learned about psychoanalysis in his undergraduate years is derivative, adulterated, and distorted. It has oftentimes been taught by people who are untrained in psychoanalysis and have an exclusively academic view of the subject.

An example of the pervasiveness of psychoanalytic concepts in the everyday thinking of psychiatric residents is the use of concepts such as "primary process." This term may have been acquired in undergraduate school, medical school, or in graduate training. In the latter it is passed on by one generation of resident to another and acquires a variety of meanings, from "loose associations" to "thought disorder" to symptoms of psychosis. Such usage exemplifies how meaning can become blurred or distorted when historical perspective is lost. In our own experience, we have not as often as we should referred our residents, in this instance, to Chapter VII of Freud's *Interpretation of Dreams* (10) for the original discussion of primary and secondary processes. Terms such as transference have become absolutely hackneyed without knowledge of Freud's paper on "The Dynamics of Transference" (11), where the concept is so simply and lucidly described.

In the immediate post-World War II era there was an enormously revived interest in psychoanalysis and considerable eagerness in reading original sources. The generation of psychiatric teachers who studied these concepts has not always had its students retrace the same steps in learning that which now seems "old hat." In our own experience we realize that in recent years we have not always provided leadership for the resident in his reading. In addition, many new areas of thought and inquiry in psychiatry have proliferated, properly claiming the resident's attention but competing with his interest in intrapsychic issues.

Some residents tend to indiscriminate and incorrect application of these concepts—as with "wild interpretation" of some of their patients' comments or behavior. Even those who come with some genuine familiarity with Freud's writings must, through clinical experience and good supervision, learn how to *apply* such knowledge. The great difference between the clinician and the one with reading knowledge of psychoanalysis is the degree of personal experience in studying patient behavior at close range and in some depth and detail. No one would presume to undertake a surgical procedure without all the preparation that leads to the point of taking the scalpel in hand, but some seem to feel that knowledge of human behavior is easily acquired and in some manner remote from patient care.

Kubie (12) in recent years has stressed the importance of careful study of individual patients in the development of a psychiatrist. He states, "The one ingredient which is essential for *becoming* a psychiatrist, as opposed to learning *about* psychiatry, is the repeated experience of being a participant in the changes which occur in one's own patients over extended periods of time." He adds, "Yet without these slow and repeated experiences with one patient at a time, men may acquire book-learning—but they can achieve neither personal nor professional maturity."

Many overlook the historical fact that psychoanalytic concepts were originally derived from clinical observations, and they seek to reverse the process in their own education—by hypothesizing *before* making observations. We have found that only through personal discovery, using his patient's productions, can a resident feel any conviction about theoretical notions. When, for example, he senses the immediacy of the transference through a patient's expression of a sexual or hostile feeling for him, he has an affective as well as a cognitive appreciation of this concept.

There is in a sense a parallel between Freud's own professional ontogenetic development and that of a psychiatric resident's professional development. The resident's experience is in many ways fortunately telescoped because of the discoveries made before him; but, like Freud, he must learn how to make observations and derive data from patients before he can understand concepts of human behavior or construct his own theories about human motives. We see the reverse in certain students who acquire knowledge of human behavior from books and courses without a concurrent experience with live clinical problems. They often have a *nouveau riche* attitude of confident and comprehensive understanding of all human problems, which stands in stark contrast to the acquired humility of the experienced clinician. An important aspect of the latter's professional development and maturation is the day-to-day living with physical disease, pain, suffering, decay and death, anxiety, guilt, and shame, which is an integral part of medical education. This kind of experience, coupled with graduated responsibility for the lives and destiny of patients, powerfully shapes the attitudes of the clinician. It not only inculcates knowledge of human adaptation and deviance, but it also enhances the erection of ego and character defenses which permit the mature clinician to make objective observations and rational judgments without being either too distant, cold, and unresponsive to the patient, or overwhelmed with maudlin pity, concern, and anxiety as a consequence of over-identification. The finely-developed and precariously maintained emotional attitude of the good clinician is laboriously and painfully acquired from life experiences. It represents an ideal, never perfectly attained—as there is always the temptation to turn away from the emotional demands of the patient, or worse, to gratify one's destructive tendencies through mishandling the problems the patient presents. The admonition, "Primum, non nocere," although an ancient one is still as crucial today; and it applies alike to the surgeon who physically invades the body and the psychiatrist who invades the mind. This is why we view with concern current trends which seek short-cuts and adulteration of psychiatric training and why we take so seriously the responsibility of training the psychiatric physician.

In considering the professional ontogeny of the psychiatric resident we must recognize the primary importance of developing a professional identity over the three-year period assigned to his training.

This is a critical matter in any specialist's development, but perhaps more difficult in some regards for a psychiatrist. Education is in great part accomplished through the student's identification with his teacher. This is uniquely so in medical-clinical education, which remains essentially based on the apprenticeship system. As expanded and sophisticated as medical knowledge has become, *being a doctor* requires emulation of the practitioner. This is not simply imitation and learning of procedure, but thinking, acting, and *feeling* like a doctor. It involves all the complicated conscious and unconscious processes of identification. As with other aspects of maturation, this process takes time, varies with different people, and cannot be artificially hastened. It also cannot be accomplished through seminar or lecture but mainly through the personal precept, day-to-day guidance, and critical demonstration of the clinical teacher. It should be emphasized that "feeling like a doctor" is not sufficient to assure a newly arrived resident in psychiatry of feeling confident and comfortable. For a number of reasons we will describe, he is bound to feel vulnerable in the face of what he fantasies is expected of him and what he has to offer patients whose requirements at this point are somewhat mysterious to him. He suspects that he must ask different questions and use different approaches than he is accustomed to in "taking" medical histories. He understands that a psychiatrist acts differently with his patients, is expected to know answers to some of life's most imponderable questions, is to be neutral and "cool" in the presence of the wildest behavior. These are some of the issues we wish to address in considering the development of a psychiatrist.

The problem of his professional identity is particularly acute for a psychiatric resident today. He hears a confusing variety of messages about the mission of psychiatry. It is not just a matter of fractionation of a field, as in super-specialization, but the many suggestions that psychiatry is not doing what it should, that it must respond to many problems in the world not traditionally thought of as within the province of medicine. We are admonished for not taking greater part in the community, in problems of the poor, in systems of delivery of health care, in third party agencies involved with health care, in political matters as remote from our daily work as Vietnam. We are urged—indeed exhorted—to become instruments of social change, and criticized for not having a "social conscience." Battle lines are drawn

between the New Left and the Establishment. As in all polemical issues, the polarization of views is more appropriate to political dispute
than to scientific debate. Seymour Halleck in the introduction to his
recent book, *The Politics of Therapy* (13), demarcates the dichotomy
of establishment thinking versus new liberation. He juxtaposes opposing views of psychiatric leaders who are at opposite poles of opinion as
to whether psychiatry should be involved in trying "to bring about
change within social or political systems." Halleck concludes, "It
appears that many American psychiatrists are still convinced that
their professional mandate is simply that of healing a form of illness
and that their therapeutic activities do not and should not have
political consequences." He believes that, "Any kind of psychiatric
intervention, even when treating a voluntary patient, will have an
impact upon the distribution of power within the various social systems in which the patient moves . . . all psychiatric intervention must
be viewed as having political consequences." He also cites the spe-
cious *reductio ad absurdum* that "psychiatric neutrality is a myth"
and dedicates his book to the destruction of this notion,

Such a line of reasoning is extraordinarily appealing to modern
youth who have rediscovered politics and become aware that the
world we live in is beset by grievous problems. What right-minded
person would not want to try to set things straight, to redress
wrongs, to help make the world a better place to live in? But the
issue for psychiatry is, aside from interested personal citizenship and
all that a dedicated individual can do in this regard, what can and
should the profession do about these matters? Rather than rush to
the barricades, we should thoughtfully examine and re-examine ourselves, our competence, our goals. For what is a physician prepared
in life? We may all be political animals, but not necessarily politicians. In our experience, physicians who have ventured into areas
where they have no competence or acquaintance have often blundered
badly and blurred in their own and others' minds their appropriate
aims in life. Furthermore, our belief is that most people whose
conscious and unconscious interests move them into medicine are
not suited for a career as a social revolutionary, a politician, or for
that matter a clergyman or engineer. Most professions are in some
way self-selecting.

Beyond this, the clinical responsibility that always rests on the
shoulders of a practitioner dictates that one be more inclined to

thoughtful consideration than impulsive action. The unremitting nature of responsibility for others' lives and welfare is a unique obligation, not shared by any other walk of life. It is both the challenge and burden of the physician. Not every one finds this to his liking; we see many examples of those who, even within our field, find it intolerable and turn away from the patient in one way or another.

Because we are accustomed to take dichotomous views of issues, we seem to find it incompatible for a man to pursue his profession, do it well, not dabble as a dilettante in other fields beyond his ken, and yet be an interested and effective citizen, have a family life, pursue hobbies, etc. There is some fallacy of thinking involved here— a notion that a man must be either "with it" or not to be counted among the living. The idea that man is a unitary force with a single identity does grave injustice to the complexity of the human personality. We all have in fact many identities, each involved with a facet of our life role, responsibilities, and interests.

Finally, Halleck's statement about "psychiatric neutrality" needs to be dealt with in passing. We agree it is a myth, but we assumed everyone knowledgeable in our field knew it, too. We are interested in where this notion originated. Elsewhere we discuss the distorted notion of the "psychoanalytic model" which leads so many residents astray. Seasoned psychoanalysts understand the importance of conducting oneself in a manner so as not to contaminate the field of the transference, in order to help the patient perceive his own feelings and projections onto the analyst. This does not imply that the analyst assumes he himself is neutral, or that the patient is completely oblivious of the analyst's human qualities and frailties.

We have found it heartening to learn over the years that of all the instruction offered the residents, including thoughtfully developed seminars, lectures and readings and clinical conferences, the exercise most prized by the resident is his regular tutorial or supervisory session—his *own,* individual time spent with his mentor, unshared with his siblings. From our description of the supervision offered in our training program we hope to demonstrate that not only is it important to graduate this supervision, by gradually increasing the level of sophistication and introducing the resident to increasingly complex problems as he develops, but also to assign a number of supervisors throughout the three-year program to give the resident a more or less individually appropriate span of models and styles.

We also recognize that the identity of the young psychiatrist is most precarious—or ill-formed—at the outset of his experience (14, 15); so this is when the greatest support must be afforded and the least demand made upon his clinical judgment. Clinical problems at this early stage should be obvious, in caricature one might say, such as flagrant psychotic states. This is the period when he needs time and assistance in making his observations. For these reasons we have felt that the proper introduction of the beginning resident is on an in-patient setting, not the clinic where more sophisticated clinical decisions must be made, often quickly and under more demanding circumstances.

Miller and Burstein (17) in a recent article state: "We recognize that the residency is but one phase in the professional development of a psychiatrist; what occurs in the residency is in part a function of what the resident brings to it in terms of past experience, and his professional identity may not be fully consolidated until some years after the completion of his residency training." Kubie, who has devoted himself to this subject in recent years, speaks of this in terms of the maturity of the psychiatrist resulting from a struggle with his own inner conflicts, the accepting of responsibilities such as marriage and parenthood, and finally the development of *clinical* maturity from "the experience of sustained relationships with patients as they fall ill and fall well again. Nothing can take the place of being a participant-observer of these fluctuating changes over weeks, months, and even years." Stressing the time and experience required in this acquisition of maturity, Kubie adds, "This is why psychiatry is no field for a young man in a hurry" (12).

Miller and Burstein's paper deals with assessment of the resident's performance, and they state that such an assessment can be made best "in relation to a clear concept of what needs to be achieved during a psychiatric residency." In this regard they speak of the basic skills of observation, understanding, and purposeful actions. "Observation means to hear, see, and feel data about the patient and oneself. . . . Such observation requires the suspension of action, a tolerance for ambiguity, and lack of closure. The observer needs an openness, a tolerance for being impinged upon by the data without fear of being overwhelmed, and the ability to be surprised." They continue, "Understanding includes both an intuitive grasp of human behavior and an ability to use a relevant, firmly established but open theory about human psychology." Finally, "Action means the ability to intervene or abstain from intervention in the light of what is observed and understood, in order to influence purposefully what is going on in the patient." Ornstein and Kalthoff (18) have spoken of the role of the physician as "the instrument of clinical psychiatric evaluation" and have described his primary functions as "observation, evocative listening and empathic-intuitive-introspective capacity."

We feel these are clear statements of the goals of a psychiatric residency program. Their achievement is a serious and difficult task which we attempt to describe from our point of view.

Not only is the nature of the clinical material in psychiatry anxiety-provoking to a new resident, raising all kinds of self-questioning and doubt within his mind; but the emotional demands the patient makes upon him are in some ways more excessive and insistent than others he has experienced to date. In addition, he does not have the props or trappings to come between him and the patient, such as the stethoscope of the internist or the instrument of the surgeon. Furthermore, touching or examining the body, he comes to realize, has different emotional connotations in psychiatry than in other medical experience, and in some instances is fraught with difficulty. Thus unprotected in his encounter with the patient, he has to regulate his distance from the patient, both physical and emotional, in various nonverbal, kinetic, and attitudinal ways. Some of these are unconscious and thus unavailable to him or his supervisor to discuss. As though this were not enough, his role vis-à-vis the patient is not clearly defined, and at first his interventions are ambiguous or emotionally conflicted. In contrast, the beginning surgical apprentice has his role and intervention clearly and unambiguously defined when he is told to hold a retractor in a certain position. His role at this point is clear and simple; he is relatively unconflicted and free to observe his mentor's activity.

Intervention in psychiatry is in great part invisible, abstract, and verbal—not visible, concrete, and palpable as compared with intervention by instrument or medication. Because of this and because most of the resident's work with his patient is done in private, we have to devise means of observing the resident with his patient and pointing out in detail what he has done, as well as to demonstrate our own expertise in interviewing patients, to provide him the necessary model. In the following chapter we discuss one method we have employed to accomplish this observation of the resident's work with his patients.

The matter of how a psychiatrist should "talk" to and with his patient is an important issue. Here, medical training has equipped the young psychiatrist in one regard—the ability to take a medical history. Although certain changes and additions are necessary to adapt the typical "history outline" to psychiatric patients, the general stance is the same. The doctor must inquire tactfully and empathically and in appropriate detail and sequence from the patient the story of his illness, his distress. We do not intend to be concerned here with such philosophical issues as whether mental illness is a myth or a reality. We are satisfied that our patients suffer from various symptoms which we regard as derived from intrapsychic conflicts and the intricate operations of a burdened mental apparatus, attempting to reconcile the demand of reality and the force of the instincts.

How this inquiry of the patient is conducted is a critical matter which is the source of considerable and varied discussion in our chapter on the Supervisory Conference, where we examine as a group, in great detail, the issues of the initial interview. In the following pages we wish to emphasize a few fundamentals involved in obtaining data from the psychiatric patient.

At this point we might describe two extremes we have observed in beginning residents, who are "talking" with patients. At one extreme is the notion that conducting an interview is somewhat similar to a social conversation. In this set, the resident and patient may lapse into a pleasant but aimless dialogue, which results in both being reasonably comfortable. It does not, however, eventuate in any systematic gathering of data from the patient nor in elucidating his problems to either himself or to the resident. The social model of two people on relatively equal footing is not applicable to the patient-physician dyad, where one is seeking help and the other attempting to render it. Some nowadays attack this latter relationship as authoritarian and lacking in egalitarianism. This is a confusion of political and medical issues and overlooks the obvious reality that the physician knows more than the patient.

At the other extreme is the resident who inappropriately adopts what he erroneously regards as the stance of the psychoanalyst. We do not understand the origin of this notion, but by it the resident apparently understands that he is to sit immobile and in stony silence, expecting the patient miraculously to tell his story in detail and without guidance. Regardless of the origin of this model and recognizing its gross misunderstanding of the technique and task of the analyst, we can appreciate its utility to the resident. It is a safe position for him in his anxious struggle to contact the patient. It affords a tight but fruitless defense against his sexual and aggressive impulses toward the patient, just as the immobility of the catatonic patient provides him with a defense against his murderous impulses. Although affording the resident some relief, such an attitude will be felt by the patient as a silent expression of hostility, disapproval, and rejection. Such an approach is just as surely perceived as an aggressive assault as if it were a physical blow.

These two extremes are cited, realizing they usually are only transitional states in the developing resident, but also to emphasize they may become professional ways of life in the absence of adequate supervision.

A common problem in our field is how we deal with the aggression we feel for our patients. We do not often talk about this or face the matter squarely by appreciating the enormous hostility that at times we feel for patients. This may arise in part from frustration of our therapeutic expectations. Some of it may be specifically engendered by a patient's character style, which stirs some particular countertransference response in us. It may also be a consequence of the more general emotional demand (object-hunger) patients make on us, and some may result from unresolved ambivalence of the psychiatrist. Being placed in a position where we must for long stretches of time be passively receptive and unable to discharge accumulated tension through motor acts available to other physicians, touching the body of the patient, employing instrumentation, or "doing things to the patient," places a great strain on the defenses against our aggression. Psychiatrists commonly deal with this by intellectualization, isolation of affect, and reaction formation, all of which may be effective in warding off the patient's demands and perception of one's own hostile feelings; but may also have the adverse result of causing us to turn away from the patient and not hear or feel his distress.

This might be epitomized in the phrase, "the patient as an enemy." In supervision one sees many examples of the vicissitudes of the patient's and psychiatrist's aggression. One sees manifestations of fear of the patient in such revealing clichés as "castrating female," "neurotic," or "manipulative, acting-out character." The fear of being manipulated by the patient,* while it has its realistic aspects, is largely a reflection of one's feeling at the mercy of the patient's hostility, or a projection of the psychiatrist's aggression toward the patient. The need to differentiate one's conflicts and symptoms from the patient's gives rise in the neophyte to certain characteristic attitudes subsumed under the adage—"There but for the grace of God go I"—and tends to induce feelings of overconfidence, lofty views of human problems, or callous and judgmental views of emotional illness. A somewhat pejorative view of psychological disability is so pervasive, even in this sophisticated age, that it inescapably affects us all. For example, in almost every psychiatrist's mind is a hierarchy of illness—it is somehow better, more respectable, less shameful to be a "case" of obsessional neurosis than paranoid schizophrenia. Perhaps because so many of us are obsessional characters, we are repelled by "untidy" forms of sickness, such as psychosis, or affronted by the "defiance" of acting-out character disorders.

The typical defenses of intellectualization, isolation of affect, and reaction-formation mentioned earlier may be seen in various reactions and attitudes toward psychiatric patients. One can listen to the most heart-rending account of human depredation delivered in the most affectless manner imaginable by a resident describing the history of his patient. The stony face, or "I'm wondering what you think?" reply to a patient's anxious question in the initial interview is another example. "It's your decision" in response to some crucial issue in the patient's life is a further instance of the psychiatrist's hostility toward the patient. The confusion of using a poorly understood psychoanalytic modality at an inappropriate time and place, such as the diagnostic interview, constitutes a serious barrier between us and the patient. Tarachow (19) rightly made the point that a patient seeking a consultation is under no obligation to us, and we have no right to make demands on him. We have to understand that the beginning psychiatrist's adoption of such a stance is not rationally chosen but a convenient defense against the aggression he feels from the pa-

---

* Cited by our first-year residents as their major source of anxiety in dealing with patients.

tient or himself. In this uncertain period of his development, he must seize on a limited repertoire of ways of relating to patients—many derived from things he's heard as to what "you're supposed to do."

The issue of object hunger, the desire of both the patient and the psychiatrist to lay claim to one another as real objects, is a most troublesome problem for all of us and difficult to convey in our teaching of the young resident. Tarachow (20) has lucidly delineated this in describing psychotherapeutic methods on a continuum from one pole of treating the patient as a real object to the other pole of taking him as an "as if" object. So many of us are in need of anaclitic relationships that the natural tendency is to treat the physician-patient relationship as a social situation in which we gratify each other emotionally. It is most difficult for a developing psychiatrist to understand that he can "help" a patient without gratifying him, or that he can ally himself with the patient without either coldly rejecting him or "being a friend." He will oscillate—sometimes getting too close to the patient, sometimes retreating too far from him. Propelled by maternal strivings (21) to nurture and rescue the patient, haunted by guilt over his aggression, and blinded by residual infantile omnipotence, his initial impulse is to rush toward the patient with missionary zeal and maudlin pity. This thrust is repulsed by the patient, who feels overwhelmed and assaulted; and the novice retreats, feeling rejected and fuming about the ingratitude of this wretch he is dedicated to "treat."

The matter of observation—the clinician's capacity to note and evaluate the myriad behavioral manifestations of his patient, quite aside from the data he collects in his formal history taking—is a cardinal issue in the development of a psychiatrist. We referred earlier to Miller and Burstein's definition of "observation" and their comment that it requires the suspension of action, a tolerance for ambiguity, and lack of closure. To describe in any comprehensive detail either the process of clinical observation, how it is taught or how it is gradually developed seems an overwhelming task. It is not a subject which lends itself to abstract discussion but rather is best elucidated by specific instances occurring in the interaction of patient and physician. It can be made manifest by the interviewer relating to an experienced observer his subjective appraisal of the patient, his accumulated impressions and interpretations of what he saw, heard and felt. In turn the mentor can correct certain impressions, add to them, point to certain omissions or distortions of perception on the part of the interviewer.

The matrix from which the clinical observer develops is his medical background—the years of training to look, observe, compare, differentiate, evaluate, which has been a pervasive theme through all his studies from microscopic anatomy to physical diagnosis, irrespective of individual discipline. Without such a basic orientation and in the absence of the requisite curiosity and capacity to engage in such inquiry, it is difficult to conceive of clinical observation ever developing adequately.

The whole question of talent is one little discussed or understood. It is something we all recognize but find difficult to define. Whatever its composition, it is a quality requisite to the developing clinician. To talent and intellectual curiosity one must add that derivative of voyeuristic interest which obviously is an ingredient in the process of observing. Finally, there must be an element of doubt and suspicion—a tendency not to accept things as they appear, but to look beneath and behind the obvious.

Given these qualities and the proper precept, the process of "learning to observe" is made possible. We have emphasized before that the apprentice-master model is eminently applicable to the training of the clinician—a means of introducing the novice to the things to look for and the ways of looking. There is no substitute for the seasoned practitioner who provides the precept. Given a variety of adequate models and the possibility of repetitive clinical experience, the conscious process of emulation and the unconscious one of identification move the resident in the direction of accumulating a series of clinical observations which become gradually compared, sorted and stored for future recall. He begins to develop a repertoire of approaches, just as he did in "talking" to the patient in order to evaluate behavior, attitudes, affective states, ideation, and many other non-verbal qualities which must be deduced by other means than asking questions or listening to the patient's speech.

This brief consideration of some of the basic issues in the professional ontogeny of the psychiatric physician leads us to discuss what we regard as the major turning point in his developing identity—the transition from the first to the second year. We will discuss later (Chapter 4) some of the details of the program and our techniques of supervision, but here we wish to comment on the transition in general terms.

Our residents spend their first year of psychiatric residency almost exclusively on the inpatient service. Their contact with outpatients is limited for the most part to the follow-up care of their inpatients. The majority of their patients have had acute or chronic psychotic reactions or severe character disturbances. On the inpatient service the resident learns to recognize the various psychiatric syndromes with emphasis on the affective disorders and the schizophrenias. Their experience with treatment deals primarily with inpatient management, drugs, electroconvulsive therapy, environmental manipulation and various supportive measures through the utilization of other hospital personnel, including the activities program. They participate in patient-staff meetings, group therapy, and family interviews.

The first-year resident has not participated, however, in the decision to admit the patient and is dealing, for the most part, with a "captive" who is available for many hours of the day and night for observation and study. The history can be taken at a leisurely pace compared with the outpatient setting, and decisions about the patient can be postponed and deliberated upon in consultation with his chief resident and floor director. In contrast, the second-year resident in the clinic is confronted with more immediate problems and the necessity to make more rapid decisions: should the patient return, if so, when, is he medically sick, should the family be seen, does he need to be admitted to the inpatient service? The resident must try to understand what the patient wants and needs and evaluate his strengths and weaknesses. In planning the patient's care, he is handicapped by his relative lack of experience in practical management of ambulatory patients and in establishing therapeutic contracts involving mutually acceptable goals.

At times, we may not have made clear to the resident the important differences between an inpatient population and those who present themselves to a clinic. Hendrick (22), in commenting on this, refers to inpatients as those "who live in a totally different environment, the hospital, among doctors and nurses and other patients, rather than the everyday world, and who are subject to ward management rather than to the ordinary rules of social conduct and responsibility."

The turning point in the resident's identification as a psychiatrist is his transition from the first to the second year. Leaving the somewhat protected and highly organized ambience of the floor team, made up of other first-year residents, a third-year resident, a senior faculty person in charge of the floor, rounding faculty, including the chairman of the department, nurses, activities people—with all of whom the first-year resident has frequent, elbow-to-elbow contact, he graduates to the second year, where either in the Emergency Division he sees his patients alone, with available consultation from a third-year resident and faculty director, or in the Outpatient Clinic he faces a new patient with his supervisor. In Chapter IV we will elaborate on a supervisory technique we have developed in recent years within the Outpatient Clinic to assist the second-year residents in this new area of experience. Here we wish to emphasize in broader terms the significance of this shift in clinical milieu from the inpatient to outpatient setting.

On the inpatient floors, with their highly structured responsibilities and roles for the various professional members of the team, their frequent meeting together, the multiple opportunities for exchange of views and the various levels of supervision, a first-year resident has a chance to sample a variety of fairly obvious behavioral deviance, much of it lending itself to ready diagnostic classification, and to gain experience in managing such cases of acute emotional illness. He can rely on tangible therapeutic modalities such as the phenothiazines and electro-convulsive treatment, which at times have almost miraculous effects in bringing to a dramatic end either an acute schizophrenic break or a psychotic depression. He also can depend to some extent on other "doctorly" devices and familiar medical knowledge while he is developing some confidence in his growing clinical judgment about "purely emotional components" of his patients' illness. He is aided in this transition by the fact that 50-60% of our inpatients have medical complications, some of them requiring active treatment and consultation with other specialists in the Medical Center. The floor environment in a sense provides a supportive "family" for the fledgling psychiatrist.

Another aid is the fact that his patient's stay and the acute phase of his illness are fairly brief. The average hospital stay of our patients is less than a month. This circumscribes the resident's contact with many of his patients, some of whom he may never see again (patients with private psychiatrists, who follow their own patients when they leave the hospital). This has the educational disadvantage of providing a cross-sectional rather than a longitudinal view of the patient's disorder, but it lightens the burden of the resident, who is learning how to interview a psychiatric patient, evaluate his diagnosis and plan his hospital treatment.

During his year's assignment to inpatient floors, the resident has a number of models for identification from the chairman of the department, the floor director, other "rounding men," to other more experienced residents. (The third-year resident has day-to-day management of the floor.) He sees these more experienced people interviewing patients, handling acute management problems, and discussing their views of etiology, symptomatology, diagnosis, prognosis— various *weltanschaungen* of the field of psychiatry, its hopes and limitations, accomplishments and disappointments. Many of the operations of these more seasoned clinicians are public and visible to the neophyte psychiatrist—an essential to learning in a field which tends to be as private as ours.

Coming from this climate into the clinic, the second-year resident experiences a sharp change. He is essentially alone and unaided by teams, other professional groups, and various devices to help ease the contact between him and his patient. He no longer examines the patient physically, usually does not have the family to help round out the history and is expected only to listen to and observe a patient he sees for very brief periods (an hour at a time), several days apart. He does have his supervisor during the initial interview to help meet the exigencies of the first encounter, draw his attention to certain critical points and help guide subsequent inquiries and approaches to the patient's problems. But he feels naked and unprepared in this task and responds often in a number of defensive ways. Many residents comment on the difference in the patients they see in the clinic and their feeling inadequate to interview outpatients. They tell us, after the first few months of their assignment in the OPD, that they never really understood how to interview a patient until experience with the clinic population. What they mean, aside from gaining experience and versatility, in our opinion, is that they have learned how to do more than gather historical data like input into a computer. They have gained some appreciation of nuance and the dynamics of interaction between patient and psychiatrist. They have begun to learn how much can be accomplished under circumstances of limited time, patient's clinical state, degree of resistance, the stage of the diagnostic study, the patient's interest and capacity to pursue the task, and a host of other factors.

At the conclusion of his second year, during which the resident has spent six months studying both adult and child (including adolescent) ambulatory patients, and six months of duty in the psychiatric emergency service, he has had a sufficiently extensive and varied clinical experience under ample supervision so that he feels a degree of confidence and acquaintance with a wide spectrum of psychiatric disorder. He has come to develop a repertoire of techniques, a set of expectations concerning prognosis and consequences of psychological interventions, and, in general, some competence in *acting* as a psychiatrist. His identity is more clear and firm. The increasing responsibility accorded to him in his third year, where he assumes management of an inpatient floor or some other unit or division of the Department, including teaching and supervision of other residents junior to him, further matures his clinical judgment and consolidates his identification as a psychiatrist.

It remains for the years immediately following his formal residency to afford him added experience. The maturing process will continue if he has had sound and substantial experience and supervision in his residency years, and if he has the necessary talent, energy, independence, and curiosity to profit from further clinical experience. The danger and possible hindrance to further development, aside from the factors mentioned above and the unresolved emotional conflicts of the psychiatrist, lie in the private nature of our work. A busy psychiatrist's practice occurs outside the scrutiny of his colleagues, and his burdened professional life affords little or no opportunity for exchange of experience and viewpoints with other practicing psychiatrists. His daily work is not as visible and understandable as is that of a surgeon, an obstetrician, or pediatrician. This may be a slightly overdrawn comparison, but taking into account the criteria of amelioration and end-points of treatment in our field, plus the privacy of the treatment itself, a psychiatrist must guard constantly against sequestration and parochialism. He may find himself drifting contentedly along life's stream with certain patients who derive emotional gratification of their "object-hunger" and do not complain they are "getting nowhere." The psychiatrist must have the intellectual curiosity and integrity to question himself constantly: What is the aim of this intervention, where is the patient heading, what is being accomplished, are we going too fast or too slow, has the relationship culminated in a comfortable and tacit mutual gratification which fails to resolve irrational conflicts? Should the treatment course be altered? If an uncovering approach was chosen, is the patient profiting or being harmed? Are therapist and patient grappling with basic issues, or creating a titillating exercise in intellectualization?

What are the safeguards against unfavorable professional development subsequent to residency training, or better, how can one help to assure continued clinical maturation, increased wisdom and competence? We would recommend as a basic foundation a personal psychoanalysis. While formal psychoanalytic training may not be necessary to achieve competence in psychotherapy, we believe personal psychoanalytic treatment gives a psychiatrist a depth of understanding of the unconscious and acquaintance with his own conflicts and emotional scotomata requisite to a thoroughgoing understanding of his patient's difficulty. Even this does not guarantee such understanding and competence; it does not prevent some psychiatrists from turning away from the emotional demands patients make on them. These sorely tax the psychiatrist's infantile omnipotence and narcissism, his need to rescue and his maternal strivings.

We regard it as highly desirable for young psychiatrists to continue after their formal training some degree of supervision and some opportunity to discuss their "cases" with other colleagues. This applies to older clinicians, too, who require opportunities to exchange with each other their professional experience. Some such opportunities exist in our organizations and societies, some have to be created by us. It is significant, however, how much of the content of our professional metings has to do with deprivative subjects—we remain chary of discussing the details of what *we do* with our patients. We must always strive to combat this tendency to defensiveness—shared, we might add, with our colleagues of other specialties—born of the uncertainty and ambiguity of our field, its means of therapeutic intervention and the results of our time-consuming and tedious work. There is no basically rational reason for feeling shame about our efforts. We have some fairly good ideas of what we can accomplish and must face honestly our less successful ventures in order to learn from our failures and frustrations. Only the intellectual rigor and scrutiny of the supervisory situation applied in some manner to our subsequent professional life can assure our own and our profession's advancement. Thus, we, as seasoned clinicians, are on the same continuum of maturation—of professional ontogeny—as our residents. We can learn from each other.

REFERENCES

1. COPE, OLIVER, *Man, Mind and Medicine*. J. B. Lippincott, Philadelphia, 1968.
2. MARINER, A. S., A Critical Look at Professional Education in the Mental Health Field. *American Psychologist*, Vol. 22, p. 271-281, 1967.
3. ENGEL, GEORGE L., Sudden Death and the "Medical Model" in Psychiatry. *Canadian Psychiatric Association Journal*, Vol. 15, pp. 527-538, 1970.
4. ENGEL, GEORGE L., Will the Crisis in Health Care Be Solved by Precipitating a Crisis in Medical Education? Address to Governors' Conference, American College of Physicians, Philadelphia, October 23, 1971.
5. ROMANO, JOHN, The Elimination of the Internship—An Act of Regression. *American Journal of Psychiatry*, Vol. 126, p. 1565-1576, 1970.
6. The Carnegie Commission on Higher Education: Higher Education and the Nation's Health, Policies for Medical and Dental Education. McGraw-Hill, New York, 1970.
7. BRENNER, CHARLES, *An Elementary Textbook of Psychoanalysis*. Doubleday Anchor Books, Garden City, New York, 1955.
8. ARLOW, JACOB A., and BRENNER, CHARLES, *Psychoanalytic Concepts and the Structural Theory*. International Universities Press, Inc., New York, 1964.
9. WAELDER, ROBERT, *Basic Theory of Psychoanalysis*. Doubleday Anchor Books, Garden City, New York, 1955.
10. FREUD, SIGMUND, Interpretation of Dreams. *Standard Edition*, Vol. IV. Hogarth Press, London, 1953.
11. FREUD, SIGMUND, Dynamics of Transference. *Standard Edition*, Vol. XIII, p. 97-108. Hogarth Press, London, 1958.
12. KUBIE, L. S., The Retreat from Patients. *Archives of General Psychiatry*, Vol. 24, p. 98-106, 1971.
13. HALLECK, SEYMOUR, *The Politics of Therapy*. Science House, Inc., New York, 1971.
14. WORBY, CYRIL M., The First-Year Psychiatric Resident and the Professional Identity Crisis. *Mental Hygiene*, Vol. 54, p. 374-377, 1970.
15. VOLKAN, V. D., and HAWKINS, D. R., The Fieldwork Method of Teaching and Learning Clinical Psychiatry. *Comprehensive Psychiatry*, Vol. 12, p. 102-115, 1971.
16. MILLER, ARTHUR A., BURSTEIN, ALVIN G., and LEIDER, R. J., Teaching and Evaluation of Diagnostic Skills. *Archives of General Psychiatry*, Vol. 24, p. 255-259, 1971.
17. MILLER, ARTHUR A., and BURSTEIN, ALVIN G., Professional Development in Psychiatric Residents. *Archives of General Psychiatry*, Vol. 20, p. 385-394, 1969.
18. ORNSTEIN, PAUL H., and KALTHOFF, ROBERT J., Toward a Conceptual Scheme for Teaching Clinical Psychiatric Evaluation. *Comprehensive Psychiatry*, Vol. 8, p. 404-426, 1967.

19. TARACHOW, SIDNEY, *An Introduction to Psychotherapy*. International Universities Press, Inc., New York, 1963.
20. TARACHOW, SIDNEY, Interpretation and Reality in Psychotherapy. *International Journal of Psychoanalysis*, Vol. 43, p. 377-387, 1962.
21. MORGAN, DAVID W., A Note on Analytic Group Psychotherapy for Therapists and Their Wives. *International Journal of Group Psychotherapy*, Vol. 21, p. 244-254, 1971.
22. HENDRICK, IVES, *Psychiatry Education Today*. International Universities Press, Inc., New York, 1965.

4

The Supervisory Program

Teaching, Freud tells us, is one of the impossible professions. The supervision of psychiatric residents—a form of teaching—is, equally, an "impossible" pursuit. Few supervisory programs continue for any extended period of time. The reason: rarely are either supervisors or residents satisfied with the design of the program, rarely can they resist, at yearly or bi-yearly intervals, tinkering with the design of the curriculum, attempting yet another solution of what are essentially insoluble problems. There is never enough time, there are never enough teachers, there are always clinical errors which inevitably escape the vigilance of the most dedicated supervisor. Nor shall we ever solve entirely the problems of accurate reporting of data, the problem of those patients in a total caseload who are never brought up or talked about, the problem of our inability as teachers to be there with advice—on the spot—when the resident most needs us. The supervisory program at Rochester has undergone repeated, sometimes drastic change. We shall describe some of them and the reasons for them when we describe our current program. Even so, the one constant factor in our training program, the one most highly and consistently valued feature of our curriculum, praised by group after group of residents over 25 years, has been the regular one-to-one relationship with a supervisor established and

A portion of this chapter has appeared in *Archives of General Psychiatry*, Vol. 23, Dec. 1970, pp. 516-523.

contracted for the broad purpose of discussing the resident's problems in learning the practice of clinical psychiatry, the evaluation and psychotherapeutic management of in- and out-patients.

Currently, our first-year residents spend their entire first year on the in-patient services. The second year is spent on the ambulatory services, including the out-patient division, emergency services, child psychiatry, community psychiatry and the courts. The third year is a year of major supervisory and administrative responsibilities for the resident, on both in-patient and ambulatory services, and of elective opportunities in various other areas of the department's activities.

First Year

Four in-patient floors, comprising 107 beds, constitute the department's in-patient services. Each floor is headed by a faculty member designated as its clinical director and a third-year house officer—the chief resident. Each floor is somewhat differently organized according to the clinical director's views on how an in-patient division should function. Each first-year resident serves for 6 months on each of two in-patient floors during which time he admits and is responsible for, in rotation with his colleagues, the care of all "division" (i.e., non-private) patients entering the hospital. Private patients—less than 50%—are cared for by the resident and the attending psychiatrist jointly. When division patients are discharged they remain the resident's patients and he remains responsible for their ambulatory care. He is *their* doctor. Private patients return, on discharge, to their private physician.

Supervision of the first-year resident consists of several different interactions. Each clinical director meets with each of the first-year residents on his division for at least one hour each week. The chief resident also spends an hour each week, in supervision, with each of his residents. When this program was first established some years ago the intention was to provide for a division of labor, with the chief resident focusing primarily on the day-to-day problems of the care of the first-year resident's in-patients while the clinical director attended to the resident's ambulatory caseload—consisting of *former* in-patients known quite intimately to both the clinical director and the resident from their stay in the hospital. In practice these separate supervisory roles were never quite so sharply divided between in-patients and ambulatory patients. Whenever a resident happens upon a particularly "difficult" patient admitted to his care, much of the supervisory time with both chief resident and clinical director is increasingly preempted by the vicissitudes of the care of that patient. One of the glaring shortcomings of any supervisory program becomes evident at such a time. Whenever a particularly complex problem arises, little supervisory time remains for other therapeutic work, and the resident goes it on his own for the most part, with all his other cases, until things begin to settle down with the problem case. It is another instance of the squeaking wheel getting the grease—sometimes all of it—with the other wheels running alongside as best they can. Generally, other time commitments on the part of both resident and faculty are too pressing to permit any significant expansion of supervisory time in these situations. It is our impression that at times, however, we get overly concerned about these kinds of imperfections in our teaching scheme. Supervisory narcissism is a fairly ubiquitous trait among clinical teachers. "Nobody can possibly do it as well as I," and "Were it not for my steady, consistent hand on the tiller, the resident's therapeutic ship would flounder on the twin rocks of inexperience and counter-transference." We tend to forget that, fortunately, we are dealing with two kinds of fairly resistant and tough "effective human organisms":

1. Patients—No matter how sick they are, they can withstand astonishing amounts of non- and mishandling, and can often find tiny grains of therapeutic benefit in the most enormous mountain of well-meaning verbal chaff.
2. Our residents who, for the most part, are well-trained physicians with the conservative, therapeutically oriented inter-personal reflexes appropriate to such training and to such a role. Most have absorbed, by the time they come to us, at least the one, all-important maxim "Primum, non nocere"— Above all, do no harm. The beginning supervisor soon learns that most of the resident's work, the overwhelmingly largest part of it, as a matter of fact, takes place outside of his ken. It makes the need all the more urgent to make the supervisory experience count. It has to count in terms of the broadest, most general applicability possible, of its content.

While attending in an ad hoc fashion to specific urgent problems in the treatment and management of particular patients, the supervisor can never hope to survey, oversee and keep in touch with all of a resident's clinical work. Using that part of the resident's case-load which the resident is willing to share with him—and those aspects of it which the resident is willing and able to share with him—the supervisor can convey general principles of therapy and management, of treatment modalities, of basic concepts of choice. He can provide a model, a living example of a possible style of patient-physician interaction.

Because of their intimate knowledge of the total patient populations on each of their separate floors, the clinical directors turned out to be ideal supervisors for beginning residents. This ideal state is disrupted when, after six months, the residents all move to one of the other three in-patient services. We have felt that this change is necessary to broaden the resident's experience. It produces problems for the supervisors, however, since the resident's ambulatory case-load is now not known to the clinical director who takes over the resident's supervision. For some time we felt that this unfamiliarity was in large part to blame for the fact that residents generally tended to be less satisfied with the second six months of their supervisory experience than they were with the first. Other factors seem to be equally or more important, as we learned gradually and sometimes painfully. Two of these are especially noteworthy since supervisors often overlook them: supervisors generally remain fixed in their own assignments for considerable periods of time, usually measured in years. The resident's rhythm of change and growth is geared to periods of six months duration. The resident perceives his first six months as a period of initiation, of learning the basic ground rules of clinical psychiatry. He looks upon the end of these six months as marking a transition from being a novice to being an experienced and full-fledged, if junior, member of the therapeutic team. The formal signpost of the end of this first developmental phase is the change from one floor to another. For the resident it is a "graduation" which he expects to be followed by some change in his status, by some perceptible recognition of his having ceased to be a raw beginner. Frequently, neither the supervisor nor the rest of the floor staff takes into account this change, this need for greater autonomy, greater responsibility—hence also the need for a change in supervisory style. The remobilization in both resident and supervisor of developmental problems of their own is fairly predictable. For the resident, problems of adolescence, the need to be optimally independent, rebelliousness, etc., once again demand adaptive solutions. For the supervisor there arise over and over again the parental problems of letting go, relinquishing control and recognizing appropriately the growing competence and therapeutic potency of the younger person.

The second problem which both supervisor and resident must confront is equally predictable, equally ubiquitous, equally and sometimes even more potentially disruptive of the supervisory relationship. The resident's relationship to his *first* faculty supervisor has a quality, an affective tone which is reminiscent of a first infatuation, is as intense, at times, and as profound in its formative effects as the imprinting phenomena described by the ethologists.

Regardless of any disclaimers the supervisor might make regarding his infallibility or the gospel truth nature of his conceptual frame of reference, for the beginning resident, His word, His person, His concepts, often take on the quality of revelations—unshakable, unchallengeable and eternal. The second supervisor, inevitably a different person—that alone is a cardinal sin in the eyes of the resident—with a different style, with an at least, somewhat different concept of what constitutes optimal patient care, with different emphasis in his teaching—this second supervisor meets then the rage, the contempt of the believer asked to convert to a rival faith. This is compounded by the anxiety generated when a scheme of action, a security-generating conceptual framework, barely assimilated by the resident, is called into question, even minimally, by the application of a somewhat different point of view. We have stated the problem in extreme terms. It exists—often in more subtle form, often almost as blatantly as described. It demands of the supervisor great tact, pedagogic skill and much patience. It is a tribute to the overall maturity of our resident staff and to the pedagogic talents of our supervisors that, for the most part, the resolution of this problem is successfully accomplished. Such resolution lays the groundwork for the development of a healthy skepticism and contributes greatly to the resident's sophistication, adds to his therapeutic armamentarium and prepares him for a broader, more pragmatic theoretical stance.

Tutorial Program (Psychotherapy Supervision) for First-Year Residents

Our first-year residents spend all of their first year of training on the in-patient floors. They are responsible for the aftercare, following discharge, to the out-patient clinic, of in-patients assigned to them. Prior to the extensive use of medication, especially the phenothiazines, many in-patients could be and were treated psychotherapeutically both in the hospital and after discharge in the Out Patient Department. This kind of care for in-patients has diminished considerably over the past 10-15 years. It has been our impression also that, perhaps due to the effectiveness of the antipsychotic drugs, in-patients, as a group, have been a good deal "sicker" than they used to be, hence less suitable for, or amenable to psychotherapeutic intervention. Other changes in in-patient care, such as increased emphasis on group therapeutic techniques, team approaches, and milieu treatment—all these have further reduced the amount of meaningful, dynamically oriented one-to-one psychotherapeutic experience of the resident on the in-patient services. As this has become more apparent we felt it necessary to create a new kind of supervised psychotherapeutic situation for the first-year resident. The best time to start this was felt to be after his first six months of in-patient experience when his initial exposure to psychiatric work has had a chance to sink in. It is at this time, too, that first-year residents generally feel the need for new and challenging kinds of work. During October, November and December a number of patients are selected through the out-patient intake procedure, suitable for insight-oriented kinds of psychotherapy. Each first-year resident is assigned such a patient with whom he is to start working during the first week in January. Each resident is also assigned to a supervisor whose task will be to tutor him in his evaluation and psychotherapeutic work with that patient for the next 12 months' period (January to January). In conjunction with the psychotherapy-tutorial, we have recently started a didactic exercise for the first-year group beginning with the academic year and continuing throughout the whole first year of training. The exercise is conducted as a seminar and is entitled: Interpersonal Therapeutics: Psychological Intervention in Psychiatric Treatment. The seminar is intended as preparation for the psychotherapy experience and continues conjointly with it, offering readings and dis-

cussion in basic problems and concepts of psychotherapeutic management. The focus is practical and clinical, rather than theoretic, with
liberal use of audiotaped material, to illustrate the problems under
discussion.

It has been our impression that, even so, this amount of experience
in supervised psychotherapy is inadequate, that incoming residents
should start some out-patient psychotherapeutic work at the very
beginning of their residency, that an insight-oriented case should be
started somewhat later during their first year, with at least one other
case to begin before the *end* of their first year. Additional supervisory
time would be required for such a program.

Supervision in the Resident's Adult Out-Patient Work in His Second Year

On entering the second year, half of our residents are assigned six
months in out-patient work with adults and children and half of
them to work in the Psychiatric Emergency Division. Here we will
concentrate on the adult out-patient experience, as the authors have
devoted a number of years in this area of the Department's activity.
We should mention that the six months of out-patient work is divided
between the adult clinic and the child and adolescent division. Our
comments will be restricted to the former experience, but it should be
noted that the clinical work with children and adolescents is carefully and individually supervised, stressing in-depth diagnostic evaluation of a limited number of patients. The six-month tour in the
emergency division, we will not attempt to describe either. The
program has been described by Atkins (1) and provides the second-
year resident with an intensive experience dealing with an acute ambulatory population. In addition to the supervisory experience in the
adult out-patient area we are about to describe, it should be mentioned that there is a seminar in psychotherapeutic work during the
entire second year. This deals conceptually with a number of issues,
and is essentially a literature review. Inasmuch as it does not, strictly
speaking, deal with clinical supervision, we will not describe it in
detail.

The setting for our supervisory work with second-year residents
and their adult ambulatory patients is the Adult Psychiatric Out-
patient Clinic of this medical center. This clinic was established for

those in the community and surrounding counties who cannot afford private professional care. It is a division of the Department of Psychiatry and affords diagnostic evaluation and therapeutic service of many types. The Clinic receives referrals from a variety of sources including about 25% who are self-referred. About 2,000 patients are served a year for a total of 15,000 visits.

Over the years we have evolved various procedures for evaluating the patients referred to us in an attempt to be more flexible and responsive and offer professional help as quickly as possible. At the present time we employ a triage method of a brief "screening" interview of every new patient by one of our senior faculty. This interview determines the subsequent destiny of the patient, be it referral to a community agency, another clinic, private doctor, or to our own clinic. Those appropriate for our care are then assigned within a week or two of the "screening interview" to a second-year resident and his supervisor. These two together make all subsequent decisions concerning the patient's evaluation and treatment. The resident assumes continuing responsibility for all such patients assigned to him for as long as he remains with us in graduate training.

Several years ago we felt a need for a different approach to the supervision of residents in the OPD (2). We were dissatisfied with the methods up to that point, which involved second-hand reporting of what transpired in the interview, reconstructed through memory and notes, or observing the interview through a one-way screen; it was an improvement on the first method, but a method which lent an air of unreality to the situation. There is also a soporific effect on the observer sitting in a dark, poorly ventilated room helplessly observing a resident struggle with a difficult patient.

We sensed the difficulty in introducing direct observation into the highly private atmosphere of a psychiatric interview. The surgeon is able to demonstrate an operative procedure to a group of residents and actually share the techniques with one or two of them. In psychiatric interviewing, however, it is difficult for a patient to reveal unguarded thoughts and feelings to relative strangers. We also realized that the private nature of the relationship between patient and doctor worked against our educational and supervisory efforts. We felt that there must be some more immediate assistance for a resident dealing with some of the difficult patients encountered in our out-patient clinic, especially with the 10% to 20% who represent urgent situations. In the previous supervisory relationship, we were always dealing with matters after the fact, the resident may have overlooked some area of inquiry, committed himself and the patient to some inappropriate course of action, or made ill-advised, at times irreversible, decisions. We could then only say, you should have done or said this or that.

At times it was very difficult to assess the clinical situation from the material presented, especially not having seen the patient. This was a consequence of inadequate data, on occasion distortion and confusion of the material through countertransference forces, or an inadequate presentation due to inexperience. When we were puzzled or unsure about some of these urgent or espcially troublesome problems, we would see the patient and find, often to our surprise, that we had an entirely different impression of the patient than we had gained from the presentation.

Occasionally untoward things happened before we had a chance to discuss the patient with the resident. Sometimes the patient would not return and was lost before an appropriate intervention could be made. This may have resulted from an unwitting rejection, a feeling on the part of the patient that he was unwanted or regarded as hopeless; other patients may have required hospitalization or were serious suicidal risks. Some left in anger and acted out their transference feelings in an impulsive self-destructive way between the initial and subsequent interviews.

Importance of the Initial Interview

The initial interview with a physician is such a momentous event, especially the first visit to a psychiatrist with all of its anxious expectation and fear of revelation, that it is often a finely balanced matter as to whether or not the patient will be willing to continue. He must be helped as tactfully and expertly as possible to move in a direction we judge helpful.

It is inner discomfort or serious hindrance of one's life that leads one to seek a means of alleviation through venting feelings and thoughts, correcting self-perceptions through another's view of him, or facing oneself with the borrowed strength of another. In addition to the distress which brings the patient to the psychiatrist, he may be besieged by other feelings: shame for asking for help and consequent diminished self-esteem, feelings of envy and rivalry, guilt and fear of losing control of his impulses (most often expressed as fear of "going crazy"). He also must cope with the social stigma and scorn still associated with the idea of consulting a psychiatrist.

The psychiatrist, in his initial contact with the patient, brings his basic knowledge of human behavior, his clinical experience with disordered behavior, his own life experience and values, his basic feeling about people, his own unresolved neurotic conflicts and his compassion, empathy and tolerance of human weakness and foibles. He must be patient, not have unrealistic expectations, be willing to help without forcing his values and judgments on the patient, and afford an unhurried and objective atmosphere. At other times he must be a man of action, particularly in those situations requiring urgent intervention.

The basic task of the initial interview is to gather enough information to form a clinical judgment of the nature and degree of the psychopathology, assess the patient's capacity to engage in a human relationship, determine his "psychological mindedness," and begin to determine what, if any, therapeutic intervention is indicated.

The patient brings to this encounter, in addition to his complaints and distress, his accumulated accomplishments and disappointments, his present situation in life, his aspirations for the future, his family situation (including neurotic problems in other members of his household), his occupation, responsibilities, and position in the community. His basic intelligence, awareness of himself, readiness to discuss himself candidly and face certain issues at this moment, his ability to articulate, and his capacity to observe the disordered aspects of his behavior are all important considerations.

Throughout the initial interview the psychiatrist should be mindful of all these factors in himself and the patient as he asks questions and listens to the patient's story. He must be willing to advance or retreat at a moment's notice depending on what he touches upon, the patient's response, his own reaction to a problem, and his assessment of what can be done. At times he has to curb his zeal and accept the fact that certain damaged personalities cannot be remade.

The psychiatrist must be prepared to deal with various manipulative efforts of the patient, who, in his competitive struggle over yielding to the therapist, may present technical problems that must be dealt with at the outset. An example that floors the novice is the patient who says, "Now, I've told you everything, doctor, you tell me what to do." The response to such a challenge is a critical matter which may significantly influence the outcome of the initial interview and the ensuing course of the patient.

In our clinic setting we deal with a great variety of problems, some of them urgent and some inappropriate. Many are not suitable for psychotherapy. The resident and his supervisor must be alert to what brings the patient: at times for a "letter to my draft board," a reluctant marital partner referred by his clergyman, someone sent by an agency who may have concern about the patient's suicidal potential, or a referral by a lawyer of his client. Many of the more obvious problems that are inappropriate for clinic care, including patients who need hospitalization or can better be cared for by family doctors or community agencies, are detected at the time of the patient's "screening" interview.

SUPERVISORY TECHNIQUE

We, therefore, decided on a simple, direct approach to the matter: we decided to have the supervisor sit with each new patient and the resident, as a third party, relatively inactive and inconspicuous, but present. Each supervisor has his own approach and style, but generally remains out of the mainstream of the interchange (unless an intervention is necessary) until the resident has finished his interview. He may then himself ask the patient a few questions, clarify some issues for the patient, or make an interpretive comment designed to test the patient's defensive structure, his psychological mindedness, or motivation.

We found "sitting in" with the residents challenging, interesting, and at times frustrating. It required a varying period of time for the resident to become more or less comfortable, having his supervisor observe the interview with the patients. Perhaps this was enhanced by the resident's expressed desire for more individual supervision. In very few instances did our presence seem to interfere significantly with either the resident or the patient. We often explained that the supervisor was present to get a first-hand view of the patient and that he would work with the resident in devising a therapeutic plan. Over the past five or six years that we have used this teaching device, we have encountered a number of difficulties. It was frustrating for a supervisor to sit quietly and observe the resident's struggle with the patient, who was in desperate need of reassurance, while the resident was stiff and ungiving. We found that the beginning resident often has a tendency to present himself as somewhat stern, unfeeling, and excessively withdrawn. We were never quite sure where this model came from, but tentatively concluded that it is a misunderstood and misapplied concept of the psychoanalytic model. While there were inherent disadvantages in the supervisor making interventions with both the resident and the patient present, in our judgment these were less hazardous than making no interventions at various crucial junctures. While we decided that the primary purposes of the supervised session were for the education of the resident, at the same time we feel that our interventions have been helpful to the patient.

The residents tended to resent our interventions, particularly initially, because they felt that the treatment of their patients was being undermined. This manifested itself in various indirect ways such as the resident who refused to sit in the supervisor's chair, or the one who complained that it was very anxiety-provoking to hear the voice of the supervisor coming over his shoulder questioning the patient. At times the resident failed to introduce the patient to the supervisor or dismissed the patient before the supervisor had a chance to ask any questions. In the following vignettes we attempt to illustrate some common problems encountered in our supervision.

DETECTION OF LATENT PSYCHOTIC TRENDS

The more sophisticated interventions of the supervisor on occasion proved burdensome to the resident because they exposed his lack of experience and ability. But, on the other hand, the more experienced supervisor might make an interpretation which brought clarity to the patient, for he was able to touch upon an emotionally charged area that the resident was fearful of entering. An example of this is a young man who came complaining, "I am dreaming at night and talking in my sleep for about five years." He added that he was nervous and not sleeping. He was a difficult person to interview, in that he was rather evasive and circumstantial, making several allusions to dreams. The resident did not pursue this topic, however. At the end of the interview, sensing that this was a critical area, the supervisor asked him what was so frightening about these dreams. He

responded that they were about "murder and sex" about "being mur-
dered, and murdering, and sex with women." The supervisor replied
by asking if sex was a problem. This led the patient to talk about
being interested in weight lifting when in his late teens and putting
a 5 lb. weight on his penis when he had an erection during masturba-
tion. This led to "straining a muscle in my crotch" and his feeling
that his penis never had been as big since then. He talked further
about the dreams, and a distinct persecutory quality emerged. It became apparent to the resident through the supervisor's line of inquiry that this man had certain psychotic qualities and serious
sexual problems, probably of a perverse nature. As a consequence of
getting some of these issues out in the open, the patient was subsequently more relaxed with the resident and confided in another
interview that he had been an active homosexual for several years.
This intervention not only clarified the diagnosis but was of therapeutic assistance in diminishing the patient's anxiety.

HESITATION TO TOUCH ON SENSITIVE EMOTIONAL ISSUES

A young man in his mid-30's who had been left by his wife three
years before spoke of feeling inadequate, of his sex life being "all
screwed up," of his marriage not working out, of drinking after their
second child was born.

In describing his loneliness since his wife left, he mentioned "to
make matters worse, I ended up having an affair with a guy, a
friend of mine." He then went on to say he had been getting more
nervous, was sleeping poorly, and having difficulty in maintaining
an erection. Further questioning revealed symptoms suggestive of a
serious depresssion. Because the resident seemed hesitant to pursue
the homosexual matter, the supervisor asked at the end of the interview for more details. The patient explained that this had occurred
several times with this one man only, that it happened in the setting
of loneliness and desperation while he and his friend, who was
married, were drinking. It consisted of the patient masturbating his
friend in the car. He then talked more about his sex life with his
wife, which had been hampered by episodes of impotence. In a discussion following the interview, the resident recognized his hesitancy
in asking the patient about homosexuality. To his surprise he noted
the patient was more relaxed at the end of the interview, having

unburdened himself with the supervisor. He learned from this experience how to make it possible for a patient to talk about a painful matter. This patient, followed subsequently by the resident, showed considerable symptomatic improvement over the next several weeks.

PANICKY PATIENT

We tried to restrict our interventions during the interview to those situations which appeared relatively urgent and where the resident momentarily was unable to handle the situation adequately. These included an inappropriate, or lack of, response to a desperate patient. For example, a 35-year-old woman with the acute onset of obsessive thoughts became panicky, fearing that she was "going crazy." She became increasingly terrified when the resident insisted on dragging her through a mental status examination, including proverbs, serial subtractions, inquiring whether she heard voices, etc. Sometimes the supervisor (as in this example) would interrupt the interview and discuss in private with the resident the difficulty he was having with the patient, indicate how to correct it, and resume the interview with the patient.

A wide range of patients is evaluated and treated in the Psychiatric Out-Patient Clinic, including a number of complicated social problems, marital conflicts and maladjustment reactions. Our experience emphasizes the necessity for our residents to sharpen their diagnostic and clinical skills, to understand the nature of psychiatric referrals, and to learn to focus on what brings a particular patient and his family to seek psychiatric assistance.

BEING ALERT TO MEDICAL COMPLICATIONS

At times it is important for the interviewing psychiatrist to be alert to medical signs and symptoms. A 19-year old young woman presented herself for diagnostic evaluation, complaining of depression and listlessness, associated with moderate disorganization and withdrawal. She had been unable to work for the previous two months and was living with her mother in the basement of an uncle's home. Her condition worsened, so that she was staying at home throughout the day, watching television, withdrawn from interpersonal contacts, and feeling hopeless. During the course of her presentation, we became aware of her loneliness, her apathy, in spite of which she had continued to make a number of efforts to gain relief of her symptoms. The patient had not been evaluated by the usual screening procedure, but had been seen by a psychiatrist and social caseworker in evaluation for a group therapeutic approach. No medical history had been obtained at that time. She felt "too desperate" for group therapy, and she was unable to remain throughout the group session, Eventually, the patient was referred to the Adult Psychiatric Out-Patient Clinic and was seen by a second-year resident and a senior supervising psychiatrist. As the initial interview proceeded, the patient, who appeared listless and depressed, mentioned in an offhand manner that she had a skin rash. The supervisor was alerted by this development and made an on-the-spot examination of the patient's skin, only to find the presence of petechial hemorrhages on both arms and legs. Further inquiry revealed bleeding tendencies, including epistaxis, menorrhagia, and gingival bleeding. Immediate medical consultation was arranged. Laboratory studies revealed a blood platelet count of 4,000. Hospitalization was arranged on the Medical Service, and a diagnosis of thrombocytopenia was made. Steroid treatment proved unsuccessful and the patient came to a splenectomy. The psychiatric symptoms abated somewhat in the hospital but later returned, and the patient subsequently required a psychiatric hospitalization.

DIFFICULT PATIENTS

There are patients who demonstrate special problems in being interviewed, and require rather bold and direct intervention. An 18-year-old girl came with a vague story, kept on her sunglasses, had her hair hanging over one eye, and kept her head turned so one could not see the other eye. She gave irrelevant answers, seemed sullen, and soon fell silent in the face of the resident's struggle to get her to talk. At this point the supervisor broke in and told the patient that we could be of no help if she did not cooperate. He asked her to turn around, look at the resident, remove her glasses, and attempt to answer his questions. She responded, became more attentive and relevant. It became apparent that she was psychotic, but with each subsequent interview with the resident she became more trustful and productive.

A man in his 20's brought in a thick sheaf of papers saying, "I thought this would give you more insight than talking to me . . . it's hard to talk about it—it's all in there—why I wrote it." He proceeded to give a meandering account of himself without much feeling, looking to the resident to take the lead. At the end the supervisor told the patient he would have to talk, that we could not do this by correspondence, and pointed to the central problem with his wife which he had touched on and which would probably be profitable to pursue. The necessity for intervention here was the need to move the patient from the defensive position of resistance in which he was thwarting a profitable line of inquiry and help him focus on what we regarded as relevant issues.

The more general situation was for the supervisor to observe the interview in its entirety and at its conclusion make certain interventions or ask questions if he so wished. For example, the supervisor might focus on an important piece of history left unclarified, or he might demonstrate interviewing technique, or he might attempt an interpretation of the patient's conflicts. It is interesting that the resident rarely makes an interpretation to his patient. He experiences a further difficulty when the supervisor attempts to make some suggestions about the care of the patient following the interview. This is no different from any other tutorial, except that our focus at this time is on the more immediate strategy for the next session, rather than on long-range goals. Generally, the second-year resident at this stage of his development is inexperienced in psychotherapeutic techniques and strategy. He needs suggestions and assistance, even though he may resent it. Although the suggestions were not always acted on effectively, they seemed to stimulate the resident towards thinking about his patients in a new way. While the residents may manifest objection to this supervisory technique initially, they have consistently commended us at the conclusion of their six months experience. With this supervisory technique the senior clinician was in a position to observe firsthand the interaction between resident and patient. Sometimes we observed a situation where the behavior or reactions of the resident seriously interfered with his learning process and the care of the patient. In certain instances the supervisor would comment on his observations of the countertransference difficulties of the resident. Our experience with this type of intervention is limited but so far appears promising. On occasion such a comment has cleared the air. For example, a supervisor might have told the resident that he was unfeeling and unsympathetic to his patient, and that his interview was a poor one, and at times he seemed angry at the patient. To receptive residents this might lead to a fruitful discussion of the countertransference. In fact, it was in those situations where a resident was able to see how his reactions affected his conduct and interventions with a given patient that some of the best learning experiences took place.

We found that with the method of supervision we have described, we could quickly assess the resident's level of understanding and provide immediate suggestions in handling the difficult clinical problems that come to our out-patient department. We were able to demonstrate effective clinical interventions and to focus upon the challenges in out-patient psychotherapy firsthand. It is our impression that it is with his out-patients that the resident begins to grasp the fundamental principles of dynamic psychiatry and to observe the clinical data from which these principles are drawn.

In an earlier chapter we have reviewed the literature on supervision. At this point we wish only to comment that very little has been said about the type of supervisory emphasis on the initial interview which we have described here. A number of authors comment on the difficulties of grasping concepts of psychotherapy in the period allotted to formal training. Arieti (3) feels there is not time in three years of residency training to learn enough of psychotherapy, and proposes further training beyond this period. Tischler (4) speaks of the difficulties of the first year of "professional transition." Rice and Thurrell (5) describe a seminar in psychological evaluation which they devised "to help bridge the gap between theoretical concepts and clinical observations." Adamson et al. (6) speak of the need for more than one supervisor during a residency, because learning interviewing skills and psychodynamic understanding of patients are essential. Escoll and Wood (7) mention, in the course of discussing their supervisory program, that on occasion they arrange a joint interview of the patient with the resident when there is some doubt about how to proceed with a given problem.

Recently I. Ziferstein (8), a psychoanalyst, reported on effects of observing psychotherapy through a one-way screen as compared with sitting in the room with the patient and psychiatrist. He was surprised to find that less distortion occurred with the latter procedure.

He said "Fewer obstacles and complications are encountered by patient, therapist, and observer if the presence of the observer is frankly acknowledged by sitting in the treatment room with patient and therapist, than when the observer is excluded behind a one-way vision screen."

Although we are not commenting on psychotherapy, we share Ziferstein's opinion. We have spoken earlier of some of our experiences with the residents. We should add that we have had relatively little difficulty with the patients. Rarely would the patient comment on the situation, and only in a very few instances would he be unable to tolerate it. Usually, the interview proceeded untroubled, and after the initial impact the patient appeared unaware of the supervisor. If he looked too much at the supervisor at the beginning, the latter had only to look away or in some other nonverbal way withdraw from active engagement with the patient. This is not to say that the presence of an observer had no effect on the patient, and this should be studied further; but it was not distracting to the point where it outweighed the pedagogic advantages to the resident and his supervisor.

We have become concerned in recent years with the decreasing emphasis on attention to clinical detail and diagnosis. We feel that only through rigorous training in this area can a resident truly understand his patient. It requires, for example, the sort of painstaking approach in the initial interview which we have attempted to document in this chapter. The resident must have the time, encouragement, and precept to study individual patients in some depth. A grasp of the clinical facts is requisite to dynamic understanding. Too often the resident is encumbered with theoretical notions, many of them inaccurate or misapplied, before he has an opportunity to make his own observations. We must be careful always to draw his attention to primary observations and to challenge such "ready-made" concepts until he has sufficient clinical experience to either refute or substantiate them himself. We feel that the ability to make good clinical observations and proper evaluation of patients cannot be learned easily, nor quickly. It is a capacity that takes some years of experience to develop. What we hope to accomplish in their six months' experience is a beginning appreciation of some of the principles involved and some awareness of their importance in the subsequent handling of an ambulatory patient. We also believe that this kind of preparation is an essential prerequisite to the understanding and practice of psychotherapy. A committee within our department devoted to studying the teaching of psychotherapy to our residents said "There must be increased emphasis upon clinical observations and how these observations lead to therapeutic interventions." They added that their findings indicated "a gap between whatever knowledge and principles the residents have, and their ability to apply this knowledge in psychotherapeutic work with patients."

There are factors on the current scene which we feel distract the resident from the careful evaluation of individual problems we regard as essential to his education. There is today a growing emphasis on group work and a parallel decline of interest in individual psychotherapy. A powerful force is community pressure on psychiatry for "delivery of service" to wider segments of the population not now served or served inadequately. We have noted a concomitant tendency to denigrate "one-to-one psychotherapy." As a consequence, the resident's attention at times is drawn to groups before he understands individuals. We feel it is basically unsound to attempt the understanding and treatment of groups before individuals. Unfortunately psychiatry is not immune to fads, and consequently that which has current favor, prestige, and power has great influence on the direction of psychiatric thought and education.

Our experience over the years leads us to believe in the importance of a substantial clinical exposure, first in the study and care of in-patients, many of whom have complicated combinations of physical and emotional components, and who can be observed intensively over a period of time under good supervision; and second, in the kind of supervised evaluation of ambulatory patients we have attempted to describe. It is the careful investigation of a number of individual patients which is an essential element in beginning development of clinical acumen and judgment. It involves mastering such essentials as how to take an adequate history, the development of interviewing techniques and skill in behavioral observation. It includes experience with a wide variety of psychopathological states and the development of appreciation for allied physical and medical factors. All this must be assimilated before the resident has a firm perspective of the "psychiatric patient," and before he is ready to apply his knowledge to wider objectives—groups, the community, and social issues. We are concerned that the young psychiatrist achieve this balance so that he is able to continue his clinical maturation as he progresses from training to practice.

The supervisory exercise as described above in detail has been one of our most successful teaching endeavors as indicated by the consistently positive response of the residents in their evaluation of the program. Almost universally they consider it to have been one of the highlights of their experience in the second year of residency. The exercise does have some shortcomings implicit in its organization and in the large amount of supervisory time required for it. Each resident sees two patients for diagnostic study each week for a period of six months—a total of approximately 50 patients whom he studies in considerable detail. For each of these he is supervised on a one-to-one basis during the first interview with the patient. Subsequent contacts with each of these patients—for whose care the resident is responsible—are not then supervised with anything like equal intensity. Often, indeed, supervision of the resident's work with these patients, after his initial interview, is catch-as-catch-can squeezed into the occasional times when a regularly scheduled patient fails to keep the first diagnostic study appointment.

Another problem arising from this system is that of the resident's caseload. This accumulates over the six-months of his out-patient assignment, as his diagnostic studies keep coming at a rate of two per week. Therapeutic decisions are, therefore, liable to be influenced measurably by the total time commitment to follow-up visits and, hence, also by the particular time in the resident's six months stint when the patient is seen: Patients seen during the early part of this period are more likely to be deemed suitable for ongoing therapy than are those seen towards the end of the six months.

Third-Year Supervision

Formal supervision during the third year of training is limited, in our program, to a tutorial of one hour per week, and to a case conference. This is chaired by a senior analyst who gives each third-year resident an opportunity to present one of his psychotherapy cases over several consecutive weekly meetings. The faculty person who conducts this conference has found a sustained interest in clinical matters over the years. This past year, at the request of several of the third-year residents, he assigned certain readings on transference and counter-transference. He was interested to observe that very few comments have been made or questions asked about this material, but the interest in their patients has remained their primary focus of interest.

In our experience third-year residents are much less intensely interested in supervisory experiences than during the first two years of training. Some, indeed, prefer an informal ad hoc kind of an arrangement with no formal or regularly scheduled appointments with a supervisor. These are usually residents who have managed to carry a minimum of psychotherapy and may not have any cases in intensive treatment during their third year. Another group, intensely interested in dynamically oriented psychotherapeutic work will receive supervision on a regular basis from one of our analytically trained faculty members.

The lack of interest in supervision on the part of the third-year resident has to do with his "coming of age," the consolidation of his identity as a psychiatrist. He feels more like a colleague in relationship to his faculty supervisor, and less like a student. This is a desirable end-point in one sense but touches on the matter with which we concluded the last chapter—what about continuing education? Such an attitude on the part of the third-year resident should not impede his interest in post-graduate ventures. As we stated earlier, such opportunities in our field are limited; and it remains for us to devise more challenging and effective means of contributing to the clinical development of the psychiatric clinician beyond his three years of formal training.

REFERENCES

1. ATKINS, R. W., Psychiatric Emergency Service. *Arch. Gen. Psych.*, 17:176-182, 1967.
2. SCHUSTER, D. B., and FREEMAN, E. N., Supervision of the Resident's Initial Interview, *Arch. Gen. Psych.*, 23:516-523, 1970.
3. ARIETI, S., Further Training in Psychotherapy. *Am. J. Psych.*, 125:96-7, 1968.
4. TISCHLER, G. L., The Beginning Resident and Supervision. *Arch. Gen. Psych.*, 19:418-22, 1968.
5. RICE, D. G., and THURRELL, R. J., Teaching Psychological Evaluation to Psychiatric Residents. *Arch. Gen. Psych.*, 19:737-42, 1968.
6. ADAMSON, J. D., PROSENA, H., and BEBCHUK, W., Training in Formal Psychotherapy in the Psychiatric Residency Program. *Canadian Psych. Assoc. J.*, 13:445-54, 1968.
7. ESCOLL, P. J., and WOOD, H. E., Perception in Residency Training: Methods and Problems. *Am. J. Psych.*, 124:187-92, 1967.
8. ZIFERSTEIN, I., Personal communication, Sept. 1969.

5

The Supervisory Conference

The authors have been active in supervising second-year residents in our out-patient clinic for a number of years. From this experience we have come to appreciate the importance of good clinical training and the problems of teaching in this area. We have participated in a variety of conferences devoted to teaching the resident something about outpatient work, yet we have spent little time discussing with each other our views of clinical supervision. There never seemed room in our crowded schedules to afford such discussion, in spite of our conviction that there was no more important subject for our consideration.

Not long ago we agreed to depart from our customary ways and devise a new type of conference. This was conceived as a "staff-development" exercise* in which faculty, without residents participating, would embark on a series of weekly meetings dedicated to examining the supervisory process. It was an interdisciplinary group (psychiatry, clinical psychology, psychiatric social work, and psychiatric nursing) and included not only people currently involved in the out-patient clinic but some who had had in-patient responsibilities. We began to meet in the early summer of 1970, and after a vacation break, continued in the fall and through May, 1971.

We began by agreeing it would be interesting and helpful to observe each other's interviewing style. This led to a discussion of interview-

---

* Largely as a result of a suggestion by a colleague, Dr. Rodney Shapiro.

ing technique, clinical evaluation, diagnosis, decision-making and the various clinical and theoretical assumptions which we held. This initial phase of the conference consolidated our original intention to focus on the supervisory process.

When the conference reconvened in September, 1970, we began by listening to a tape of a patient interview conducted by a resident. We decided to use a variety of such tape-recorded interviews and supervisory sessions as a focal point for our discussion, and we also decided to record these group discussions for future study. Toward the end of the conference in the Spring of 1971, the authors decided on using some of the material we had recorded for the substance of this chapter.

A problem arises in reading typescripts of recorded informal discussion—they suffer as does a foreign language in translation. We do not speak as we write: to convey meaning to each other in conversation, we rely heavily on non-verbal cues—bodily movements, facial expression, tone of voice, various expressions of emotion. Syntax and organization of thought suffer in unrehearsed speech. In an attempt to overcome this problem we have edited the material of the conference—not by rephrasing participants' comments—but by eliminating awkward grammar and distracting mannerisms of speech, omitting tangential or irrelevant comments, and finally by selecting only portions of the total dialogue. These selections have been made and topically arranged to illustrate various aspects and issues of the supervisory situation, which we have referred to earlier in our review of the literature and in developing our own views of supervision.

Because these were informal discussions, not prepared speeches, the conference dialogue tends at times to be discursive, even repetitious. For the same reason, the participants did not always stick to a theme and usually came to no tidy conclusions at the end of each session. We hope, nonetheless, that we have been successful in preserving something of the informal atmosphere of colleagues exchanging views and debating issues in a friendly but searching way. We are aware that this sort of unguarded conversation is rather revealing—as are candid snapshots. We do not sound profound, at times in fact we are banal; but we are paying careful attention to the clinical details we feel are important to emphasize in the education of a psychiatric clinician.

In previous chapters we have attempted to enunciate basic prin-

ciples and fundamental issues involved in the supervisor's task and
the resident's growth and maturation. It is our hope that the following vignettes with their clinical examples will serve to amplify and
exemplify these principles and fundamentals through the detailed
consideration of them by the conference participants.* Much of our
work with residents—as is the case in all clinical teaching—follows
the model of the apprentice-master process of learning. The interchanges between a resident and his supervisor are so infinitely complex as to virtually defy description and categorization. How can one
do justice, for example, to describing how an experienced clinician
conducts a masterful interview? How does one define in general or
abstract terms the process of clinical observation or the act of psychological intervention? Through these recorded interchanges between patient and resident, resident and his supervisor and among
conference members, however, we are able to illustrate some of these
important issues.

Finally, we want to add that we found this type of conference
stimulating and helpful—and perhaps long overdue. Up to this point
we had not had an adequate forum for supervisors in the adult OPD
area to discuss among themselves their work with second-year residents. We trust this account will give some sense of our philosophy
and working concepts and be of help to others engaged in the highly
important work of clinical supervision of psychiatric residents.

THE INITIAL ENCOUNTER WITH A NEW PATIENT

We have chosen this topic, which actually came up in our first
conference, to introduce our conference discussions, because we feel
strongly that the initial interview is a crucial issue. As we elaborated
in the preceding chapter, it is a critical moment in the life of the
patient who confronts a psychiatrist (and himself) for the first time.
It is a time of great stress for the neophyte psychiatrist also, demanding all the skill and resourcefulness he can muster. In the following
interchange a resident, who faced this problem early in his OPD
experience, was additionally burdened by learning something in ad-

---

* Participants, other than the authors, are indicated only by an initial in the
following text. Residents are likewise unidentified. We have already acknowledged
by name the members of this conference. By agreement of all concerned, only
the authors are taking responsibility for their remarks.

vance about his patient which further increased his anxiety. We will see how his concern about his patient, some of it thought to be irrational, distorted his relationship with the patient and consequently his capacity to gather certain critical data. We attempt to examine in some detail the interactions between patient and resident in order to illustrate some of the strategies employed by both patient and doctor. A major point stressed in the conference discussion is the necessity of gathering sufficient historical information from the patient in order to arrive at a clinical diagnostic impression so that we can arrange a rational therapeutic approach. We also comment on the nature of interviewing experience in the first year of psychiatric residency (on the in-patient service) and how this does not always prepare a resident for his subsequent out-patient experience.

The week before we began recording these conference sessions, we had begun to listen to a tape of one of our second-year residents (hereafter referred to as Dr. X) interviewing a young deputy sheriff from a neighboring county. It was apparent to us from the discussion between Dr. X and his supervisor, Dr. Thaler, prior to their seeing the patient (they had reviewed his medical record), that Dr. X was anxious about seeing his patient. He spoke of how an intervention with a man like this would affect many people, because of his position as a police offcer. He also revealed some of his bias about the patient's occupation and consequent view of the world. Dr. Thaler, in addition, expressed his concern about the patient's problem of passivity and possible development of paranoid trends, thus adding, perhaps, to Dr. X's concern.

The patient had always before been treated by medical men in our Emergency Department, but due to an increased frequency of visits to the "E.D.," he was referred by one medical house officer to the Adult Psychiatric Clinic. He had been "screened" by one of our senior faculty and referred for diagnostic study to Dr. X and his supervisor, Dr. Otto Thaler.

Just before seeing the patient, Dr. X said to his supervisor that he was "going to make it a short interview, because I'm uncomfortable just with what I know." When the patient came to the interview, Dr. X asked him what he saw as his problem. The patient replied that he didn't know, that doctors had conducted many tests on him which were "all okay." He went on to describe his back pain and "spasms" which he thought might possibly be a result of nervous tension. He said further that they were like "attacks" that often came on during the night. At this point he said to Dr. X that he didn't know anything about his job (being a psychiatrist) but added that these attacks seemed to come "in a time when I'd have my dream cycle." He stated that when these came on it scared him and made him fearful that "it might be something serious." He went on to discuss something of his work, implying a relationship between symptoms and tension arising from his job. He said that he had wanted to go into juvenile police work, "in the prevention area," but could not get this kind of assignment.

We did not get further in our discussion that day, but we resolved to tape our conference discussion from that point on, in order to capture the dialogue which focused on the supervisory process as exemplified by this resident's case.

Dr. Thaler: We began last time with a patient interview by a second-year resident. The patient, Mr. F, is a man in his early thirties, married and a recent father of his first child, a boy, who I think will feature fairly heavily in the problem that this man has.

D: I thought it was a relative's child and this patient adopted it.

Dr. Thaler: No, they had the baby. In addition they had adopted, took in, two foster children of a relative who died. He presented with all kinds of physical complaints associated with anxiety—at times, back pain, primarily with vague hypochondriacal ruminations about whether this could be a heart attack or could it be this or that. He had been seen in the Emergency Division several times.

C: Do these symptoms date from the birth of the child?

Dr. Thaler: This is what we found out eventually, but this hadn't come out at the beginning. One of the things that emerged in terms of the interview itself was that Dr. X (resident) did not very specifically pursue the onset of symptoms and the nature of them, and this came up in my supplementary interview of the patient—the relationship between the onset and the birth of this baby.

Dr. Schuster: Couldn't we make a speculation about this kind of symptom and its onset in this setting—that this man probably has a significant passive-feminine identification.

Dr. Thaler: Right, and I think we actually suspected it when we looked at the introductory note. Remember we were talking about that the first time. I made some comments about caution in terms of the interview. This man is a sheriff's deputy, and he felt that part of the onset of these symptoms was often connected with his being out on some kind of a stressful assignment. I think this is about where we stopped.

Dr. Schuster: One of the initial points of a couple of weeks ago I remember was that some were concerned that you, with your caution about this man's passivity, might have interfered with the resident's spontaneity or his own way of proceeding.

A: I don't know if this is a general feeling, but it came up last week that this patient, maybe as a defense against his passive trends, is quite controlling, and this seemed to anger Dr. X who in turn became very controlling. We have a contest between resident and patient. It also implies that Otto didn't stifle Dr. X's spontaneity, because he certainly doesn't lack spontaneity in the interview.

Dr. Thaler: A part of my initial, more extensive than usual, instructions had to do with my perception of his anxiety about the patient. He was anxious about this particular interview.

B: We also talked about facing new patients with the concept of the approach to the problem, and the approach to the patient's symptoms whether in a problem solving manner or whether in a taking-care kind of approach.

Dr. Thaler: Yeah, I think one of the things we were wondering about was what, after all, is the goal of the diagnostic study, and what within that goal is the aim of supervision? We wondered whether supervision should focus primarily on diagnosis, or on the interaction between the resident and the patient. We came up, I think, with the idea that it should be a complementary back and forth kind of situation. Diagnosis may not be the major concern of the resident, because he wants to know what do I do now, what is going to be demanded of me by this patient. I have found that my discussion with the resident after his interview is usually focused around what happens next. What do we do after this? I think we also realize that the time for doing this, at the end of the interview, is usually very short. You don't have very much time to discuss diagnosis, interviewing techniques, the resident's good or critical points in his conducting the interview, and in addition to help him to carry on from there. That is a lot of very major tasks that one has to juggle.

B: In this same regard I was talking to a resident yesterday who said that he feels that he tends to fall back on being kind, thoughtful, the taking-care of approach to his patients more often when he doesn't know what to do than when he does know what to do. When he does know what to do, he gets at solving the problem with the patient.

Dr. Thaler: When in doubt be kind. That's not a bad rule of thumb.

Dr. Schuster: One better rule would be, when in doubt keep your mouth shut.

C: I've always felt with my residents that somewhere early in the relationship I focus on some of the techniques that Carl Rogers presented early in his career, in terms of nondirective methods. I try to teach the notion that when you don't know what to do, be nondirective. I think this would be better than being kind, because you lose nothing—you give nothing up. When you're kind, I think sometimes you give things up in the treatment that you can't get back, or you take a position with the patient which is basically unhelpful. I mean, if the goal for the patient is to grow up and take care of himself. That's what I mean by something you can't get back. I think it's important in the tutorial to talk about things like that, what do you do when you don't know what to do.

Dr. Thaler: Okay now we'll listen to a little bit more of the interview. D, you made a comment to me after the last time which I wish you would repeat now, because I thought it was an important comment in terms of supervising a medically trained resident.

D: The comment that I made after what we had heard of this interview from Dr. X was that he did not sound like a doctor or a psychiatrist. It sounded to me like any social worker could have taken that same material, sat there and said "uh huh" and never moved into an area of being medical. I think this is not right, the training of a resident is to be a doctor, a psychiatrist, and not fulfill the function that other professionals can.

Dr. Thaler: I think particularly with this case. Again I tried to point this out to Dr. X in my supplementary interview of the patient. In this case there were very specific and potentially major physical symptoms he failed to pursue.

C: Except that he knew the patient had had extensive workups. The patient had been told by physicians that these symptoms were not physical.

Dr. Thaler: Yeah, he'd had a couple of EKGs in the ED and they were negative, and he'd had a physical examination which was said to be negative.

C: Oh, so he hadn't been thoroughly worked up.

Dr. Thaler: No.

Dr. Schuster: Even if he had, unless you're absolutely certain as to the quality of the workup. . . .

C: Couldn't he assume that these had been dealt with and explored?

Dr. Thaler: No—only in the grossest sense, in terms of his being fairly sure there was no serious coronary disease.

> *Pt.*: This has a lot to do with it, because I get aw-fully concerned over the youth, and I think we've got to reach them at a lot younger level than we are today. None of us are God, and we can't control this thing, but I feel that I could do a lot more and be a lot more effective in that area. You can't properly handle the situation, and you pass it off a lot of times, and you can't spend the time you need. This causes frustrations I'm sure. I think that's got quite a bit to do with it.

Dr. Thaler: He's talking, I think, about his police work and how he turns out to be not a typical "stereotype" of the deputy sheriff cop. He's interested in the sociological problems, in pursuing things, why people act like they do.

> *Dr. X*: You mean you can't really rest easy unless you can do things as you think they should be done.

> *Pt.*: I don't think I'm perfect. I don't feel I've got all the answers to the problems or anything like this, but I feel that a lot of the problems I'm working with are problems of society, and I think that these things should be nipped in the bud and we're not doing it.

A: I think the patient is also saying "you're not the only smart alec around here."

Dr. Schuster: Do you think this was annoying Dr. X?"

Dr. Thaler: Yes and no. I think we talked last time about something similar—something came up about the dream cycle.

C: Yeah, the patient said he wakes up sometimes at night with an anxiety attack or with a pain, and he thought it must be part of the dream cycle, or something like that.

Dr. Sandt: He knew the theory of dream deprivation. He was missing out on his REM sleep. He actually said that.

Dr. Thaler: And Dr. X quickly said, "Oh yeah, yeah."

C: He was feeling a little bit put upon to think that the patient knew something he wasn't supposed to know.

> *Pt.*: I think it's going to cost us as taxpayers a whole lot more to try to nip it in the bud than to let it go. It's also going to save a lot of kids. I try to put this across, but they don't want to buy it.

Dr. Sandt: The patient also knows the sociological aspect of police work.

Dr. Thaler: Dr. X thought this is going to be a typical dumb, country cop. Then this guy starts coming on about how these kids really are not all bad, and it's society and all this sort of thing. Dr. X who feels very much that way himself felt this produced a positive affect in him toward the patient. It changed his view of the patient.

Dr. Schuster: That's an important point because Dr. X should understand that he's going to be in the best position to make an evaluation of the patient if he maintains some degree of neutrality.

Dr. Thaler: He's not aligning himself with the patient.

Dr. Schuster: He's being sucked right in at that point, you know, by the content, the patient's view of life. This will result potentially, at least, in Dr. X not being attuned to certain other things the patient will talk about.

C: Aside from Dr. X's ultimate and predictable feeling of betrayal when he finds out that what he was just listening to was only the first layer, and maybe it ain't really so, he's going to feel betrayed by the patient because he's been sucked in.

Dr. Thaler: And also we have to think about the patient's motivation in coming on that way toward Dr. X who wears a beard and all—you know—there are all kinds of other implications, and we talked about that later, too. Dr. X felt somewhat ill at ease about seeing this guy who's a big guy, he's about 6' 4", he's huge. Again he had this stereotype, this is a country sheriff's deputy, and here I am little Dr. X with my beard and all, and he wondered how is this cop going to respond to me? He'll see me as a hippy type.

A: It's very clear that most patients make incredible efforts to please the therapist or the interviewer, and we know this from research, they watch for very subtle cues of reward: This man has a need to assert himself and to proceed, which I think is healthy in him. What he's defending against may not be so healthy. So what happened is, he started off competing with the psychiatrist, dreams and sleep stuff, and Dr. X is very anxious about that—very controlling and said "I know!" Then the patient switched and didn't compete with him but tried to talk values which he felt more sure about, and Dr. X fell into the other part of the trap. So a steady process of interaction is developing between them:

> *Pt.*: Our county has, you might say, one part-time juvenile officer for the whole county. The State Police don't have any, or anything like this. This is the one thing that's eating at me, and I'm only going to be here so long and I feel I'm here and not doing what I think could be done. This is going to cost us as taxpayers a whole lot of money to try to nip it in the bud.

> *Dr. X*: So sometimes people don't see things your way.

> *Pt.*: Yeah, I don't feel that people have to see things my way, I mean I could be wrong. We're all wrong at times.

> *Dr. X*: Do you ever get a feeling that people on the job, let's say, or in the county are really not going to listen to you at all and are sort of not sympathetic with you in the least, no matter what you said they wouldn't listen to you?

> *Pt.*: No, I don't feel they treat me unreasonably. I understand their problems. I know that a lot of times they put themselves first. Politics, I don't like politicians. I don't know if that will help any in my feeling, and I know that this is one thing that bothers me is that I don't believe there is true justice, and I agree. I am a police officer and I like long sideburns, and I like bell-bottom pants, and I don't consider you are a creep if you wear them. And I agree with a lot of the things that are going on today outside, and we would have to put down if we were called upon.

A: I think we should raise the point that Dr. X is very naive. If he were dealing with a country policeman he'd actually be in a better position, because these people are usually so dedicated to authority that they agree with everything you say. They're ideal patients. This man is much more subtle and far more dangerous in a way, in that he's oppositional in a much more complex way. He lured Dr. X into agreeing with him, then he said no. He's very skillful, much too skillful for what Dr. X is doing.

> *Pt.*: Maybe they have a right to do some of these things. I think I'm in sympathy with them and it gives you torn, mixed emotions. Drug addiction and things like this, for example.

Dr. Thaler: One curious thing, here he's talking about sideburns and bellbottoms, and he didn't talk about beards. (Laughter) It would have been the other obvious thing to mention.

D: The thing that impresses me about Dr. X and this patient is that if Dr. X had only said "Tell me about —— County." Now this policeman is talking about an urban, or Rochester environment, and it has nothing to do with his county. It's an intellectualization, and Dr. X is just going right along with it.

Dr. Schuster: He's very skillful in picking out the areas of Dr. X's interest and arranging things to interest the therapist.

> *Pt.*: Half of us are drug addicts right now ourselves, including myself. The only thing is that I go about it legally, where maybe some of the poor kids, I'm using these same things, escape mechanisms, tranquilizers and things like this to try to put down my anxieties where the kids in high school and colleges. . . .

Dr. Thaler: I think that's kind of beautiful. He's telling about revolt within himself and the measures he uses to put down the instinctual revolt that he's experiencing. He's hurting.

Dr. Sandt: He's a proponent of his point of view. That's what one might well expect, and also a defender of his point of view, and a persuader of the listener. This is the first interview, and I think you have to let the patient present this pretty much in his own style.

Dr. Thaler: I think this gives us an idea of his style. If you pick it up as that, I think it's a very valuable piece of material, but if you're sucked into content. . . .

Dr. Sandt: Dr. X seems to be picking it up as a buyer of this material.

Dr. Thaler: No, I think you underestimate him. We'll have a chance later to listen to his and my discussion, and I think he picks up the style.

Dr. Schuster: By now he *could* be saying to the patient, "Well, what is it that's bothering you?"

Dr. Thaler: Yeah, he's in a sense wasting time. I think actually in terms of the supervision, the problem is to point out to the resident that now that he has an idea of the patient's style, get some data. That's what this interview is for, not to listen endlessly to the patient's intellectualizations.

A: What do you do when a patient won't allow you to get a word in? X doesn't know what to do, so he's letting him go on and on.

Dr. Sandt: Why do you need to get a word in anyway? What's this business that the patient's not allowed his own pace to be allowed to present himself? It strikes me as premature to decide that. The patient should be allowed to continue without all the affective displays of empathy.

Dr. Thaler: But it isn't a question of how long, in other words the diagnostic interview, in a sense, is a set task. You have an hour to find out what's wrong with him.

> *Pt.*: Where the kids in high school and colleges have maybe the same types of anxieties do it illegally, maybe because they can't afford to do it legally. Maybe they don't want to, I don't know.

> *Dr. X*: What medicines are you taking now?

> *Pt.*: Well, I was taking Valium.

> *Dr. X*: Are you taking any now?

> *Pt.*: Dr. W. from G—gave me a medicine which is three layers, three different colors, and I don't know what the composition of it is. It's supposed to act the same as Valium.

Dr. X.: So it's like a sandwich.

Pt.: Yeah, it's like a sandwich, and it's, I guess, a muscle relaxer.

Dr. Thaler: He's again being sidetracked, he's trying to figure out what medication he's taking and he's gotten a pill that has three different colored layers, a multiple tranquilizer. We were trying to figure out what it was, but you will hear a lengthy diatribe. He's gotten me to get the PDR out and look it up.

Dr. Sandt: Did he have the medicine with him?

Dr. Thaler: No.

Pt.: And it's probably got some kind of tranquilizer in it.

Dr. X: Which are you taking now?

Pt.: I'm taking that.

Dr. X: You're taking that rather than the Valium.

Pt.: I think this helps keep it down.

Dr. X: How much do you take? How many pills do you take a day?

Pt.: One every three hours is what he directed. Sometimes I take one every four or five hours. If it starts to bother me, or I start to get up tight. I think a lot of it is muscular. I don't know because . . .

Dr. X: If it comes on, do you take a couple because you're feeling tense?

Pt.: No, not unless I'm directed to. I think that over a period, that I took the Valium for quite a while, and I think that I would be somewhat addicted. If someone, let's just say, says you can't take this any more, I will not give you any more prescriptions, I don't know what that would be like.

Dr. X: You'd feel uncomfortable.

Pt.: I would probably feel uncomfortable.

Dr. X: So, right now you're only taking that one pill.

Pt.: Yeah, I didn't want to mix any more than I had to.

Dr. X: And you're taking one every three hours or so. Do you know what the name of the pill is?

Pt.: I don't know what it is.

Dr. X: Is it Librax?

Pt.: I've taken Librax but that's not it. It's something new and he didn't tell me what it was.

Dr. X: Do you have the bottle with you now?

Pt.: I don't right now.

Dr. X: So you're not carrying the pills with you now.

Pt.: I've got some here—well they gave me Darvon and. . . .

Dr. X: Do you have some in your pockets right now? Can I take a look at them?

Pt.: Sure. These are the ones I took before though. I haven't taken these since I've been taking the other ones, except the doctor told me if I had one of these attacks— these are the 5 mg. Valium and these are the Darvons here.

Dr. X: And what you're taking now is different from that?

Pt.: Yeah, the one that I'm taking now. . . . I haven't taken the Darvon since I had the last real bad spasmatic attack.

Dr. X: So you don't take the Darvon regularly.

Pt.: I don't take the Darvon at all, hardly, except for the one time.

Dr. X: What are the colors of the pill, do you remember?

Pt.: White, blue and pink, I think.

Dr. X: White, blue and pink. Do we have a PDR? (to Dr. Thaler)

Pt.: If you've got a book, I could probably show you.

Dr. X: Let me see if I can find it for you.

Pt.: The prescription is on record at P's Drug Store at G— I could probably find out what it is.

Dr. Thaler: (Laughter) You know we laugh at this—again it doesn't take more than a couple, three minutes altogether, but what can we identify? Is this terribly bad? (to look up the medicine in the patient's presence) Does it make any difference? Or is it merely one of those little tangles you get into, and then move out of again?

A: I see it as a benign collusion between the two of them to avoid the interview.

Dr. Sandt: This is a tranquilization of the interview. (Laughter)

Dr. Thaler: One thing occurs to me that we probably should address ourselves to. I think we notice a lot of mistakes that the resident makes, and I have a feeling that as we listen to ourselves, we will notice a lot of mistakes too. But in spite of that, most of these guys do pretty well with their patients over the long haul. I wonder whether we can also identify whether it is a good thing to point out to the resident what he is doing right and why it is working in spite of the fact that he's doing so much wrong.

Dr. Schuster: Of course, one of the underlying issues here is the way this operates irrespectively of how a resident behaves with the patient. There is a tremendous object hunger that everybody has, and if you gratify that—even if you do it clumsily, you're meeting a basic inner need of the patient.

Dr. Thaler: In therapy I think one sees that a patient will forgive you over and over.

A: No matter how stupid you are.

Dr. Sandt: Also the vehicle is the idiom which the patient has come to see as supportive, like a discussion of medication with the doctor which is a nice safe supportive area for the patient. So Dr. X is gratifying him. He's maintaining a role, maintaining a sort of stereotypic kind of response system, and the whole thing strikes me as supportive.

C: The only thing I don't understand about this sequence is what was so intense about this experience that X had enough—the threat or frustration or tension or anxiety he was experiencing is not apparent, nor was the patient controlling the interview. The patient also has a style that interacts with Dr. X as a relatively impatient person. He has a very plodding, monotonic manner. The thing that impressed me that I would regard as somewhat significant in terms of ultimately getting to it in the supervision with Dr. X is, what was it he really had enough of—so much so that he went to fairly drastic extremes? I don't think it's typical to haul a book off the shelf and sit there with the patient. I mean it's not within the average expectable mistakes a resident makes.

Dr. Schuster: Well, we know that his attitude, feeling toward the patient preceded his appearance. I mean he had some concern before he saw the man, right?

Dr. Thaler: See, he was concerned about this patient, and all he knew about him. I think he was more concerned when he saw his bulk. Then he had this experience of discovering he wasn't really a typical cop. In addition he has told me he has a special interest in drugs. Now I don't know what that means. I finally took the book away from him and said "I'll look for the pictures, and if I find it I'll let you know"; and he went on with the interview.

C: The question is what would Dr. X have said to a later question like, "Look, you could have asked the patient to bring in the bottle of pills. You would have found out everything you had to know from that, or from calling the pharmacist if it were that important. So what were you trying to accomplish by engaging with the patient in this kind of thing?"

Dr. Thaler: Another factor is the presence of the supervisor and X's reverberating memories of previous in-patient service where you always try to identify what drugs the patient's been getting. He may have done some of this for me to make sure that I know that *he* knows the importance of knowing what the patient's medications were.

Dr. Schuster: I'd be interested in his response to this question: "What is the outline in your mind in taking a history from a psychiatric patient?" I get the feeling that he does not have a clear notion of the path he is pursuing here.

C: I agree with you, and I wanted to bring up three points in the last few minutes of that interview that he never responded to when the patient was talking in terms of taking the pills: when he "gets up tight" was one time, "to keep it down" was the second time and the third time I don't recall; but on each occasion the patient was presenting a clue to a relationship between psychological events experienced, feelings, and taking the drug. In each of those instances Dr. X had a chance to explore two things—first the fact that the patient came in after a history of focusing on whatever symptomatology he has had. Second the relationship between his feelings and the medications. The patient is aware that these are supposed to do something for him. This would have kept Dr. X in the right arena, namely, "What are you taking the drugs for? You are aware that it has to do with feelings." He misses this and keeps saying, "What *is* the medicine you're taking?" In a dependent patient like this, how many chances is Dr. X going to get? I think that relates to a concluding question—what are you trying to get at in the first interview?

Dr. Thaler: One of the problems I think is that we try to teach the taking of an associative anamnesis, in other words in the course of an hour or two you take the patient's lead in doing an open-ended interview. If you pick up the proper leads, you can get all the historical data you want to. But the resident has to understand this. He assumes if you let the patient talk, he'll tell you everything. This is not so. The patient will tell very little of what you want to know, because he will try to get away from it.

Dr. Sandt: I call it the explanatory model. I think I'd leap at the same kind of thing you're talking about. In the interview I'd try to get from the patient his explanation for this and how he puts this together in his head, because that's where you're going to cut in. If he explains this on the basis of a somatic issue, then you have to start with that as a substrate; but I agree that there's a little clue here that this fellow doesn't have to be started with on that kind of level. You cut in at another level then, of psychological sophistication, if you want to call it that, or the explanatory model can start being explicit.

C: One of the things that also might have given X an opportunity to explore the issue of how psychologically minded this guy is, aside from getting clues to the nature of the guy's difficulties, would be information that will tell him something about how therapy is likely to proceed. This could be assessed by ultimately raising the question with the patient, "So you do have some idea that these symptoms are connected with feelings," and see what he does with this.

B: Don't we have to ask why doesn't he do this? Assume that he, as all of us, needs to feel like he's doing something significant in taking care of a patient, helping, doing something that's helpful— that's what gives us our role. Why is there something amiss with the way he goes about trying to do something helpful?

C: I have a private hypothesis about that. Dr. X was trying to develop a safety play. In the back of his mind is a feeling about this patient I still don't quite understand, which led him to feel that he was not going to approach this patient psychotherapeutically. In case he couldn't, and since he does have to assume responsibility for this guy, he is looking for a reserve play—I am going to treat this guy with drugs. What drug has he had, can I try a phenothiazine? If he's had some "crummy" superficial tranquilizers, then we can go to the big bomb. I think this is true, and I think he was establishing a small nucleus of control for himself, of how he could treat this guy without moving further in the direction of making him anxious.

B: To let the patient talk about his feelings is to relinquish the control.

Dr. Schuster: I also submit in response to B's earlier comment that the best way to be helpful to the patient in the first interview is to assist the patient in giving the information necessary for us to make certain decisions as to whether we can be helpful after the first interview, or whether we cannot. In other words, this need to be helpful, this maternal striving that's in all of us along with other factors involved in our interest in "helping patients," has to be curbed initially. I think we have not as yet obtained the chief complaint, and that should be possible within the first moment or two. I don't think we have to wait ten minutes to find that out. Following that, you want a lucid exposition of the present illness. That's the next step in my mind. Then you move on to other things.

B: When I said helpful I didn't mean helpful in the maternal sense. I meant helpful in the sense that we are competent in our jobs to be able to do something constructive. We all have a need to be successful, I think, and therefore we want the patient to get better—not because we don't want to take care of him, but because we want to be good. We want to be successful.

C: I think what he was doing was preparing a cop-out for himself.

Dr. Sandt: You can regulate the intensity of the relationship very nicely by giving somebody a pill.

Dr. Thaler: Ever since we've had tranquilizers, which has only been about ten years, this is what's been happening. I think it is one of the reasons why so few people are in psychotherapy today. The first thing that happens when a patient comes to an in-patient floor, they shoot him full of drugs.

B: I think the reason he pulls the cop-out is because he's afraid he's not going to be successful. He doesn't know how to be successful. He's intimidated by this.

C: I agree absolutely, and I don't understand it. The patient, as we listen to him, has not been emitting flagrantly threatening kinds of stimuli. There are patients that scare me, too, but different kinds of things scare each of us.

Dr. Schuster: He's not surly, impatient, he's not silent and stubborn, he's not overtly paranoid. He's a rather affable fellow.

C: Even at a more superficial level he's not scary. You don't get the feeling that if he walks out the door now he's going to go kill himself. He's not presenting with emergent problems. He's not acute, so what's scaring Dr. X?

Dr. Thaler: Let's listen, then, to the patient.

Pt.: I started off having these pains. It's been since I've been in police work. I can't deny that.

Dr. X: You mean you were feeling better before you started the police work.

Pt.: I spent five years in the Army and then I spent one year as an electronics technician. Then I went on the police force, and I was always very idealistic about police and police work. I see a lot of things there that really bother me. It probably would be hard to explain to someone who's not familiar with it. The lack of what you really feel if you believe in the Constitution or anything as it's written, the lack of true justice in many cases and the lack of manpower and lack of cooperation between units and departments.

A: I think we've allowed Dr. X enough time to obtain information about the patient's problems. I'm wondering whether Dr. X seems to need some kind of repertoire to help him. One thing that might be most useful for him is this sort of statement to the patient, "I'm going to have to interrupt you from time to time," which doesn't say I'm going to defeat you. The patient would usually like it, if Dr. X would say, "What you're saying is helpful, but I don't know very much about you, and I need to know more."

A's interjection at this point signalled a shift in our discussion to our concern for the resident who is struggling to get pertinent historical information from the patient, why he has problems doing this and how we can teach him to be more effective in this important task. Our main interest here is in helping the resident to arrive at a clear diagnostic impression of the patient through an orderly and coherent history-taking procedure. In the following we point out some of the differences in taking a history on an in-patient service as compared with the clinic.

Dr. Schuster: He's thrashing around looking for the right thing to discuss.

Dr. Thaler: The simplest thing to do is not to do anything and just let this fellow roll over you.

A: You've got to lead the patient. You've got to show that you can understand, and you can guide him. Dr. X doesn't know how to do this; he doesn't know how to intervene. He intervened in a most inappropriate way at one point when he commented about the medication—it came out of the blue. It wasn't related to something in the interview, so he needs some sort of repertoire. Even at this point if he had some remarks he could use with a patient who won't let him get a word in.

B: Well this takes me back to problem solving. If you help the resident to keep comfortably focused on what is the symptom, why do you think you have the symptom? What are the problems that you are faced with that have led to this? Then a lot of this can be avoided.

Dr. Schuster: How would you do that here, though?

B: I think you could say, "I understand that these are concerns that you have." Rather than get at the problem, the patient displays his problem in talk. If you see that, I don't necessarily think you have to interpret it at the time; but you could keep getting at how does this affect you? How are you feeling in the face of these problems?

Dr. Schuster: Well, just to put it in the context of supervision, how would you arrange that? Would you interrupt Dr. X at this point?

B: Oh no.

Dr. Thaler: I agree. This is something to discuss when you are through, but the question is when and how to say that again in the short amount of time available.

Dr. Schuster: In this case you'd have to write off this first hour and talk with him about it.

D: He misses a lot the patient says that he could use for further clarification.

B: I don't know why he does. Is it in his training? I mean, if he was going about examining somebody's chest because he complains of a cough, he would stick with the problem, he would listen, feel and examine. Now he has let this person wander.

Dr. Schuster: I think we suspect that it's a combination of some internal problem, something within his personality, and some deficiency in his technical skills.

B: Are you sure there isn't something in the way we teach psychiatry that encourages a person not to stick to the problem?

A: We talked about this enough for it to become apparent that a resident doesn't know how to interview, because he never learns how to interview on an in-patient service where you have a captive audience, a patient you can see in your own time at any time. It's a different situation. They never learn how to interview.

B: They learn how to do a medical interview.

C: If you're on the in-patient service, and a resident comes to a patient sitting in a room, the criterion that applies to the adequacy of his work is what gets in the chart. Whether that was obtained after

8 hours of interview, or after one, nobody ever knows. I know that Dr. X could sit there with this guy for about 8 hours, and, ultimately, I have no doubt, write a diagnostic workup that's quite adequate. We'd say here's a bright young man who's learned psychiatry. But that's the issue. Nobody ever sat in with him on his initial interviews with a patient on the ward, and nobody ever noticed whether he went in at 9:00 in the morning and saw the patient for an hour and at 1:00 when he had another free hour and then at 8:00, because he decided he didn't have enough information, and because he's got to get something in the chart. Then at 1:00 the next afternoon and at 4:00 and at 6:00. Nobody sat with him, and nobody knew how long it took him and how many millions of words came out before he boiled it down to a rather good history.

B: Wouldn't that be a passive position for the patient and totally active one for the doctor, in which he gets a bulk of information, from which he draws conclusions and makes formulations and a diagnosis? To my way of thinking that is totally anti-therapeutic.

C: I'm not disagreeing with you at all. I'm saying that it is a style that is easy to develop, and probably the one that you're likely to develop on an in-patient service if you don't have somebody looking over your shoulder. You asked why don't you do this with a physical exam. In your training in physical examinations in the beginning you usually *do* have somebody looking over your shoulder and somebody who says, "Now look, you were supposed to be listening to the heart, why the hell weren't you? You go here, and then you go there and there, and that's the sequence in which you listen." Nobody has ever shown him for a whole year.

B: You mean no one has ever shown him how to conduct an interview? By psychiatric interview you mean different than what is taught on the floors, which is a fact-finding medical interview.

C: The resident loses nothing by taking four hours to get what he should have gotten in an hour. You've got the patients on the floor, and he can go in to see them any time he wants to.

D: I think what impresses me at this point is, I'm wondering if he is picking up or can be taught significant landmarks to be looking for. Now, here this man said he has been in the Army. Further questioning about that part of his life would be very informative on how he handles authority figures, how he handled that block of time in his life, what circumstances put him there.

C: The patient gave him a response which was even more primary. He said this all started when he "got on the cops," and Dr. X never picked it up. *What* all started when he got on the cops?

B: I want to get back to this thing, because it seems to me that the model that's developed on the floors is very different from the model that is suggested from psychotherapy, and it has to do with the difference between psychosis or physical illness and emotional disorder other than that caused by some physical problem. On the floors the medical model, I would say, predominates. In the outpatient department the therapeutic, psychotherapeutic model, predominates.

A: I think it's unwise that first-year residents start on an in-patient floor, because they get lost in the details and are put in a double-bind situation. They are told that they're physicians, therefore they're in charge. Yet they know nothing. They can't admit they know nothing, because their self-esteem is at stake, so they play games. When you get to know what goes on with the personnel on an in-patient floor, as I do because I'm now a supervisor there, it's incredible the games that go on among the staff. The therapeutic achievements there are usually miraculously incidental, because it's a management problem. I don't understand your mystification at this. The residents are put in this spot, and they have to go back to the one resource they have—medical training, so they can use drugs and quote medical things. They are insensitive to patients' needs. I've seen this in group therapy. They don't hear, they've never been taught to hear. Then they come into the OPD, where by circumstance they are forced to make dispositions about human beings who come in for an hour and disappear again. They can't put them in seclusion, they can't control them. I don't think Dr. X is particularly bad. I haven't heard any second-year resident sounding as if he knows how to interview.

Dr. Schuster: I would submit, though, that if they had learned how to take a proper history they wouldn't be having this trouble in the second year. I do not agree with B that the way you take a history as a psychiatrist and a physician is poles apart. I think the extrapolation from the medical history to the psychiatric history is not an extreme one. I think you start just as you do with a medical illness, with the chief complaint, then you develop the present illness and look into the family history.

B: The psychotherapeutic interview has to be a joint project, because the medical history is not a joint product or joint effort. If you want the patient to grow up and solve his own problems you cannot approach him as if you were someone who is going to do it for him.

C: The model that Dan is presenting isn't that, it doesn't necessarily include the kind of taking over that you're talking about. It's a modification of this. The point is that the resident must have some framework. He knows he has to take a history, he knows he has to review certain systems, he knows in the physical examination he looks at certain organ systems of the body, he examines signs of adequate or inadequate function. It's perfectly possible to use that as the conceptual framework without taking over for the patient.

B: How?

C: Well, I think Dan is pointing out the notion of what is the chief complaint, what brings you here, what bothers you now, how and when did this start, what is this like? When the patient says "I feel up tight" what does up tight mean for him, how does he experience this? Those are not questions that necessarily take over from the patient. They are the things that the interviewer would like to know.

B: That's true, I agree with all of that, but at some point you're going to have to say to the patient, "Well, given these things, this is what you should do."

Dr. Schuster: That's later, after you know enough.

B: I know, but at some point this crossroads must come.

C: It doesn't even have to be sooner or later. It can occur in the context of the screening interview. In a 15-minute screening interview of a neurotic patient who looked like she might be a reasonable intensive psychotherapy case. Even in the 15 minutes it's possible in the course of getting very superficial information. You ask the patient, "I wonder why you smiled when you said that?" simply to use it as a test question. Is the patient capable of some kind of introspective reflection, would she try to come up with a psychologically based statement about her relationship between her expressive behavior and the content of what she's saying? It's possible to create microcosmic, little micro-therapeutic episodes even in the briefest interview.

B: But let's define what micro-psychotherapeutic activities are.

Because they are not passive on the part of the patient nor active taking care of medical problems.

C: No, but you can say to the resident, "Look, I'm getting information from the patient. Part of what I wanted to know is, were you able to make some kind of tentative prediction about how the patient is going to respond to a certain style of treatment? The best way to do this is to emit a stimulus and see what happens." It's just a tiny little test, and it's in the context of the diagnostic interview without necessarily beginning psychotherapy.

B: Isn't it fundamentally that you're saying to this other individual, "What do you think?" Isn't it supporting the development of himself?

C: That can occur in this context by asking him what he feels when he's "up tight" and what it is that makes him think it started with the police, and what was the difference between the police and non-police. I don't know if this guy is married, I don't know if he has any children yet, I don't know what his relationship with his wife is yet, I don't know anything about his sexual functioning yet. I don't know how he handles aggression, except from what I can gather from the interaction in the interview. When are we going to find out all these things? It's not taking over from the patient to ask him to give you information about himself.

Dr. Schuster: And also I think you're overlooking something else, B. A patient comes to the doctor or the psychotherapist, because he knows, and has the right to hope, that the doctor knows something more about this condition than he does. In other words that "authority" relationship exists in his mind—he's not just going to another friend.

A: One analogy to the medical interview would be the framework —in other words the feeding of information and sorting it out. The one difficulty with Dr. X is that he doesn't know what to believe in. He's said to me, "I don't believe in psychoanalysis, I don't know if I believe in behavior therapy." He knows a little about each, and he's left with an incredible vacuum.

Dr. Sandt: He's not very different from many other residents.

A: So what happens to a poor resident who has a smattering of knowledge about any framework theory.

Dr. Thaler: This is one of the things to be considered in terms of the lack of any structure that is presented in his first year.

C: Isn't that part of the training of the resident, to test out different belief systems and then start learning?

Dr. Schuster: You'd hope he'd leave the first year with some framework.

PEDAGOGY VERSUS THERAPY

This is an issue which recurred throughout many of our discussions. It is central to the supervisory process and has been commented on by many authors. It has pervaded the medical ethos for centuries and has to do with "Physician, heal thyself"—or more precisely, the intimate relationship between the physician's unresolved neurotic conflicts and how he looks at and reacts to his patient. In the supervisory context, the task is one of the supervisor's dealing with the resident's countertransference while keeping in mind, hopefully, his own. In this section we continue with the resident and patient just presented. We speculate here on how Dr. X copes with his anxiety engendered by his patient and how we can help him in this struggle. In helping him, some felt we must move toward a therapeutic stance with the resident, while others in the conference believed we must draw a sharp line between therapy and teaching. The following comments illustrate the difficulty in drawing this line but also the importance of recognizing the issues involved.

At this point in the interview, Dr. X had been questioning the patient about his tension and anxiety. The patient began discussing some relationships between "his trouble unwinding" and his work. Dr. X abruptly veered off from this topic and began asking him about the doctor who had prescribed medicine for his tension. In discussing his doctor's impression that his symptoms were a consequence of anxiety, the patient said, "I hate to just give everything up because of this (his symptoms). That's why I'm here, I guess."

> *Dr. X*: Do you ever feel like giving up? At the end of your rope?
>
> *Pt.*: No, not at all. Did I ever think about committing hara-kiri or something like that? No.
>
> *Dr. X*: You worry more about the other—that you might have a heart attack.

> *Pt.*: I worry more about the other, and I think a lot about my family and things—if something should happen to me. I don't know if that's a normal worry or an abnormal worry but I think about that.

> *Dr. X*: Do you ever feel bad enough to think about suicide? You know, I mean really down.

Dr. Sandt: It's quite clear that any time someone is depressed, Dr. X will respond much more givingly. Any time somebody comes up out of that, he's really quite anxious; so it does seem almost as if he bludgeons him into feeling depressed, and sometimes a little seductively. He's apparently unable to ask directly, "have you ever felt?", the seductive tone really makes the patient wonder what the devil happened. You can just see him swiveling emotionally. This solicitude really puts the patient off.

> *Pt.*: I never have (long pause). There was one time, a long time ago when I was in the Army, when I thought about it, but not really seriously.

> *Dr. X*: You never tried anything.

A: There's no doubt that patients by virtue of their own malfunctioning are very sensitive to what pleases the therapist. This is one of their problems. One of the things I often have noticed is the patient who pleases the resident because he is sick and helpless and wants to be liked. As soon as the patient starts becoming well and autonomous and functioning and can disagree and be assertive, many residents become threatened and send out very strong cues—"be sick again, and I'll like you." I think it has profound implications for the teaching of therapy, but it comes up even in the diagnostic study phase. Clearly Dr. X is saying, "I feel most comfortable with you when you're sick, so you stay sick, and I'll like you." This is the message, not worded but clearly coming across, and I think it's an important point.

Dr. Sandt: One way you can deal with that as a supervisor is to try to help the resident pick out the areas of "good functioning versus bad functioning" then you don't have to judge the patient as a "sick person." This will allow you less areas of threat for the resident. So where are the areas in which the patient functions better and the areas that he doesn't function so well? With this patient imminent collapse is suggested, and Dr. X responds by asking have you ever thought about suicide.

Dr. Thaler: Some part of this I think you may be right about— the underlying motivation which the interviewer is not aware of, but part of this may also be at a more superficial level, a clumsiness of technique. In other words it is appropriate to establish the severity of a patient's depression the first time you see him. You *do* want to find out if this guy is going to kill himself before you see him again. But here it was done in a very abrupt sort of way. Where do you tackle this kind of an error or this kind of situation? Do you tackle it in terms of saying to the resident, "Look at your technique."? It seems as though there was a very abrupt kind of transition from one topic to another, all of a sudden you clobber this patient with the idea he is about to kill himself. Do you say to the resident, "Now what is there about you that makes you interject this particular comment right here?"

A: What you could ask is how did you feel about this man, and he may be able to admit that he is afraid of this huge hulking brute. "Is there any way in which you feel comfortable dealing with this huge hulking brute?" "Yeah, when he's sick and miserable and pathetic, I feel strong." If you can lead him to that, what he's doing will make sense to him. It seems to me he admitted his own fear of this huge policeman right from the beginning. If a huge hulking brute comes toward you, you have some apprehension. Then the patient says, "I'm needy, and I'm sick, and I'm helpless," and you're not going to feel so frightened.

Dr. Sandt: I think just confronting the resident with that is not right. You have to talk about where you are with him, what hour you're in, just as if he were the patient—where you are in terms of a relationship with that resident, how long you've been meeting. If this is the first hour you've supervised that resident, it's no time to talk about *his* dynamics. You just know you're not going to confront him with any of this. You ask very, very indirect questions about how things went in the interview, what his feeling about it was. You reassure him by saying the first interview can be expanded later, and that sort of thing.

A: Dr. X is saying, "We will find ground on which I won't be anxious with you. I won't be anxious if you need me and you're helpless and you're sick." There are very few residents in the beginning who feel comfortable unless their patients are very sick, and I think that's often destructive, because that's the message the patient gets. He knows this is the one way he can get somewhere in the relationship with his doctor—to be very sick. It's a paradox, and I've seen it a lot.

Dr. Sandt: That's the story with any psychiatric patient. They have to convince you that they're sick enough to "need a psychiatrist" which is a double-bind for the patient to begin with. He never can present himself as a functioning person until he's sure you will accept him, that he's sick enough to need a psychiatrist, As I said, there are two ways to deal with this, one is dealing with the resident and hoping he can send the message to the patient that it's all right to be okay in certain areas, and two is working on problem areas rather than treating the patient as a totally shot-down person. An interesting vignette parallel to the story of this man. This morning we had a diagnostic interview, a person with almost an identical personality style, an ex-Marine who's full of acting-out impulsive things, mostly with cars; but it turns out that he's had thoughts of joining the police. He's had 30 jobs in two years, and one of the things he'd like to be is a policeman and ride a motorcycle around. He likes war movies, and X said I just knew you'd want to be a policeman. I had thought this, too, but he couldn't stop himself from telling the patient. It was incredible. He just popped it right into the interview. He smiled when the fellow said "policeman," you know, like that's great, and congratulations on his own perception. It was incredible, and the upshot of the whole thing that just tore the whole interview was that this patient goes trap shooting. Last weekend Dr. X was trap shooting, and he recognized that the patient was somebody he had seen trap shooting at the same place, and that the two of them might meet trap shooting some day. The issue with the patient was control of his aggression. It was really a fantastic interview, but what I'm saying is that what was great about it was that this fellow was to Dr. X as the patient we have been discussing. Apparently Dr. X had put the patient's aggression into a context of control, called trap shooting, which somehow reassured him.

B: I agree with what you've been saying about his need to control the situation because of his own anxiety, but another aspect of it might be that rather than his needing to see the patient as sick, it may be simply that he needs to feel that he has something to offer, that he can be a doctor, he can control the situation and has some knowledge. Therefore, the questions that he would ask would make the patient fit into a mold which Dr. X could then feel that he could do something about, that he could identify, he could label, he could feel competent to do something.

Dr. Thaler: I think that as always there are multiple determinants: who's one up and who's one down, and the other is the maternal needs of the therapist who must feel that he is somebody who has something to give, and that the other person is someone who needs and will be fulfilled by what he is giving.

B: But these are also possibly paternal in the sense that he needs to feel like he's able and competent and can do something. I just want to clarify this aspect of it—to put the patient down so that he'll be less afraid of him could be almost a total self-absorption, that Dr. X is just fighting for his own sense of worth, and the patient suffers because of it. It's not really anti-patient it's pro Dr. X, but it winds up being anti-patient.

A: But even on the most trivial level it's bad, because it may be faulty technique. It's always faulty technique if the interviewer introduces a new topic. If he directs this man in a very neutral fashion, and the man comes up with some talk about depression, it would be meaningful to respond to that; but for him to suddenly introduce, "Are you suicidal, or are you depressed, and when are you going to commit suicide?" is obviously X's problem, not the patient's.

Dr. Thaler: I think the whole area of teaching how to do an associative anamnesis is one that we're very much lacking. I've tried to demonstrate this periodically in some of the interviews, for example when the patient asked, "Do you want to know about the family, or was it my work?" What better place to say, "Well tell me about your family." You can even direct it by saying, "I've heard a lot about your work, but I haven't heard much about your family."

B: I would agree with A, I think that it would be better to try to deal with X about his feelings about it rather than to point out what this is doing to the patient. You can help him with his feelings— it will only make him feel worse to see what he's doing to the patient and make him all the more anxious and therefore all the more controlling. I think that there should be in our discussions about supervision and tutorials a definite emphasis on dealing with the resident and his problems. I have a feeling from what I've heard from residents that in the past you go to see a psychiatrist or go to an analyst in order to be treated, that you don't deal with your personal problems in your tutorials or in your supervision.

Dr. Thaler: Well, I think that may be one of the most difficult and delicate problems of supervision. I personally feel quite strongly that it's terribly important not to get the therapeutic and the pedagogic roles mixed up, and while it may be clear in your mind you also have to be sure that it's clear in the resident's mind as to what you're there for—that you're there to teach him how to do something well or better than he's able to do it, but not to engage him in a therapeutic relationship.

B: But a therapeutic relationship exists all the time with everybody anyway.

Dr. Thaler: No, I don't believe that.

Dr. Sandt: Our contract isn't that explicit with the resident.

A: What about contracts with the supervisor? You've got to start working that through, because it becomes very tricky.

Dr. Thaler: I wish I had on tape what Dr. X said to me at our last meeting. I received one of the most glowing adulatory testimonials that I have ever heard from a resident, and I love to be praised, but it was almost embarrassing. He indicated there was something about the way he felt I was dealing with him in contrast to some other contacts he had had, which produced some very intense responses in him.

B: Well, so what are you saying?

Dr. Thaler: I'm testifying to the potential intensity of the relationship, and how careful one has to be in dealing with this kind of thing. After all, this man has been meeting alone with me for three hours a week for three months in a row. He and I, in a really not very explicitly defined relationship, in which he reveals a lot more about himself than I do, just as in therapy. He reveals many many things about himself. He reveals sort of the inmost secrets of his skills and nonskills, of who he is as a psychiatrist, how he is with other people, his ignorance. He appreciated particularly, he told me, the fact that I was not harsh with him in my criticisms. How to deal with that whole business of criticism is one thing I've rarely seen or heard anything about, the whole idea of how do you criticize somebody. What is the whole dynamics of this business between you and the resident? Obviously he's there to be criticized, and he knows it, but how you do it may determine how much he can benefit by your criticism and how much he will suffer from it.

Dr. Schuster: Well, B's question is important. It is one that's difficult to answer—the separation of the pedagogic from the therapeutic role. I think one of the main points here is the limitation on what one can point out effectively to the resident as to his problems or his counter-transference. I think we're sharply limited by what he can see, that's the whole thing. It's a little simpler if somebody's in psychoanalytic training, and the supervisor of a case can say, "You seem to be having some trouble with this specific problem—you ought to think about that in your analysis." That means he can at least have another place where he can approach this problem.

B: Why can't you do that in a supervisory or in a tutorial?

Dr. Schuster: Because he's not in treatment.

B: Well, but you might talk to a friend about such a problem or your spouse about this.

Dr. Schuster: Well, I'll give you an example. Yesterday a resident interviewed a patient, and it was pretty obvious to me that he was very angry with the patient, not without reason; so I pointed it out to him. I don't think it was the way I pointed it out, but he couldn't see it at all. We talked about it at some length, and finally I gave up, because there was no point in pursuing it. It's a wonder he didn't get punched in the nose by this patient. It was so blatant that everybody else in the group could see it.

B: So you did try to point it out.

Dr. Schuster: Yeah, but I say this is an example of the limitation I spoke of.

B: But that doesn't mean that the approach isn't a valid one, even though it didn't work in that instance.

Dr. Thaler: That's the difference between a therapeutic and a pedagogic relationship. In other words, in a pedagogic relationship you can tell the resident, "It seems to me, as I listened to you, that you were being angry with the patient." The resident says, "I don't see that, I wasn't angry with the patient." So you can pursue it further. You can ask, "Well, how did you feel? What was going on as you were talking to the patient?" That still seems to be a pedagogic exploration. When he still doesn't see, however, can you then ask, "Well would you associate to this, or how is it with you

and your father?" If it happens again and again, then you can say
to the person, "Look, it seems to me that these interviews aren't
going too well, because each time I detect a rage toward the patient which you can't see. Maybe you ought to look into this with
somebody else."

B: Yes, but the patient might say to you or the resident might
say to you—either one—"Isn't it possible that you're detecting
anger in me because of your problems? I really don't feel angry, and
the fact that you asked me to free associate to my father doesn't
necessarily mean that you're right."

A: But you're just proving why supervision shouldn't be therapy.
This is exactly what happens in therapy. You try to work through
resistances and countertransference. Nor can you assume that a
resident is asking you to be his therapist.

B: You're all assuming that you're right, that he *was* angry.

Dr. Thaler: Well I think that I have good reason to assume so
by virtue of my lesser involvement and my greater experience. Also,
I do tape most of the things we do. We can then go back over the
tape, and we can both listen to it and figure out what each did
and said.

Dr. Schuster: I don't think it's that the supervisor is always right,
and the resident is always wrong; but I think you must have a basic
operating assumption that the task of the supervisor is to try to help
the resident, and the reason he can help him is because he's had
more experience. It doesn't mean he's infallible, but we have to
assume they're not equal in terms of their ability, experience, knowledge, etc.

Dr. Thaler: And aren't you supposed to instruct them?

Dr. Schuster: I'm sympathetic to what you're saying. I'm just
saying it has limitations. I remember one particular resident some
years ago who was generally regarded as a disaster, and he came
into the OPD for six months because nobody else wanted him. I
sat with him for every single interview he had with his patients
over many weeks. I told him such things as, "How can you talk to
an adolescent like that, so stuffy and remote, you sound like you're
giving a lecture." I really hammered on him, but I must say that he
did finally come around.

Dr. Thaler: But you didn't tell him.

Dr. Schuster: I didn't tell him what his psychopathology was, I just told him *what he was doing,* as I saw it, and he was educable to a degree. He could see finally what he was doing, and he changed.

B: Because you did involve yourself with him and his problems.

Dr. Schuster: I didn't think of it in any way that was unpedagogic. I didn't regard it as therapy.

B: Don't you think it was?

Dr. Schuster: If that's the outcome, that's fine, but my intent was not to direct my attention to his intrapsychic conflicts. They are his problems. My attention was focused entirely on what he was doing with his patients. If that set him to thinking afterwards, "Now I wonder why I behaved that way," fine!

B: Well, I guess what we're struggling with is a question of where and how do you define the limit. Where does it change from pedagogy to therapy?

Dr. Schuster: I guess that's one of the main differentiations— *what* you're doing rather than *why* you're doing it.

B: Could you give an example of that?

Dr. Schuster: Well, the example I gave. My focus was on *what* he was doing, not *why* he was doing it that way.

Dr. Thaler: In other words, if he was stuffy with the adolescent, you tell him you're being stuffy with the adolescent, but you don't explore with him why he needs to be that up-tight with this adolescent patient. You don't inquire about his own background, his life, his own relationship with his parents or his relationship with me.

B: All right, I have said to the resident, it seems like you're being stuffy with the adolescent, you might think about *why* you need to be this way.

Dr. Schuster: That's going one step beyond, isn't it—one step in the direction of *why*?

Dr. Thaler: Now what happens is you're giving him an invitation.

B: That's right.

Dr. Thaler: If he comes back the next time and says to you, "Dr. B, I have thought about this, and I had a dream the other night and in this dream such and such occurred." What are you going to do about it?

B: Talk to him about it, right then and there.

A: There's a patient waiting outside the door.

B: If you can't right then, you can another time.

A: This is the dilemma, you've not contracted a time, he's not paying you, he hasn't chosen you as a therapist, all sorts of problems arise. What happens at the end of the three months when he has a dependent transference with you? Do you say, "Well, that's the end of our supervision, or that's the end of our therapy?"

B: Couldn't that be discussed then? What concerns me is that you're afraid to get involved, that you're afraid that you're not going to be able to get out of it.

Dr. Sandt: That's one aspect from the point of view of the supervisor, but what about from the point of view of the resident who also feels somewhat trapped into an unpleasant contract.

B: Look, if it became a problem all I think I'm saying is, allow a little more flexibility in this direction. If this became a problem, or if it looked like all you were talking about was the resident's problems, then couldn't you tell the resident, "Perhaps this is something you should go into in more detail." Not to do this at all denies the resident the opportunity to talk with any of the people who have had experience in these areas with things that they are concerned about, about themselves and their relationship to people including their patients. Where else are they going to do it unless they go formally to a psychiatrist? I mean if you had a good friend on the staff, let's say, and you couldn't understand why you were reacting a certain way to a patient, you'd talk to him about it if you felt he could be helpful to you.

Dr. Schuster: I'd only respond to that by saying it isn't a question of being flexible. It's a question of how much you want to extend yourself in a therapeutic direction and how essential that is to the pedagogic situation. Also what potential assistance you're going to be to the resident and how much you want to get involved in that sort of thing. Some people might be more phobic about it than others, I grant you, but I think the main question is, is it necessary to go in that direction?

A: I think we keep lowering the boundary between therapy and understanding, and I think any good supervisor doesn't follow very rigid lines. Understanding does help the resident reflect, does help him to become more open, but you use your judgment as to whether to take it further. I see it as potentially destructive, that one can easily become paternal and intrusive and get second-year residents, who are very vulnerable, by the way, to depend on you. I've seen it at other psychiatric centers, and it leads to a good deal of acting-out of problems. I can give you a concrete instance in Dr. Y whom I supervised. This resident had many problems with patients, and I have made him aware of some of them; but I can't pursue it because I see him needing years of therapy to change his character. I'm not prepared to say you should go into analysis. He may see me as being helpful but it doesn't work in the long run, because my contract, as supervisor, doesn't go beyond six months. That doesn't mean that in the supervision I don't try to deal with his own difficulties in communicating with patients, as when they say they are going to commit suicide, and he won't hear it. This is what happened three times. I'm willing to point that out. Y may say it's his problem that he's not hearing this, but what he does about it, is up to him. After all, he's an adult.

B: I agree that it has limits, but you don't have to shut it off. I mean after you say therapy is different from understanding, I don't quite understand. I don't quite understand what is therapy?

A: Therapy is a contract—it's a business contract in which you've contracted some X number of hours for a therapist. No one has told a resident his supervisor would be his therapist. So it's intrusive for me to say I'll be your therapist. In therapy the patient pays a certain amount of money in return for the time of the therapist, and the therapy is conducted according to certain ground rules and limits.

B: That's a very good answer, but therapy also goes on between people without any contract. You talk to a resident about problems that exist in a relationship, and that is the same thing you do when you're under contract for psychotherapy—I mean similar things do take place, and it just so happens that in one instance you're getting paid. I think I'm arguing that I hate to see a definite line set.

Dr. Thaler: I think there is—you're saying there isn't much difference, and we may agree, but I think it's important to see where we don't agree. This doesn't mean that either you are right or I am, but I don't agree with you. I feel rather strongly that the more definite line we can set the better off we are. In a definition of therapy, the contract is the crucial part of the definition, because the contract defines the responsibilities of each party and makes it as explicit as it is possible to make it. One person has certain responsibilities, and the other person has other responsibilities. There are certain things they can expect of each other, and their relationship is primarily focused on the work that they do together, on the problems of the one individual, the patient.

B: Yes but I'm afraid that the so called contract is a protective device which the psychiatrist has created in order to keep the patient at bay.

Dr. Thaler: That may be part of it, and I think that's appropriate, because it defines the realities of the situation. If you don't have certain limits to the possibilities of the relationship, how many patients could you deal with? The contract protects the patient, too, against the psychiatrist.

Dr. Sandt: The contract serves more functions than safety I think. It serves a focal purpose, too, so that we don't wander around saying you and I are really relating, because every now and then a wave length of our empathy is on the same channel exactly. It seems to me that it serves not just for clarification and focus, but it's methodological, too. You're setting up a style in which you two are going to relate. I think it has other functions than safety, and I agree with your thrust. Your point really is that human beings relate whether they're on contract with each other or not. But the purpose for which they relate is so different than everyday life. I find it easier to make the contract for these reasons, rather than for safety.

Dr. Schuster: Also, B, I think we owe it to ourselves to be as precise as we can about these things in an imprecise field. Therefore, I agree with Otto that a line should be drawn more clearly rather than less. I think you're confusing therapy with being helpful. For example, I think a friend talking with another friend can be helpful, but that isn't psychotherapy in my book. It's an *analogous* situation, because one is talking over his problems with the other. This might be helpful to the person and have a therapeutic effect, therapeutic with a small "t," in the adjectival sense. I believe we owe it to ourselves to try to define what it is we do with our patients as precisely as we possibly can. Granted that the whole thing is subject to much imprecision. A considerable factor in all this is the point Tarachow made that everybody is hungry for objects; and in the therapeutic situation you have to be aware of the continuum from the one extreme where you and the patient take each other as real objects to the other extreme where you eschew this kind of involvement with the patient, and it is more of an "as if" relationship. You have to resist the patient's demand upon you to take you as a real object and your own needs to lay claim to the patient in this manner.

Dr. Sandt: We could be talking about the supervisory needs of all the supervisors. There is also the popularity issue, the seducibility of residents in the first place, what it means to be in a position where your point of view is really sort of the way you live, almost a substitute for your own values and therefore your own self. All those projected things. I heard that from Dr. X the first day when he said, "Now I don't believe in psychotherapy, behavioral therapy is the answer. I just want you to know that I have that point of view."

Dr. Thaler: I think also that if you're going to be a therapist, the therapeutic contract involves the deliberate exertion of a skill and you're going to undertake to do a skillful job. That's your major task. Now the kind of job you do with a patient, I think, is different from the kind of focal job you undertake as a pedagog, as a teacher or as a friend.

B: There's an overlapping.

Dr. Thaler: Of course, there's always this, you know human behavior is very hard to classify.

Dr. Sandt: Yeah, but I think what we're really after is some technique or technical skills, and you can keep calling attention to those, and if that's not working then you'd better start thinking about some other things.

Dr. Thaler: I often make this explicit with my tutees particularly when we start a tutorial arrangement. I usually tell the tutee, "I am here to teach you something about psychotherapy. I'm not going to be your therapist. If I point out certain things that I perceive about your behavior it will be in terms of what I observe you doing with or to the patient. Why you're doing this is your business, and if you feel you ought to do something else about it, you can make arrangements for it."

B: Suppose you thought by talking about a certain aspect of a resident's problem in one of your tutorial sessions, or three of your tutorial sessions, that you could actually help the person make a change that was beneficial to him and give him some insight. Does he have to go to a psychiatrist and pay for it to get that interpretation?

Dr. Thaler: If I can make the change by *instructing* him I would do it, and if I could say, "Look try to be different," or "It seems to me this is what you can do to make a different kind of situation of this." If it were to involve an interpretation, I would not make an interpretation—it's not my business. As a matter of fact if somebody did it to me I would get very angry.

B: Well, suppose the resident says to you: "Dr. Thaler, I don't understand why I react that way."

Dr. Thaler: Then I would say, "Try to think about it, and if you can figure it out and change, fine; and if you have trouble with it then maybe you ought to get some help from somebody else."

Dr. Sandt: I think that last line should be very, very carefully considered. I think you're in an awfully tough position when you say it sounds like that problem is getting so much in your way that you really better get some help about it. The way that's perceived by the resident is, God, you mean, Dr. Thaler, that I'm so sick that—you know that kind of thing.

Dr. Thaler: Well if it is so, then you should say so.

Dr. Sandt: I don't think you have to say that, is what I'm saying.

Dr. Schuster: That's a tough question, and it's hard to answer that. I would tend to shy away from answering.

C: I dont' think a resident's ever asked me that.

B: Residents have said something like, "I'm sure I do this because I remember I reacted the same way to my father," and I have said, "Well, so you see that connection. Maybe that does have an influence on how you react in the situation."

Dr. Thaler: But you don't say tell me about your father.

B: No, but I don't say I won't talk about it. I say that's worth talking about.

Dr. Schuster: I think that's going a step beyond.

Dr. Thaler: I think we've articulated our views on this, and maybe we ought to go on.

At this point we returned to the interview with the patient, exhausting for the moment the question of pedagogy or therapy.

THE SUPPLEMENTARY INTERVIEW OF THE PATIENT BY THE RESIDENT'S SUPERVISOR

In Chapter IV we spoke briefly of the usefulness of the supervisor's interventions at the conclusion of the resident's initial interview of

his patient. Here we continue with Dr. X and his patient and his
supervisor's supplementary interview of this man. Dr. Thaler began
with a detailed inquiry of the patient's symptoms in order to demonstrate to Dr. X the relationship between the patient's symptomatology
and certain important events in his life. Again, he was stressing one
of the issues we regard as cardinal—without a carefully pursued
history of the present illness we cannot establish diagnosis and
therapy. This inevitably led to a discussion of the so-called "medical model" and its applicability to the work of a psychiatrist. This
case served as a good illustration of this issue, as he had a number
of bodily symptoms which posed a diagnostic problem as to whether
they were of physical or psychological origin.

At this point in the conference we listened to the closing remarks
of Dr. X and his patient and then went on to Dr. Thaler's brief
supplementary interview of the patient. The ensuing discussion of
the conference participants focused on certain principles of history-
taking and clinical observation.

Pt.: I'm doing my job as it should be done.

Dr. X: You want to do things right.

Pt.: I want to do things right.

Dr. X: That's a good idea.

Pt.: I want to do my job as I thought it was to be done and
doing it properly and not causing any trouble.

Dr. X: I think that's a very good idea. I think that's
a good sign that you are concerned and responsible and
want to make sure that things are okay and are as they
should be, or as best they can be.

Pt.: The main thing that bothers me is that I go along
and work, and I would like to work 10 or 12 hours a day,
as long as I felt I was accomplishing something. The
thing of it is that it's a bad system. Pains start in my
back. I didn't know what was causing them, and they
(doctors) didn't, and you get to thinking about all
sorts of diseases. I suppose I get that on my mind at

times, too, and I suppose that if things continue it could over a period of time lead to depression and that. . . .

Dr. X: I think your future can be a little bit more comfortable than in the past. I think we may be able to manage to make you feel better, to understand the problem better. I want to have a few more meetings with you to get to know the problem a little bit more. Okay? I think Dr. Thaler might like to ask you a few things now.

Dr. Thaler: I usually explain to the resident that I would like to ask a few questions at the end.

Dr. Thaler: Could you tell me what physical things have been bothering you?

Pt.: Pain in my back, and then they go around into my chest.

Dr. Thaler: I'm going to ask you about the chest pain but I'd like to ask you first what all is involved. The back pain is one thing, what else?

Pt.: And then the chest—I get the chest pains and then I get nervous, I think. I mean I start to get up-tight and then when I feel these coming on . . .

Dr. Thaler: The back pain and the chest pain go together.

Pt.: Well sort of. It starts in the back and comes up through my chest.

Dr. Thaler: I see—it starts in the back and then they come and involve your chest also. Have you ever had the chest pain without the back pain?

Pt.: Once or twice I know of I got the chest pain, and then I started to worry.

Dr. Thaler: I understand you also have some stomach trouble. Is that separate?

Pt.: This comes along a lot of times with it. I used to get it at first. I used to wake up in the night with terrible indigestion.

Dr. Thaler: That's what I was wondering, you'd wake up with heartburn and you've had colitis.

Pt.: Colitis which comes and goes.

Dr. Thaler: Who called it colitis?

Pt.: My doctor.

Dr. Thaler: Your doctor called it colitis.

Pt.: Yeah.

Dr. Thaler: Did you bleed with it?

Pt.: Yeah, I had some passage of blood—bright red.

Dr. Thaler: How long did that go on?

Pt.: Well I've had it for quite a while. It seems to come more often in the spring of the year.

Dr. Thaler: Is there anything else, any other part of your body that's troubling you—your back, your chest, the stomach trouble and sometimes the colitis. No headaches?

Pt.: My hands get clammy, and I get cold sweats. When I sleep I sweat a lot.

Dr. Thaler: Now what you call attacks. They're always the same with the pain in the back and going to the chest. When was the last attack?

Pt.: The last was a few weeks ago. I can't remember the exact dates. It was around 10:00. I was patrolling.

Dr. Thaler: So you'd been out for most of the time on your shift.

> *Pt.*: It hadn't been very busy. As a matter of fact it was a little less busy than usual.

> *Dr. Thaler*: Can you recall as much detail as possible just how this came about?

> *Pt.*: I had just come in for a soft drink at the station. I think I had transported a prisoner from court.

Dr. Thaler: One reason I was pursuing the interview this way was because I wanted to point out to Dr. X the detailed relationship between the various pains and physical symptoms and the patient's own perception of what they were. This is why I asked about the colitis and who called it colitis, because some patients name their own symptoms or medicine. Then the patient had been talking about attacks earlier, so I wanted to ask him the nature of these attacks and also the set in which the attacks occur. In the interview with Dr. X I had not learned about all these points, so I wanted to touch on them.

B: You say the important things that he missed. In *your* opinion these were important. Well then, what are the fundamental things that always should be asked?

Dr. Thaler: I think that's basic. In terms of the focus of our discussions, perhaps we should arrive at some point of consensus as to what it is we are trying to teach and get at in the supervisory interviews. Implied in all this, of course, is that I have a certain view as to what is important to get in the initial interview, what kind of data we need in order to make some kind of rational disposition of the situation by the time we have seen the patient for one hour.

B: What could you say is important in general and why are you pursuing these things here?

Dr. Thaler: Why am I pursuing these lines? Well, certainly one of my thoughts is that on the first interview it is important to know two primary things—one, what is the patient's reason for coming or what is the chief complaint, and two, some fairly clear idea as to what is the course and nature of the development of his present illness. These are the two basic items I would think are important in order to make some intelligent determination as to what happens next.

Dr. Schuster: Here you were pursuing the present illness, trying to get the temporal relationships.

Dr. Thaler: First of all trying to get it in logical terms and what he is experiencing that brings him finally to ask for help—first medical help then psychiatric help. Secondly, in what set is this taking place? When did he have these attacks that he is just now talking about? People say, well, I've had this many times, and they can't recall the first time; but when we ask about the last time it is most vivid in their minds, so we can get some idea of the setting.

B: I think what you're doing here is what we so often see with residents, they keep jumping around. Perhaps it's because in emotional problems things are less defined and concrete, but what often happens is that the resident starts out well intentioned along the same lines as you were doing now and ends up quickly. The present illness often comes out fast, and then the patient goes into a silence or pause.

Dr. Thaler: Yeah, often the second question is "tell me about your childhood" which is irrelevant in terms of the first interview.

B: There was a lot of this going on in this interview. What you seem to be doing here is pursuing in detail, very precise and careful . . .

Dr. Thaler: I think one confusion that exists is concerning what is known as an associative anamnesis, in other words, an open-ended technique in the interviewing, and the confusion in the resident's mind that this is not compatible with an orderly approach to the problem. You can't have in your mind a completely orderly idea as to what constitutes an optimal kind of historical investigation into the patient's problem but it's possible to have some organization in your mind as to what this eventually leads to. They believe you can't get that kind of information by doing an open-ended interview. I think one of my points was to demonstrate that you can do an open-ended interview and at the same time have a framework and get specific kinds of data that you feel are important.

B: What do you mean by an open-ended interview?

Dr. Thaler: Well, you listened to my questions. For instance, to ask a patient, "Can you tell me something about the setting in which this occurred?" is an open-ended question. To say to the patient,

"Did you have a pain in your chest?" is not an open-ended question. Any question in which the patient answers yes or no is not an open-ended question. Any question that forces the patient to respond in his own terms and to bring out what is in his mind and not in yours is an open-ended question.

Dr. Schuster: Your kind of interview is really a combination, and that is where the confusion arises in residents' and students' minds. They hear a so-called open-ended interview being conducted, and they think that's the only way you can interview a patient. You just say "uh huh" and let the patient go on and on. You cannot do that in the initial interview of many psychiatric patients, I don't think.

B: If a person comes to you; and your job is to try to help him without using certain words like chief complaint and present illness, suppose you use words like problem—what is the problem for which you want help? You are open-ended in the sense that you want to solve the problem, and solving the problem I assume always has to do with the patient's participation. Wouldn't that be a fundamental in which we'd all agree, that the concept of psychiatry or psychotherapy, I should say, implies that the patient must be an integral part of it. He can't be a passive recipient, or he doesn't change, doesn't grow up, he doesn't solve the problem. Well anyway, assuming that you then say what is the problem and then pursue it in an open-ended way, eventually you will come to the point—what do you think caused it, because you can't solve a problem without knowing the reason why it developed. Then I think the last stage is what can you do about changing the causes of this.

Dr. Thaler: Well, what's different about that, except the words? You're identifying the problem and assuming, I should think, that the patient comes to you because he thinks you know more about problem solving than he does, or he wouldn't need you. Hopefully you have been trained and are skillful in solving certain problems more effectively than the patient could by himself. Now, you have to identify what the problem is, the circumstances of how it arose, which again is just another way of saying you have to get to know the present illness.

B: I know but I'm trying to look at it almost more fundamentally.

Dr. Thaler: I don't get hung up on this business about the medical model.

B: Maybe you don't but I do, and a lot of people do.

Dr. Thaler: I don't think it matters very much whether you call it a "present illness" or whether you prefer to call it a "problem." As long as you approach the situation in a rational, intelligent, useful and meaningful way. . . .

Dr. Schuster: I'm interested in what your problem is in this, B. Why do you object to the use of these medical terms? You said you feel it should be more fundamental. What do you mean by that?

B: I wanted to talk about how you pursue the problem with the patient, because I'd like to talk about words like, do you do it logically, do you do it with using the conscious mind of the patient? It does seem to me that you go about this in a logical progression of solving the problem. The concept of problem-solving is fundamental, and yet in the end the patient has to be able to do this on his own— be able to solve his own problems. Therefore, how we go about solving the problem is awfully important, because you don't want the patient to be dependent on you in the end; you want him to have learned the technique of problem solving, the process of doing it.

Dr. Schuster: I think you're several steps ahead of us—first we have to identify the problem.

B: I know I'm several steps ahead, because of this concept of medical model. If you begin taking over and do not just pursue it logically with the patient and begin directing the interview, then you're destroying the ultimate goal, which is that the patient himself be able to do this.

Dr. Schuster: I don't think it's that tenuous. I mean, you can shift gears with a patient. For example, if you find that you're intruding too much on a patient by asking certain things that make him too anxious, then you retreat. But you do it skillfully, and you haven't destroyed the relationship at this point. I don't see how else you can identify the problem without asking questions. That doesn't mean you are directing the patient.

B: I know, but I mean it's how you ask the question.

Dr. Schuster: Why sure, you're right.

B: And shouldn't the questions be asked logically and open-endedly as Otto was suggesting? I mean if you pursue any problem logically you'll come to the right conclusion.

Dr. Schuster: Well, I'm all for being logical as much as I can, but I'm not sure what you mean by logical. For example, one very good reason for not abandoning medical knowledge in taking a history, in my opinion, is that at the outset I never know what I'm confronted with. When a patient comes to me and says he has back pain, because I'm a doctor, I'm going to think of other possibilities than psychological ones. I'm not going to assume that there's nothing but a psychological problem here. The very fact that over 50% of the patients on our in-patient floors have some kind of medical complication is enough of a warning to all of us that we still have to consider medical possibilities. So until I identify the problem and feel confident I'm dealing with almost purely emotional or psychological problems, I can't shift gears, I don't think.

B: Well then would you say that if you are convinced that it's truly psychological that you would do it this way?

Dr. Schuster: I think in the first place that it's too dichotomized. I don't think it's this way or that way, I think you have various blends. You can be both open-ended and directive in the same interview. You can ask questions, and you can retreat and let the patient take over. It's constantly fluctuating. I think the essence of a good interview is flexibility, and we needn't commit ourselves to some hard and fast course.

B: The reason that I keep hammering at this is, for example, I just finished talking to a resident who presented me with some paper that says that psychotherapy is no more effective than talking to a minister or a friend. Therefore, a lot of people feel that the whole of psychotherapy is a mish-mash, that nobody really knows what they are doing or why they are doing it. I think probably that a decade from now we'll probably all look back at this time as a very, very beginning of floundering around in understanding this concept of psychotherapy, or what makes a person happy or fulfilled, or however you want to put it. If possible, I think one of the things we should be trying to do here would be to take certain stands even though we may have to veer from them for certain reasons, as you suggest. At times we have to shift back and forth; I'm sure in practice that's true, but in principle—do we have certain principles that we wouldn't veer at all from if we were able to do so? That's what I'm driving at. Can we then give these to residents so they can have something to hold on to and feel that this is not a mish-mash but a principle?

Dr. Thaler: I think that's essentially the sort of thing we are trying to arrive at here over the course of our discussions—mainly what are some of the basic things we want to convey to our residents.

(We returned to the interview with the patient.)

> *Dr. Thaler*: So you were patrolling by yourself. What time in your shift was it?
>
> *Pt.*: It was about 10:00.
>
> *Dr. Thaler*: So you'd been out close to the end of your shift. How had it been going?
>
> *Pt.*: There hadn't been anything too much going on. As a matter of fact maybe it was a little less than usual. I think sometimes the quiet bothers me more.
>
> *Dr. Thaler*: When things are quiet it bothers you more than not. Can you recall in as much detail as possible just how this came on?
>
> *Pt.*: I stopped into the station, I don't know if I was transporting a prisoner or what.
>
> *Dr. Thaler*: You picked up somebody.
>
> *Pt.*: I picked up a prisoner from court.
>
> *Dr. Thaler*: Is this the sort of routine thing you do?
>
> *Pt.*: Oh yeah, a lot of times we transport somebody or commit them. I was in the station, and I went to the men's room. I bent down to the sink. When I did that I felt something like a pain.

B: I think in contrast to what Dr. X did, that you are pursuing something logically in an open-ended way, and I think that what he was doing was asking questions.

Dr. Thaler: Yeah, but he was also asking questions without a pattern.

B: Well, even let's suppose they had a pattern. It would still be bad, because he asked questions based on the problem.

Dr. Schuster: It's not whether or not you ask questions, it's what kind of questions you ask. Dr. X was skipping all around, here and there, with no pattern to it. He didn't pursue anything—no trend emerged from it. Now we're beginning to see and feel something about this man's life and what's going on. The skeleton is being filled out. I had no idea or feeling about this fellow before this.

B: It's allowing the patient to do it. He's doing it here; Otto is just supporting his doing it, whereas Dr. X was directing it or doing it for him which creates a passivity in the patient.

Dr. Schuster: To put it another way, he was turning him off and Otto isn't.

Dr. Thaler: In terms of technique I'm simply repeating what the patient said. "So you went to the bathroom," and he goes on in that direction.

> *Pt.*: Then I began to feel a sharp pain. Afterwards I went out and felt like I was going to pass out. When I felt that, I thought maybe I should take a Valium.

Dr. Thaler: I connected it with taking this prisoner. What about this prisoner? Could there be something specific to this particular person or the problem of that particular person that he had been responding to? I really didn't know, so I was waiting for more supportive data.

> *Pt.*: Yeah, It was the back that was hurting, and it started to get worse, so I turned around and came back in.

Dr. Thaler: How long did you last with it?

> *Pt.*: Oh, it lasted maybe an hour.

Dr. Thaler: So you were hurting for an hour before you came in.

Dr. Sandt: You said how long did you last, and he said how long did it last. What was in the question concerning his endurance which he dodged? The issue about what sort of ability you have to be a stoic or a spartan is involved in this guy.

Dr. Thaler: Yes, he mentioned it. He said in spite of the pain he went out.

Dr. Sandt: It's interesting he chose not to answer in that direction.

Dr. Schuster: Otto had in mind how long did the pain last, and he had in mind how long could he take it.

> *Pt.:* I figured I was out, and the way I was I really wasn't too much good to myself. I couldn't be any good to somebody else, so I might as well get in the office and get the car off the road and not have them depend on me.

> *Dr. Thaler:* It was getting that bad.

> *Pt.:* Yeah, so I came in and . . .

> *Dr. Thaler:* What were you feeling at that time?

> *Pt.:* I was mad and disgusted because it had come on, and I had to come in.

A: What I'd like to ask you—it's clear that that incident—something in that circumstance of bringing the prisoner in might be provoking symptoms. You obviously had some sense of that too. Was the prisoner male, female, old, young, what was the charge? Did you have some sort of reason why you didn't pursue it?

Dr. Thaler: I'm not sure if I asked him a question later or not. If I didn't pursue it, which is possible, I can't say at the moment. It seems logical that one should.

A: Something about his style emerges here. Namely, that he gets his symptoms, then he says I feel angry for having the symptoms. I would figure it the other way around—he's got symptoms because he's angry. I feel that incident may have been very important.

Dr. Thaler: Another possibility seems to be the feeling he states, that while it may be related to the incident it also deals with his being angry at himself—in the sense of a discrepancy between his self-image which is that of a tough cop and the event which is that of a guy who succumbs to backache.

Dr. Sandt: His standard is that his body should not give way under anything. I think your pursuit is worth pointing out, that retrospectively whatever you have in mind is that it's hard to be that conscious about why you're pursuing one course. But you would say one thing to Dr. X, that you're interested in information. You're pursuing what happened very much like a detective. The choice of the point at which one asks "How did you feel then?" is important. You could have asked him how he felt at a lot of places in the interview.

(We return to the interview.)

> *Dr. Thaler*: Show me where it hurts. Does it ever hurt in your side?
>
> *Pt.*: It starts here and comes up to my chest.
>
> *Dr. Thaler*: Do you get the pain on one side more than the other, or is it in both sides?
>
> *Pt.*: Sometimes the right side.
>
> *Dr. Thaler*: What sort of a sensation is it?
>
> *Pt.*: It's a real bad pain—you mean sting or what?
>
> *Dr. Thaler*: What adjective would you use?
>
> *Pt.*: Tightness, like a charlie horse.
>
> *Dr. Thaler*: Do you feel the muscles go tight in your back?
>
> *Pt.*: I don't feel the muscles tighten up, I can't move.
>
> *Dr. Thaler*: Is the pain sharp or dull?
>
> *Pt.*: Not dull enough.

Dr. Schuster: This raises another issue we haven't talked about. Otto uses the word "adjective," and it occurred to me, I wonder if he knows what is meant. This is an important problem for residents, learning how to talk to patients at different levels than their own. That's very difficult for all of us. We tend to be accustomed to talking to each other and communicating in a certain syntax and using certain vocabulary. Then we get to talking with patients who may not have the same level of understanding, and we have to modify it. This is one of the things you see medical students and residents doing all the time, asking complicated questions with medical vocabulary such as, "Do you have angina pectoris?"

Pt.: It's a good pain.

Dr. Thaler: It's a *good* pain. (He said it's a good pain and I emphasized this and I wanted X to hear this so I repeated it.) Does the pain feel like it's outside on the surface or does it feel like it's deep inside you?

Pt.: It feels more deep, feels more interior.

Dr. Thaler: Does it concentrate in any one part eventually?

Pt.: Well, it's sort of—I took the Darvon and I slept and I take hot baths and I massage with hot packs and it seems to work it out of me. It really exhausts me by the time it's over.

Dr. Thaler: It's obviously not a localized pain. Would it go to one spot or is it just sort of all over?

Pt.: I don't really know, I'll say it's not in one specific area, but it is worse in the back and through here.

Dr. Thaler: The problem here is he thought I wanted a specific answer. When I gave him two choices, is it in one spot or all over he wonders what is it this guy wants to hear? Would he rather hear it's in one spot, or would it please him better that it's all over? It also indicates to me that it's not a localized pain. If somebody has a localized pain, and you ask him, he's bound to say it's right here.

Dr. Thaler: Do you remember anything else about the kind of a day?

Pt.: I can't remember prior to coming to work. I know it (the pain) causes a lot of family tension.

Dr. Thaler: Is it like that all the time?

B: It seems to me there's quite an emphasis on your part in obtaining details of physical complaints, when I assume that you believe that the problems he has are emotional ones. What, for instance, would prevent you from cutting through and saying, "Do you feel that some of these problems that you're experiencing have to do with emotional problems that you have, problems of your living or your life that are affecting you?"

Dr. Thaler: Well, I thought that it was too early for that. Now let's assume for the moment—I think part of this was my need to establish fairly firmly in my own mind that this man was not experiencing coronary pain. Now even though it had been coronary pain, I still would have been interested to know what brings it on, whether it's coronary pain or whether it's the result of an emotional problem, with no organic background. The next step, then, is to establish the situation in which the discomfort arises. I think one would handle it differently if he had said, "Well you know, come to think of it, it is a severe crushing pain, and sometimes I feel it in my left arm." I think I would have been a little bit more cautious about pursuing the circumstances and having him recall and relive the circumstances under which the pain arises.

A: I want to ask a question which has intrigued me. I think it touches on many issues. It's curious that to a psychologist working with many residents this issue of symptoms becomes very important. I'll grant you that I'm not medically trained. It's also a point that I might have a bias toward in my profession. This is what I want to say. I believe that as a psychiatrist you have a certain job. This job could be put in various layman terms—that you are an emotional-problem doctor or a mind doctor, as opposed to a dentist or an obstetrician or whatever. So if a patient comes to see you, then it's principally because of that. Now if he comes with a long list of symptoms, my bias is to say "Why don't you see a doctor?" Which means he's got to say to you "Well, okay, I have these symptoms, and I can see a doctor, but what about my problem?" I think that one of the things I see in residents is that as soon as there is any anxiety they collaborate with the patient to pretend that there's a medical problem. I'm wondering if it must be really hard for you, the physician, when a patient is presenting an intriguing possibility, maybe a coronary, for you to resist saying, "Well, I hear you have these symptoms, and they may be serious, but you should see an internist about them."

Dr. Thaler: I have a different opinion. I don't see this as a difficulty. I see it as an extra dimension that I can deal with, and I view the human organism holistically. I reject any kind of dichotomizing or mind-body relations. This is perhaps what medical training teaches us—never to take anybody else's previous examinations or data for granted; always get your own information. First of all, we know that even if the previous physician has done everything he was supposed to do, we know that patients don't always tell everything the first time. The patient, on the other hand, may come for emotional problems—it's his idea that's what he's got, but he doesn't know. He's not an expert to decide this, nor is the general practitioner who sent him. If I say to him, "Go back to your doctor," he's going to say "Well, I've just been to my doctor, and he told me to come here."

Dr. Schuster: Well, it is bad if it results in a collaboration to avoid a psychological implication.

A: I just want to find out, because I agree with the whole listening point of view. I think it's important to hear the symptoms in terms of relating them to a framework we have, which is that life events may be precipitants. I think it's a tricky thing for you to say, "Well, how do we know we can trust the doctor?"; you see, that's presumptuous. How does he know he can trust *you?* I think you as a psychiatrist are then assuming a role which is inappropriate. You're saying that a heart physician may not really know, but I can find out more than he can—that's very tricky.

Dr. Thaler: That's not the point. It's not that I can't trust the doctor. Even if I know him, or if he's my own physician I know that the next guy often gets more data than the first guy regardless of his competency, so it's my job.

A: But he hasn't come to you as a body physician—to put it in crude terms.

Dr. Thaler: He's come to me as a physician, which means I'm supposed to take care of whatever ails him and refer him if necessary. I will refer him back if I feel it's really somatic.

C: I think there's another reason for a psychiatrist's being interested, and that has to do with the fact that the patient takes his symptoms quite seriously, notwithstanding the possibility that the psychiatrist will ultimately want to come to a conclusion with the patient that in some ways these are tied up with emotional variables. I think it would be a constructive communication if he were to say to the patient, "I do want to hear about your pain," because all too often the opposite side of the coin obtains, where the patient comes out of the interview convinced that his doctor's not interested in the nature of his experience. Whether the pain is emotionally based or not, damn it, it hurts this guy. Recently I saw a young girl whose symptoms were vomiting, back pain and stomach pain. I'd seen her for testing, and during the course of the testing she said, "Look, there's one thing I want you to know, it really hurts." So I said "Why do you say this to me?" and she said, "Because I think the doctor thinks I'm putting it on, that I'm imagining it." Then she made a very interesting statement. She said, "Look, maybe I bring this on, but when it comes on it hurts."

A: I think there's a subtle thing here which I haven't expressed. I'm not disinterested in the symptoms or anything else. He may be talking about the anguish he feels, because his pet has run away. I'm interested. What I'm saying is, I'm here to understand you as a person, and I'll hear what you've got to say whether it's the pain in your body or the anguish about something else, but I'm not here to make a physical disposition leading to my treating you physically. This is what I mean, and this is often not conveyed by a resident, because he hopes it *will* be a physical symptom he can treat. I think that's inappropriate.

Dr. Thaler: I agree with that, but I think where we seem to need to clarify our viewpoints is that I would not say that the resident should pursue the physical symptoms with conviction they are physical symptoms that he can treat. Now, what he should do then if he's convinced there is a physical symptom that needs treating, is arrange for it to be taken care of by the patient's physician. There is, of course, the danger of collusion between the patient and the psychiatrist to focus on the symptom. I think where this is most commonly seen is in conversion hysteria where the patient comes with some physical complaint of paralysis or whatever it is and says, "Shouldn't I have another X-ray?" Here it's important to say "Look, you've had all the examinations that are necessary. I've talked with your doctor who's done all this, and that's not your problem. Now, let's get on with our work."

A: I want to very briefly give you an example of how medicine can be a major communication. This is a patient who every time you talk about anything in his life says, "Well, I'm fine." Now he's been to see four psychiatrists and every one of them fell right into this and spent months talking about the chemistry of giving him one drug after another and getting nowhere. Being forewarned, I listened sympathetically to this and then I said, "Well, you know I'm a psychologist. I don't know anything about this. Is there anything else I can do for you?" He had a big smile on his face, and I said, "You're smiling." He said, "Yeah, you're the first person not to argue with me about the chemistry." I replied, "You may be right, but what else can I do for you?" Then he conceded, "Well, I'm a little anxious," and he got very panicky. This is what happens with many residents, they get lost trying to argue the patient out of the chemical business, and it doesn't work; or else they say we'll try this drug or that drug.

Dr. Thaler: I think that's a perfectly appropriate response that you made, and which I might have made also in the same way. I might have said, "Well, if it's chemical there isn't much I can do about that, but what else can we do here?" So what you're really saying is that one has to be able to recognize the physical complaint as a resistance and deal with it as such, and that's where the psychiatrist has it over another medical practitioner who may not recognize the psychological implications.

> *Pt.*: I think my family right now is suffering because of these spasms.

> *Dr. Thaler*: When was the very first time you had an attack?

> *Pt.*: It was about two or three years ago. It was after I had been on the Department for quite a while. It was very hot, in the summer. I'd worked hard, and it was a 4-12 shift.

Dr. Thaler: Another thing which X has not asked about was when did his symptoms start. What was the setting in which they started? It turns out that 2 or 3 years, ago, when I got down to specific dates, was approximately the time that his child was born and when the whole thing started.

Dr. Schuster: I was curious about what he meant about this pain increasing tension within the family.

Dr. Thaler: I think the fact that he complains that he hurts and is sick periodically.

A: It could also mean that his symptoms are a weapon against the family.

Dr. Thaler: Interestingly enough one of the most significant statements he made we didn't get on tape. He made it, as patients often do, on his way out. He said something about there are other men in the force who have problems in the family, and it turned out later he meant his wife. He said they take a drink, or they run away, or they take up with other women. He said, "You know, I don't want this to destroy my family."

> *Dr. Thaler:* How long had you been with the police by then?
>
> *Pt.:* I'd been with them for two summers, but I'd been bothered by colitis before this. I'd never been bothered by colitis until I was going for the State Police and got notice that I'd passed the written test and that I'd have to lose 15 or 20 pounds in about a month. I went on a real crash diet, and that's when the colitis developed.
>
> *Dr. Thaler:* When you first had this attack you said it woke you out of a sleep. Do you remember if you had been having dreams?
>
> *Pt.:* I don't remember with the first one if I had or not, but I know that I had the upset stomach which I get when things are tense.
>
> *Dr. Thaler:* Can you tell me about a dream like the ones you've been having?
>
> *Pt.:* Yes, I can tell you about two.

B: Well, aren't you now doing what X did—jumping around?

Dr. Thaler: I am jumping around a little bit, because I had a number of things I wanted to get at. Actually he had told me that he had awakened from a sleep with the first pain, but I wanted to focus on that because X hadn't talked about it. There was another issue I wanted to bring up, too, before we stopped, and that was about the Army. I wanted to get that data, because I felt it was useful to know what his Army experience was like in terms of how it was different from the police experience. Why didn't he have symptoms when he was in the Army? I picked up a number of points during X's interview which I felt he didn't pursue, although he should have. I pursue them both to instruct him as well as to get some information which I need. I'm not conducting my own initial interview. I feel this is a different kind of a set, so I had three issues I wanted to get at: 1. I wanted to find out more about this incident in detail; 2. I wanted to find out about the onset of this incident; and 3. I wanted to hear something about the dream. Incidentally, I had noticed over several diagnostic interviews I've had with X that three or four of these patients spontaneously reported having had dreams on the night before they came to the interview. I began to get interested in this, and I also wanted to know something about his Army experience. I'd have to interrupt him and ask a question, but I knew what questions I was going to ask. This may be a matter for discussion as to whether one should do this at all, should one do it for this purpose, what's in it for the patient, is it for teaching? So many issues can arise with this sort of thing.

A: You're under pressure of time, because you have little time and a pedagogic role.

Dr. Thaler: I *was* under pressure. I usually have between 15 and 20 minutes to ask what I feel I need to know.

B: Well, I think that there's a problem of his passivity in his relationship to both of you. He is compliantly responding to a number of questions that are put to him rather than getting at what he feels are some of the reasons for why he feels the way he does. I don't know about your interview, because you had certain things in mind and you had to get to them so you jump in at this point.

Dr. Thaler: Your thoughts are that it would have been better not to do this.

C: Well, I don't agree with you, B, because I think in that last sentence before we stopped was the first time that he referred to the therapist with the word "you." He said "I'll tell *you* two of them" after Otto asked about the dream. He seems more spontaneous, and it seems to be a signal of a relationship, a kind of bond, between the interviewer and the patient.

Dr. Schuster: Just because he uses the word "you"?

C: Yeah, "I'll tell *you*." I mean it's an acknowledgment of the therapist. You see the patient sits there for an hour, and he simply responds to the questions. Then for the first time he says I'll tell *you* something.

B: But he's been telling you something all the way along.

C: But the fact that he says, "I'll tell *you* two of them," indicates he's going beyond a passive response.

B: I think he's saying I'll tell you, because he's in deeper in passivity.

C: Passivity is an interesting notion, because the patient is there to talk to the doctor, and he is the source of information. The doctor is listening in a diagnostic interview. If the patient came in and said in effect, "Now shut up, I'm going to tell you what's wrong with me" and tried to control the interview we'd get upset by that.

Dr. Thaler: I think what C is saying is the phrase that he used is a sign that there is an engagement developing. It would be interesting to have a video tape of this. The quality of the patient's voice does change gradually over the course of my interview. He becomes more animated. I was physically, motorically, kinetically communicating in a very different way. X was sitting back like this, and I was leaning forward talking to the patient; and we were having a two-way conversation and all sorts of things were going on nonverbally.

D: Otto, speaking now of the supervisory relationship in a time sequence of the 50 minutes, how long is your portion of this interview?

Dr. Thaler: About 10 or 15 minutes. I usually ask the resident to interview the patient for ¾ of an hour or so, then I interview for the balance of the hour. I feel usually to talk with the patient for an hour is enough for the patient, much beyond that is tiring. Then we have another half hour to discuss the case.

D: When I listen now to your action in this interview, I wonder if you're moving in almost to take over and wrap things up. Could you not have let Dr. X close off the first interview, and then given him suggestions for the second interview?

Dr. Thaler: That's another question in terms of how would you conduct this, I mean, it's simply another way of doing it.

A: I want to come back to the animation of the patient. You saw this as engagement. My hunch as to what's happened is this: he was giving you this long, enlightened, monologue of his physical symptoms, and now he was trying out a different sort of thing. Maybe he felt you weren't going to get to talking like a doctor, so he reminded you. He said his family's tense. Finally when you came in with this dream, he saw it as a refreshing break. It's like both of you have been getting nowhere, so let's talk about the real stuff. That's why he became animated with you. This is what he wants to get off his chest. He's had a series of doctors that he's given this monologue to before he came here.

(We return to Dr. Thaler's interview.)

> *Pt.*: Yeah, I can tell you about one, I'll tell you about two (dreams). The first one I had when I was working. There was myself and a partner, another police officer. We were trying to apprehend two guys just like on television, and we were being fired at.

> *Dr. Thaler*: Has that happened to you before?

> *Pt.*: Have I been shot at before?

> *Dr. Thaler*: Yeah.

> *Pt.*: I've never been shot at. We were going to go up a hill, and somehow we got up the hill. We got them up against the wall, and I was frisking one of them, and I had the gun, and I bent over. I bent over to frisk down one pant leg, and when I did he spun around and grabbed for the gun as I came up. The guy was standing right there with it like it was real, ready to pull the trigger. This was it, there was no out, and I woke up.

> *Dr. Thaler*: Just as he was pulling the trigger?

> *Pt.*: Yeah, I woke up, and I was in a sweat.

Dr. Thaler: It's a very vivid memory.

Pt.: Yeah, like it really happened.

Dr. Thaler: When was this?

Pt.: It was maybe a month or two ago. Then I just had another one. We had an accident. An oil truck went down a side road, so we followed and somebody jumped from the oil truck. There were two guys in the truck, and it turned out that we were trying to apprehend these guys for something. Then when I got to this point of apprehension I woke up.

Dr. Thaler: Is there any one dream that comes back over and over again?

Pt.: The last few have been about apprehending somebody.

Dr. Thaler: When you were in the service were you engaged in combat?

Pt.: I wasn't in combat, I was on a Nike site, but we were actually in a combat situation—we were tactical.

Dr. Thaler: Now I'm going on to the next question which I had in mind which involved mainly his experiences in the service.

Dr. Thaler: Where was this?

Pt.: This was in Germany during the Berlin Crisis. But we were tactical all the time. It was the same for us as if it was war time. We weren't a non-tactical unit like the rest of them. We used to have unidentified aircraft and stuff, and I had 12 men under me.

Dr. Thaler: During the time you were in the Army did you ever have any troubles of this sort?

Pt.: The only time we had problems was every time we got an unidentified aircraft, we assumed it was an enemy aircraft. Actually it wasn't a case where you say we're pretending. This was the actual thing. All that time

we didn't know if it was an enemy aircraft, or what
it was. We actually were hooked straight up to the
missiles and everything. We were ready to fire on the
aircraft until we got identification. We used to get them
quite often.

Dr. Thaler: Did you experience any difficulties like
you do now?

Pt.: I didn't have time I guess, maybe.

Dr. Thaler: No pains, no sweats, no stomach trouble
or anything like that?

Pt.: No.

Dr. Thaler: So that didn't seem to bother you as much
as some of what's going on right now?

Pt.: Yeah, it didn't seem to bother me then. I knew
that possibly any thing could happen during the Berlin Crisis. We were the first target if anything had
happened; and I knew that maybe some day it could
happen. I know that the pressure was there. There was
a tremendous amount of pressure.

Dr. Thaler: The interesting thing to me was that he was in a very
tense situation there with the crisis and the missiles and all that,
and he was about to begin World War III, and yet there were no
symptoms. But the symptoms began after the birth of his child.
That's the fantastic thing. Here the whole fate of the world is in
balance, and he doesn't have symptoms!
D: There was an *external* danger, which was more comfortable.
Dr. Thaler: Sure, and I thought it was important for the resident to see the difference between that situation and how well
the patient handled it and the present situation in which he falls
apart.

Dr. Thaler: When did you get out of the service?

Pt.: I got out of the service about five years ago.

Dr. Thaler: Did you consider staying in?

Pt.: Yeah, I passed the O.C.S. test and everything, and I was going to Officer Candidate School; and I turned it down, because I decided to get out.

Dr. Thaler: Can you tell me why?

Pt.: Yeah, I'd seen some things in there. Situations where first and second lieutenants had gotten blamed for things that maybe they were responsible for but weren't *directly* responsible for, and in my estimation I don't think that they were responsible. I think that somebody else should have gotten the ax, but they got the ax because the commanding officer had to put it in his report that he had taken action, so he gave somebody else the ax.

Dr. Thaler: So you felt there was injustice?

Pt.: Yeah, I felt that it was indeed an injustice, and I figured that if I was put in a command position at any time and I had to do something like that in order to save face, I'd rather look for something else to do. I can't take dirty politics and stuff like that. This is the type of thing that really gets me.

Dr. Thaler: You're very strong on that.

Pt.: Very much so. I believe in honesty.

Dr. Thaler: So to see that sort of thing happening must have hurt?

Pt.: Sure it hurts. Just like it hurts now to see it happening.

Dr. Thaler: At that time what you did was to quit?

Pt.: Yeah, I got out and left it, but my wife was sort of tired travelling at that time, too. She was with me at that time.

Dr. Thaler: How long have you been married?

Pt.: I've been married since 1960.

Dr. Thaler: Children?

Pt.: I have one now.

Dr. Thaler: How old?

Pt.: Two or two and a half—well, will be three in December.

Dr. Thaler: You see all these data Dr. X didn't get in the first interview. How long the patient has been married, he didn't know anything about the marriage, and the other things which you really need to know.

Dr. Sandt: It's the birth of the child. There was a hint before that what sent this man into anxiety was the birth of a child. Now you want to know how long they were married before the birth of that child, the postponement index for the anxiety. Why didn't he have a child for that long, was it really on the basis of anxiety?

Dr. Thaler: Boy or girl?

Pt.: (long pause) Boy.

Dr. Thaler: I asked him whether it was a boy or a girl, and he wasn't saying which it was very quickly.

Dr. Sandt: Well, you already know that his problem is the child. The whole business of the sex of that child is important.

Dr. Thaler: It's interesting asking this kind of a question. I was talking with some first-year residents about an interview that one of them did—a first interview, the first time the resident saw the patient on the ward. After the interview was done, he knew nothing about the patient. I inquired "Why didn't you ask?", and his response was "You're not supposed to ask any direct questions."

Dr. Sandt: Where do they learn this? I don't know any textbook that tells you that.

Dr. Thaler: It's really a myth or fantasy. I know, because I've been on the in-patient service. We don't teach that, I don't teach that. It all has to do with the medical model. You're not supposed to use the medical model.

Dr. Sandt: No, but I'm saying that a medical model doesn't have to be a checklist of organ systems.

Dr. Thaler: One of the things I'm trying to demonstrate with the interviews I conduct is the associative anamnestic technique. In other words, a patient mentions his wife, then you ask about the wife. As you go along you get it all, but you also have to ask about his marriage and all that.

Dr. Sandt: That's relevant, you know the whole thing is to get it in some kind of organized manner.

Dr. Thaler: If he says we got married last week, and he's got an anxiety attack that's one thing. But to be married for five years, and to have an anxiety attack five years later, that's another thing!

Dr. Sandt: How did they respond to this after you pointed it out?

Dr. Thaler: With astonishment and gratitude. They were relieved. "You mean we can really ask questions?"

D: I think sometimes the residents feel that to ask a direct question means being too intrusive.

Dr. Thaler: It's not being open-ended. Their idea of being open-ended is that you never ask anybody anything. From watching these guys behind the screen doing interviews I know that the easiest thing for them is to sit there and say, "yes, go on—you seem to be upset about this, please go on." It's not the way for them to get any specific data. It's a strange thing. I don't understand it, but that's what they all feel. I think part of it is that they don't really know what to do, and the easiest thing is to do nothing.

Dr. Schuster: But if they hadn't been through an internship, I would be a little less surprised. They've been on an internship where they've had to get medical histories and have had to ask patients direct questions.

Dr. Thaler: But also they come here with a strong fantasy of what it is to be a psychiatrist, and many of them think it's totally different from what they've done up until now. Secondly, they have in their minds this model of the reflective, Buddha-like, mirror-image type guy who never says anything.

(We return to the patient's response to Dr. Thaler's question, "Boy or girl?" in which he paused and replied, Boy.)

Dr. Sandt: Did you get that? You could almost see him checking it out.

Dr. Thaler: He hesitated for a shorter period of time when he was asked about the age than he did with the sex.

Dr. Thaler: How is it with you and the boy?

Pt.: Pretty tight, pretty tight, close together. We waited 8 years.

Dr. Thaler: You waited 8 years because you had to, or . . .

Pt.: Finally he came along and . . .

Dr. Thaler: That was good for you.

Pt.: That was good for me, but I think these things that we talked about, like the fact that you might walk up to a car and get shot or something like that—I didn't really think too much about it until he came along.

Dr. Thaler: That didn't worry you until he came along?

Dr. Schuster: What did he mean about he and the child were tight?

Dr. Thaler: Tight, they're very close. Although that's a very interesting way to speak of it.

Dr. Sandt: That's very interesting and he said it a couple of times.

D: I was thinking "up-tight," you know.

Dr. Thaler: They're very close, but he gets up tight about that.

Dr. Sandt: That's what he's really saying.

Pt.: Now I got two foster kids too. My first cousin died in an auto accident about three years ago, and then their mother died from ill health.

Dr. Sandt: That covers all the modes of death—accident and ill health.

Dr. Thaler: What's also been going on currently is that this cousin died, and the cousin's wife died, and he's taken the couple's two children into the home. I don't think he's adopted them, but he's taking care of them.

Dr. Schuster: That's about the same time they had their own child.

Dr. Sandt: Yes, that's all gone on. He's really very responsible now. A lot of people are dependent upon him.

Dr. Thaler: Interestingly, one of the major things we didn't get down on tape he said as he left the office. "You know there are other guys that I know who take care of their tensions in a different way, they run around with women, they get drunk, they do this, they do that." He then added, "I don't want to destroy my family."

What I did at this point was set up a second time with the patient. Usually Dr. X does the second one by himself, but I thought I had noticed that he was having a lot of trouble with this patient. There were some things that I think we really didn't go into that we had intended to. In the patient's presence I said that I would like to set up another appointment together with him.

> *Dr. Thaler*: I'd like to get some dates straight in my own mind about your problems. When was the onset of your attacks? How can you pinpoint the date?
>
> *Pt.*: It was about July or August of 1966.
>
> *Dr. Thaler*: 1966 or 1967?
>
> *Pt.*: 1966.
>
> *Dr. Thaler*: Four years ago?
>
> *Pt.*: Well let's see—I got out in 1965, about 1967.
>
> *Dr. Thaler*: Three years ago.
>
> *Pt.*: Yeah. He (his son) was born on December 23, 1967.

Dr. Thaler: I was trying to demonstrate to the resident the need for precision. You've got to know whether it was three years or four years ago. It makes a difference in terms of the event that preceeds it. If it was four years ago the wife wasn't even pregnant yet. It turns out it was three years ago at a time when the wife was almost ready to deliver. This is so impressive to the resident, to see this time relationship demonstrated. I think we talked the other day about whether you should do a supplementary interview or not. We did not need to discuss the reason why I asked these questions, it was obvious. One of the more effective ways of teaching with this particular resident was to do these supplementary interviews. All he'd have to do was hear what I was asking, which he hadn't, and he got the message:

> *Dr. Thaler*: When did this thing happen with your cousin? When you adopted the kids.
>
> *Pt.*: This was just recently. We didn't adopt them. I took them in. I saw the position they were in, so I went to the Social Services, and now I've got them as foster children.
>
> *Dr. Thaler*: How long have you had them?
>
> *Pt.*: Since last January.
>
> *Dr. Thaler*: Well, we're going to have to stop now.

Before the patient left, Dr. Thaler arranged to see him a second time with Dr. X. He did this because of the difficulties Dr. X was having with the patient, and because time didn't permit him to obtain all the information he needed to help X proceed wih this case. Dr. Thaler then spent a few minutes discussing his initial impressions of this patient.

> *Dr. Thaler*: Dr. X had seen (in the out-patient area) so many things that he'd never seen before. This was one example of the kind of situation he hadn't come across before. You don't see this kind of thing on an in-patient floor, and he was constantly in a state of astonishment at the very different clinical material that he was now seeing in the clinic.
>
> *Dr. Thaler*: Does something strike you about the dates?
>
> *Dr. X*: Yeah, and I think he hesitated when he said what sex the child is. It was this time when his wife was pregnant.

Dr. Thaler: Yeah, you see it's very interesting because first he said it was 2½ to 3 years ago that was the onset. After he'd talked about the boy, he makes it 4 years, then says no, it's really 3 years. It was just as the wife began to show that she was pregnant. His symptoms started in August, and she delivered in December of 1967. There are all kinds of things involved. It reminds me of the retreads in Korea. These were the guys during the Korean War who were recalled from the reserves for active duty in Korea. Many of these fellows had been remembered as officers of great distinction during World War II. They mustered out, went in the reserves, they got married, had families, started businesses and then they were called back into the service in Korea. Within a very short period of time they decompensated. The difference now was that these people had established their relationships, they were responsible for families, and it was a totally different ball game. They could not tolerate the stress of combat under those circumstances, and I have a hunch that this may be what's going on with this guy. In other words, there was one point earlier in the interview when he said "maybe I am" then he said, "lack self-confidence." What he was going to say is maybe I am yellow. This guy with all his needs to defend against passivity, then has combat dreams. I have a feeling that this man is ashamed, that he is scared now, because of a different life situation, of getting hurt. He has no way of getting out, because his self-respect does not allow him to quit the police. I wonder whether one could help him at that level, no deeper than that, to recognize some of these feelings and perhaps find something else for him to do in life.

Dr. X: I'm worried about this patient, I think he was not telling the truth.

Dr. Thaler: Well, he may have been. He denies a lot. This guy—I jotted down some of the way he talks—and really one of his major defenses has been denial. "I don't think I'm God, I don't think I'm perfect, I don't feel people have to see this my way, I don't like politicians, there is no true justice," and everything he was talking about was in the negative. He was denying all kinds of stuff.

Dr. Thaler: One of the problems, as I listened to myself here, was the lack of organization. I was excited about the situation of this very interesting patient, and I was talking off the top of my head. I would appreciate some comments about that. In other words, on the one hand I think the supervisor's enthusiasm for the case may be very impressive to the resident. I think it has been to Dr. X. On the other hand, are these the things that are most necessary to talk about with the resident at the end of an interview? In a sense we were free associating to the material, and I'm now asking for comments, because as I listened to myself I felt a lack of organization in my comments to the resident. What is most needed to talk about with him after the entire interview?

Dr. Schuster: Well, before we get to that I would be curious about your reaction and his reaction to the patient. Your enthusiasm and his astonishment. What do you think grabbed him about this patient?

Dr. Thaler: Well I think for one thing he had expected something quite different. You remember earlier before we even started, he was concerned he was going to be a typical cop. Particularly this resident, he's trying to make an effort to be "with it," to be with the times. So he felt concerned, I think, about his own countertransference feelings. And what happens in the interview—a cop comes and talks about his own concern about justice, and how he doesn't like to do things that are unjust, and how he's concerned about young people.

Dr. Schuster: It kind of jarred Dr. X.

Dr. Thaler: Now he's developed a very positive feeling toward this patient. Also he's noticed that although the guy was a big and heavy man, he was quite passive, and he didn't threaten him at all. Dr. X expected to be afraid of him. It turned out that this man was anything but somebody to be afraid of. Also I think his getting the idea that maybe he could help the patient was important. In the beginning he was afraid this might be a very difficult, threatening patient who was not suitable for treatment. He now changes his mind about that and says this is somebody I can help.

DEVELOPMENTAL PROBLEMS OF THE PSYCHIATRIC RESIDENT

This section begins with Dr. Thaler discussing with Dr. X his patient and the interview. The first aspect taken up by the conference was Dr. X's perception of the patient as suicidal. Some members of the conference found it difficult to understand what there was about the patient that impressed the resident as "suicidal." This led us into a discussion of how to handle the resident's misperception of the patient—what counter-transference factors may have been at work. This in turn brought us to discuss some of the developmental aspects of a psychiatric resident in training—particularly his struggle to master interviewing techniques. We touch on the confusion in the young psychiatrist's mind over such matters as the "open-ended interview," the "psychoanalytic model," the concept of "neutrality," and various approaches to the interview situation.

(We return to Dr. Thaler's supervision of the case with Dr. X.)

> Dr. X: I'm worried about this guy. I thing he's suicidal.
>
> Dr. Thaler: Very depressed?
>
> Dr. X: I think he was not telling the truth.

Dr. Schuster: What was your estimate of the patient's suicidal potential?

Dr. Thaler: I wasn't concerned.

Dr. Schuster: I wasn't impressed that he was suicidal as we listened to the interview. What made X have that impression?

Dr. Thaler: Well, I'm not sure. I think it has to do again with some of the things we brought out before about his whole approach to this man. Remember first he was scared of him, now he's scared for him.

Dr. Schuster: From a pedagogic standpoint would it be any help to halt at that point and ask him what led him to this estimate of the patient?

Dr. Thaler: Yeah, I think so. I'm not sure, but my last comment was that I wasn't as worried about suicide as he. I don't know whether I elicited more from him on why he thought that or not. If I didn't, I should have.

Dr. Schuster: You think it's part of his being afraid of this patient.

Dr. Thaler: Yeah, I think so. First he was afraid of him and now he's protecting him.

Dr. Schuster: What's so striking to me all the way through in this particular case is there's nothing, or not much, that comes through in the verbal content that gives us an explanation of X's reaction and attitude toward the patient. There must have been a lot in other than the verbal production, like the appearance of the patient and his non-verbal behavioral attributes. Dr. X ends up feeling the aggression he attributed to this man has to be shifted from homicidal impulses to suicidal ones.

Dr. Thaler: If you had more time would you tend to elicit or convey some of the things you've just said about his changing attitude toward the patient?

Dr. Schuster: Yeah, I think so. I think I'd start by asking why do you think this patient is suicidal? Then I might say that I don't see this.

Dr. Thaler: But will you then tell him, "It seems to me that you have switched gears here. You were first concerned about the patient's aggression towards you."

Dr. Schuster: Well I might or might not depending upon how he took the initial question.

C: Well I think I'd be least inclined to do that. I might go as far as to say, "You may want to think about why it was necessary for you to see him as suicidal."

Dr. Thaler: Think of it at a number of levels. One could say, "Look, the data do not indicate that he's suicidal." The next step would be to ask, "What are your data?" He might say I thought this and this and this. You reply by asking does this add up to a psychotic depression, and he would have to say no. The next step then would be to ask, "Then, why did you have to see him as suicidal?"

B: Then what would likely come out would be the anxiety that every resident, and I think probably every doctor feels: am I going to be able to help this fellow? Am I going to be able to do something that's going to make me feel like I've fulfilled my role in life as a psychiatrist? That's a common anxiety and something all of us feel.

Dr. Schuster: I tend to feel that one has to go a little farther here than one ordinarily would, simply because the entire handling of this case hinges on what appears to us to be a largely irrational countertransference reaction on the resident's part. He cannot see the things that we feel are important for him to see about this patient. So I do feel compelled to go farther. Maybe you could put it to him simply by saying, "There's something about this patient that bugs you more than I think it should."

B: The implication is there when you use the word counter-transference.

Dr. Schuster: I wouldn't use that term to him.

B: Well it may not even be counter-transference. It may simply be that this is a threatening situation to any young, inexperienced person trying to face. . . .

C: Most of us feel that's not why X handled it the way he did. I mean, what you're saying is probably true and is probably present in virtually any young, new resident; but we don't really believe that that's what it was here. I think he was scared to death of this guy, this big man. I think he was angry with him.

B: Why? Why was he scared of this big man?

C: I don't know X well enough to tell you that, but I could guess a little. I think it was pretty obvious from the interview that X had a lot of private feelings that colored his perception about some things about the patient.

Dr. Schuster: What you're saying, B, is applicable to a first-year resident who's on an in-patient floor with a lot of crazy people, a really frightening kind of psychotic patient. Then everybody would share this anxiety you speak about.

B: Haven't you experienced the feeling with a new patient who might not be a policeman but let's say a very prominent person in the community, the wife of a psychiatrist, a feeling of added worry.

Dr. Thaler: I think that in terms of our clinical perception as supervisors that we all seem to be agreeing that this is more than a kind of normative anxiety produced by your VIP.

A: We're omitting something very important—the anxiety may or may not be normative, that's hard to say, but what is clear is that whatever is upsetting X has led to distortion. Once that happens, I think you can call it counter-transference. If it's counter-transference, you want to get at that. One of the things I always do at some point after the first interview is to say to the resident, "How did you feel about this *person*, not *patient*?" That gets it out of the framework where he can stop talking about the patient and talk about what this person was like for him. "Well, he was kind of aggressive, and I don't really like that sort of person." Maybe that would lead him a little.

Dr. Thaler: That is very useful. I've done that a lot on the floors when I've been dealing with groups of students and residents. I've interviewed a patient and usually my first question is, "How do you feel about this person?" Then they say he's a schizophrenic. "That's not what I'm asking. How do you feel, what's your gut response to this interview?" The question that we're struggling with, and it's an important one, is what is the borderline between our pedagogic job and therapeutic intervention?

C: Well, what's the most you could expect as a consequence of your intervention in the direction of some exploration of X's behavior in this situation?

Dr. Thaler: What you could expect I think is for him to recognize an attitude of which he was not aware up until that point, not its genetic roots, but the mere fact that he was performing or doing something in a way different than expected. Play the tape back to him and tell him this is where you were angry.

C: What would be the next level of awareness that anybody could expect of him?

Dr. Thaler: The next level would be for him to have some recognition of why he felt that way. In other words, "It must be because I have this stereotype about cops."

C: I think you can end by saying, "Maybe you'd like to think about this." It suggests to the resident that it would be worth some exploration on his part and also respects the issue of privacy, because too far you cannot go.

Dr. Thaler: But even a statement of maybe you ought to think about that is potentially a pretty explosive thing to say, because he may interpret this as your saying, "Look, you know you've got a problem, maybe you ought to get therapy."

C: He may want to think more about it. If the resident comes to that inference from what I say, then I would say there is a significant personal addition to the content of my statement to make him think about whether he should have therapy.

Dr. Schuster: He might say, "Come to think about it I have an awful lot of trouble with certain kinds of patients."

C: But if he were to ask, "Are you telling me I need to go into therapy?" as a consequence of that remark, then I'd think he's added enough of his own projection into my comment for me to think maybe he should. He's made a big leap from, "I want you to think more about why you did this," to "Are you telling me I need therapy?" There was one other thing I wanted to see if the group had any ideas about. After the kind of thing we've spoken about, it would be worthwhile exploring with the resident as to whether he can recognize in himself some cues as to when he's going to *begin* to deviate, to retreat to rigid and stereotyped and perseverative kinds of human behaviors which inevitably lead to not seeing the data. I'm not sure about this, but every once in a while there is a resident who happens to get something like this, and you may not get very far with any insight on his part as to why he felt the may he did; but he can pretty clearly acknowledge that he knew he was behaving differently. "I know it wasn't going right, I can see myself asking questions I never ask other patients, and I didn't know why." I think you can help a resident to be responsive to feeling cues in himself.

Dr. Schuster: You mean he can see something happened?

C: That he can begin to recognize or to anticipate this is going to be an interview where he really has to watch his step, or he'll start getting off the track.

Dr. Thaler: I think in the course of three months of supervision he *was* able to differentiate. He knows he's doing better now than before.

C: I think a psychiatric interview is like any other skill that we learn; it's a combination of a fairly gut level style that you develop, which gets augmented by the specifics of the patient sitting in front of you. It is that which is reasonably characteristic, habitual, a part of yourself, a style of interviewing and orientation to the patient that gets modified in terms of specific content of what you explore, specific things you look for, etc. I think the times when the patient comes in, and for whatever reason, the interviewer gets anxious, uncomfortable or begins to perceive in a distorted fashion, he can no longer use what may be for him a very tentative style or framework of how you go about exploring with the patient what his difficulty is. So you begin to interact with the patient in uncharacteristic ways. For example, what I would consider uncharacteristic for psychiatric interviewing was when he began to interact with the person's views on medical matters. What does that mean to me? It means that you try to understand X has regressed from the level of function as a psychiatrist to a level of function that he found comfortable or learned earlier, a level he has had more practice at, that of the medical student on the medical floor. I suppose if he got more and more anxious, the interview might become characteristic of some quite different situation, it might regress into some sort of quasi-personal or social level.

B: You said something that is one of the problems we should be dealing with here, that the resident in interviewing a new psychiatric patient relates to him on a certain baseline level represented by his own personality, and superimposed on that are specialized skills that he is learning to understand. Now I think that a lot of residents do not start with what is their natural self. I think they start with some idea of what they think a psychiatrist should be like.

C: Oh, I'm sure that's right.

B: So I think we ought to discuss that, too, because it is at least their understanding that a psychiatrist should relate to a patient with this concept of neutrality.

Dr. Schuster: One example of that is the misapplication of the psychoanalytic model that many residents use.

Dr. Thaler: I've seen this recently very strikingly in observing first-year residents interviewing. What I've done the last few weeks is to have a first-year resident interview a patient recently admitted. This is his first contact with the patient. One after another the interviews that I have seen have been the kind of interviews that would not even be appropriate in a long, on-going therapeutic, non-directive relationship. The patient may be psychotic, dissociated, grinning inappropriately, etc. All the interviewer is doing is reflecting the affect and questioning the patient. He questions him about why he is laughing when what he's saying isn't laughable. This goes on without any attempt to get historical data.

C: Well the stereotypes about what you do as a psychiatrist come from all kinds of fragmented experiences in medical school. They observe an interview by a psychoanalyst, or maybe they saw it in the movies, I don't know, or they've read Freud, and they misapply a model that's not appropriate to this setting.

Dr. Thaler: When they're performing behind a screen, they get so anxious they forget what little outline they have in mind as to what data they should get. They revert to this fantasied image they have of what a psychiatrist ought to be like. The simplest thing to do is to say nothing.

B: It's a way to protect themselves.

Dr. Thaler: Yeah, they hide behind this mask.

Dr. Schuster: In the course of time this "neutrality" can be employed in the service of aggression. I've seen residents who have let patients suffer while they maintain this noble, objective stance of not interfering.

C: I see it very much as a cop-out. I really see it as an effort to say, "Look, I'm doing what I think is right. If the patient is incapable of responding, well, that's his problem, because he's a sick man."

Dr. Schuster: Another example in the same category of behavior is the response when the patient asks a question, and the resident responds, "Well, that's your decision. I wouldn't want to interfere in your life," leaving the poor patient hanging from the ropes. This again is a misapplication of neutrality. It isn't neutral at all.

B: This then brings in the concept of treatment through learning. If the relationship between the doctor and the patient is supposed to be a vignette of all other relationships, then there is no other relationship in which one person tells the other person everything about himself and meets with no feedback, no exchange. I think it is a principle of psychoanalysis which supports the concept of learning through self-reflection, based on the distortions that occur in a relationship with a psychiatrist. Now you can say that they carry this idea down erroneously. It seems to me that the concept is erroneous. It's more than just a misapplication of a proper concept.

Dr. Schuster: I don't agree with that. I think it's a misapplication of a *technique,* which has its own place. No responsible psychoanalyst would suggest that this technique be used to interview patients in the initial consultation.

B: I realize that, Dan, but you see if psychoanalysis is held up as the *sine qua non* of being a psychiatrist, then even if the resident realizes that it's inappropriate to his task, he says if I could do what is really best, I'd be doing this.

C: We're not holding up to the residents a model and saying: "Some day when you grow up you, too, can be a psychoanalyst, and only then will you be able to effectively treat patients."

Dr. Thaler: One can be non-directive and not intrusive, in the sense of not intruding one's own problems into the therapeutic situation, without being inactive. I think one can be extremely active and conduct a totally non-directive, open-ended interview. This is one of the basic things residents don't understand. They think that open-ended means you're silent, that you say nothing.

C: I regret your use of the word non-directive, because that sure as hell ain't what non-directive means.

Dr. Thaler: Well, instruct me.

C: I don't think non-directive in any way, shape or form carries the notion of neutrality.

Dr. Schuster: Don't you think that was the original implication, that you were not interfering with the patient, just letting him grow up by himself without. . . . ?

C: Non-directive implies, it seems to me, quite a few things. In terms of interviewing style, it implies the therapist's not choosing the direction of the patient's associations and not communicating to the patient any judgments of the therapist. One of its primary characteristics always was the profound appreciation of the patient's feelings, and I would regard this as quite different from the sense of neutrality.

Dr. Thaler: I don't think in psychoanalysis neutrality means idle, that you're not at all involved or concerned about the patient's feelings. I think what we should do is abandon that word all together and call it non-judgmental. You don't convey to the patient that you think he's a cad because he does this or that, or conversely that you feel terrible pity for him because he's done something else, but rather that you understand his feelings, and you're here to help.

C: Yeah, I think that neutral should mean that the therapist does not attempt to lead or push or direct the patient into either decisions about himself or decisions about the way he behaves in the outside world.

Dr. Thaler: Also that he doesn't take sides. For instance, when the patient reports a conflict with her husband and says my husband is this, that, and the other thing, the therapist is neutral in the sense that he doesn't say to the patient, "Well I agree with you, that's a terrible thing for him to do."

Dr. Schuster: He may have to go to the other extreme, to the extreme of "activity" by making an interpretation that she is comparing the husband unfavorably with the therapist and that this is leading to an impulse to act out something. To come back to Rogers, I think the initial implication in his work was that non-direction was not only empathic, but there was a certain preciousness about it, that you mustn't say anything but "uh-huh" or reflect the patient's comment.

C: It was naive . . .

Dr. Schuster: A prescription.

C: Yeah, there was a prescription for only three real kinds of responses that the interviewer could make. He could either, "uh-huh," or he could reflect the patient's feelings, or he could restate the content of what the patient said.

Dr. Schuster: You merely did these three things and let the patient go on, and somehow he would get better.

C: Of course that's not so. Nobody could ever accuse Carl Rogers, in terms of the work he's doing today, of being concrete.

Dr. Thaler: That system is probably rigidly and concretely applied by the novice and those who didn't have enough brains to think farther than what we're complaining about now, in terms of our residents flying the so-called psychoanalytic flag. In teaching the resident I try to show how you can be very active, indeed, and yet remain open-ended and non-judgmental.

B: Well, I'd like to challenge that. I mean I'm not sure about it myself—this idea of non-judgmental and non-directive. That concept can come dangerously close to the concept of laissez-faire. Whatever you want to do, whatever you feel is right for yourself is the thing that we as psychiatrists should do—help free yourself to do what you feel is right for yourself. Now if that happens to be deep dependency, that's your bag, you do it.

Dr. Thaler: That's utterly wrong. The definition of psychological freedom in the psychoanalytic model, as far as I understand it, is the capacity for rational choice. The goal of treatment is to help the patient reach the point at which he is the master in his own ego-house, where he's not driven by irrational impulses but has the capacity to make rational choices on the basis of the data that are coming in from the environment itself. That's very different from saying to a patient, "If you want to be totally dependent that's your bag." If you are going to do insight treatment, then I think it would be up to *you* if he's totally passive, which means that he's driven by his passive dependent needs, to get him to the point where he can perceive the neurotic aspects of this and hopefully modify his behavior accordingly.

B: So self-determination is where we would take a stand.

Dr. Schuster: I remember one of my analytic supervisors saying that the end result of the analysis of somebody's hostility shouldn't be that he become a rude person, but hopefully that he'd understand the genetic roots of his anger and not have to repetitively express his anger toward infantile objects. It is a popular misconception, too, that psychoanalysis stands for unbridled hedonism.

Dr. Thaler: In terms of this non-judgmental and non-directive issue, it's an ideal. It can be applied in such a rigid, concrete fashion that it doesn't make any sense. However, I'm saying that if one deviates from that ideal, one should have a good clinical reason for it. For instance with adolescents at times you have to say, "Look, you're acting like a horse's ass, cut it out."

Dr. Schuster: Well I think we kid ourselves, too. I think what you're saying is that in the treatment situation you're trying to attain an atmosphere of neutrality which means you're consciously trying not to intrude on the patient with your own judgments and morality and view of life. For example, a patient I had in analysis who was approaching termination started engaging in a variety of symptomatic acts, including becoming involved in a number of extramarital affairs which was quite unlike him. It seemed obvious to me that this was part of the transference situation in the termination setting, that it was an attempt to substitute objects for loss of me. It had to do with a very deep oral problem which eventually emerged in the ensuing months. He said, "I think that you're being very judgmental about this, I can just hear you saying cut it out." In a sense he was right, but I couldn't say anything, because I wanted to give him a chance to see if he couldn't discover for himself what was impelling this. He did, but after he got himself into considerable difficulty. That's what I think Otto is trying to say.

B: It all sounds very reasonable, and it may come up again. I have this certain doubt that creeps in from time to time about this concept. Is there a definite philosophy to which we adhere? Or is our role simply to let that person's ego emerge and be what it wants to be, whatever that may happen to be?

C: I think that it's only the very, very special case in which the last part of what you're saying ever takes place, and that is in the psychoanalytic situation, at least as I've seen it. In every other situation, it seems to me, that may be approached but never achieved. There's no way you can keep a patient from using you for a model for identification, for example, in a therapeutic situation that is not psychoanalysis. That's an absolute statement. I could modify it to make it more perfect. It would be in my mind extremely difficult, if not impossible, to prevent the therapist from becoming a very important part of any patient's future efforts at adaptation or growth except in the psychoanalytic situation.

B: Shouldn't we also be talking here about what our philosophy should be? In other words, if all the patients in our lives are going to be part of us, then shouldn't we be something . . . ?

C: We are, I think we are. I've always taken that as so much of a given that you don't even talk about it. For anyone to say that the therapist doesn't communicate aspects of his own value systems to the patient is ridiculous.

Dr. Schuster: That's where we're naive.

C: I was thinking about it today when I selected a tie to wear. Any patient who walks into the office and sees you wearing a certain tie is getting a communication. He's going to deal with it in some way, and if he's not in analysis it's very unlikely that it will ever come up. It's incorporated in some kind of framework. The clothes you wear, the pictures you have on your wall, all of these things, unless you define the situation as such while lying on the couch where he can associate to a thought he had about the picture you had on your wall, that stuff is never going to come up, or rarely. There is so much about you, the way you talk, the way you look, the way our office is, everything about you, the words you use, the information about your own background and cultural heritage. All of this stuff which very rarely if ever comes up in any kind of psychotherapeutic situation except a very, very special one.

Dr. Thaler: I think what B is asking is, should we articulate for our residents some kind of ideal value system?

B: In the sense particularly I'm thinking of, in light of concepts such as dependence versus independence, activity versus passivity, autonomy versus dominance.

Dr. Thaler: Well, what do you think?

B: I think we should, and I think that we all remain dependent in various ways, and I think we have to accept that. But we accept it as something that we *have* to accept rather than something that is a goal to be attained.

Dr. Schuster: I think you tend to talk about these things in an ideal state as though there was such a thing as perfect health; it's too black and white. For example, your dependent issue; of course we're all frail, and we're all dependent to a degree but . . .

B: Is there a principle toward which we should all be striving? Granted that it's limitless, granted. . . . Is it acceptance?

C: In my mind the goal of the psychological treatment of the patient is to facilitate his adaptation to his world. Not the *only* goal.

Dr. Schuster: And then the activists are hot on your trail saying you're forcing people to adapt to this tyrannical, unjust social system.

Dr. Thaler: That depends on how you define adaptation. You have to distinguish between adaptation and adjustment. Adaptation means a mutual fit between the environment and the organism, while adjustment is a sociological term. Adaptation is a biological term.

A: I think we're looking at many facets of something basic, and that's the relationship. We all have a different philosophy of what we see as therapeutic. I was thinking while you were talking that I guess mine is a more inter-personal one. My set towards a new patient is simply: this person is having difficulty with the human world, not with objects, but with the human world. Maybe what I can offer this person is a relationship which he needs, or he wouldn't even be coming to therapy, that is somehow different from all his previous relationships. In other words, all his previous relationships have been engaged in at a price. He's either had to give up his autonomy to a parent, please other people, use other people, whatever. Maybe I can offer a different kind of experience; one in which I will try to understand the person without using the person, without saying you've got to please me or be like me and allow that person to use me or for me to be like that person. That is the primary goal. All these other things are just facets. My primary goal is understanding without exploitation, and I don't think a good therapist does exploit. We do not use patients, and we don't let the patients use themselves. This will offer that freedom which they never experienced yet in a relationship—that is a basic trust.

B: There's no such thing as basic trust.

A: I think there is. That is where you can trust the therapist to be strong enough to understand you rather than use you or to be used by you. That to me is so crucial that it's the making of therapy.

B: What other relationship in life is like that?

A: I think there are none. That *should* have been the primary relationship, because that's really why they're sick.

B: Mothers use children.

A: That's why they come into treatment because they've gotten their ounce of affection for a heavy price. The beginning therapist doesn't know this, and he will use patients. He will ask the patient to love him, and he will need to feel love for the patient. Good therapists whom I've seen do not do that. They are self-sufficient and can accept without judging. . . .

Dr. Thaler: This is also, again, why you have to have a therapeutic situation and a therapeutic contract, because in real life nobody can sustain this sort of thing. It's only in a therapeutic situation where with training the therapist can tolerate this kind of basically non-gratifying contact.

B: But don't you see that the patient's going to come into treatment and have this marvelous unrealistic relationship, and unless that's at some point resolved, it could be very frustrating to the patient.

A: It's frustrating because he comes in with a lifetime of sick expectations, and you spend months with his trying to praise you, please you. Then when it's not working, he gets furious but realizes that it gives him freedom. He can be himself. He doesn't need to be a model to you. At the same time he'll make what we call manipulation attempts to get you to react, and he sees that that doesn't work. It's a relief after the anger that he can start being himself. You accept him for himself, not what he should be.

B: Granted. But he needs to see at some point that you, too, are a person like any other person who is not all self-sacrificing to the nourishment and development. . . .

A: You're not self-sacrificing, you're charging him money.

Dr. Thaler: He knows you're not self-sacrificing, because you refuse to gratify him outside a therapeutic situation. If he says let's go have a cup of coffee, you refuse.

Dr. Schuster: Of course, this all comes back to the point made earlier about Tarachow's concept of the continuum from one extreme of accepting the person as a real object—the object hunger he speaks of where the therapist lays claim to the patient as a real object for gratification—to the other extreme we try to attain in psychoanalysis, where you eschew this tendency and do not lay claim to each other as objects. Instead we regard the patient as an "as if" object; so the patient can eventually see what's going on. I think that's one reason why the family situation is really not at all comparable to the therapeutic situation. . . .

C: But I think what you said, B, represents only one point along the continuum of psychotherapeutic relationship. I don't think that you would argue that's the way it is with every patient you treat. Some of the aspects of this I see as universally applicable, but if I think of my own psychotherapeutic ventures I don't think I could say that that's my set with every patient. For instance, I'm well aware of the fact that with some patients I do use a notion, like my approval of what they do, deliberately. I do try to become a certain kind of object to them—that is, I'm thinking specifically of a young schizophrenic girl whom I treated for a long time. I very carefully want to continue to be perceived by her as someone who thinks very highly of her, loves her. I want her to think of me as a very benign, warm person. Not someone who can lean back to say you don't have to gratify me but someone who has said to her you do gratify me by the way you grow and change. I get a great deal of pleasure out of seeing you now compared to the way you were when you were huddled in a corner of my office in a catatonic stupor. There's a big difference in you now, and boy I like it.

PEDAGOGY VERSUS THERAPY REVISITED

Several months after our discussion of "pedagogy versus therapy" in relation to Dr. X and his patient, we returned to this theme. In this case a resident had a "problem" with his supervisor. Through a misunderstanding, the supervisor had not scheduled as much time weekly with his resident as was customary for other supervisors. The resident had been reluctant to confront his mentor with this situation, and the unspoken tension between them created difficulties in their working together and interfered with the resident's relationship with a family he was treating. In discussing this instance, the conference participants returned to the controversial boundary between helping a resident with his patient and helping him with his personal problems.

Dr. Schuster: When you speak about personal problems, what do you have in mind? When you made your comment to him about sensing some resentment on his part (about not getting as much supervisory time as he felt entitled to) that could be a personal problem. As it turned out, it was partly a realistic matter, the differential in time between what he had and what others had, and partly it was his own personality responding to that situation. You mean getting into things such as B suggested, his marriage and all this sort of business?

A: Well, I found in his work with this family that he wasn't helping them. He was depressed and passive and withdrawn, and that concerned me because it was affecting them. So I felt maybe something was going on that was handicapping him in his work with the family. That could lead to anything. If it led to his feelings about his father, or something like that, then I'd say I'm not in a position to deal with that. Maybe he needs some therapy; but if he's angry with me because I didn't give him more than two hours, I'm going to deal with that.

Dr. Thaler: I think we've talked about this much earlier, and, B, I can agree that the resident should have a chance to talk to his tutor if he feels that some personal problem is troubling him and possibly interfering with his work. Then you can say, "If you have problems with your wife which you feel you can't work out yourself, maybe you ought to go see someone for treatment." Would you undertake then to help him resolve the problem with his wife? Would that be a proper function of the tutor?

B: I think it would if he wanted to.

Dr. Thaler: In the tutorial?

B: I think I would listen to the problem.

Dr. Thaler: Yeah, listening to the problem, B, and doing a therapeutic job with it is a different thing.

B: Well, suppose it's something that could be discussed within that hour?

Dr. Schuster: What would be the point in listening if you weren't going to deal with it?

Dr. Thaler: What if it takes 10 hours to resolve? What happens to the tutorial then?

B: It stands in abeyance for 10 hours.

Dr. Thaler: I can't see that. Where's your therapeutic contract?

B: What is a therapeutic contract?

Dr. Schuster: Well, let's not get into the contract business. Let's look at it another way. One is always hard put to separate the pedagogic from the therapeutic in this whole matter of supervision, but we do have the machinery or the system for personal consultation and, if necessary, psychotherapy, within the department. So why would it be necessary for you to get involved in the first place?

B: I would say in answer to that—let's suppose I know you, and because I know you and respect you I want to talk to you about it. I don't want to be referred to some person on the staff, whom I may not respect.

Dr. Schuster: That's hard for me to separate from the rational factors.

Dr. Thaler: Suppose this guy needs psychoanalytic work, are you going to meet with him five times a week?

B: No, I think I would try to do the reasonable thing. I wouldn't go on and on. All I say is that I think it's wrong to shut the door on it, and also it's wrong to do everything that's needed.

Dr, Schuster: My middle ground there would be that I personally don't think that it's going to be helpful to a resident in learning from his tutorial, if the thing becomes a diversion into his own problems. That doesn't mean that if he started telling me he was very troubled about something that I'd say, "Shut up, I don't want to hear you." But I think if it became apparent to me that he wanted some kind of help, then I would say, "I think you ought to go through the proper channels and get what help you need."

B: Why not take care of it if it looks like it's something you can do?

Dr. Schuster: Because your job as a tutor is not to be a personal psychotherapist. It's just not practical, in my opinion, in terms of time and energy and . . .

B: Why, Dan? I really don't understand that. Why is it impractical to be both?

Dr. Schuster: It's a matter of time to begin with, and what you're supposed to be doing as a tutor is to teach this man something— not about himself.

B: What is more important as a psychiatrist than to understand yourself fully?

Dr. Schuster: Oh, I couldn't agree more, but that's done somewhere else. You have a division of responsibility and a division of labor so to speak, and for many reasons that division should be more or less honored. Also you mustn't overlook the fact that if you get involved with somebody personally like this, your role changes. He looks at you differently, and there are some things then that you'll be inhibited in discussing with him about his work. In other words, I don't see how you can wear two hats at the same time.

Dr. Thaler: I think there is a basic difference of opinion here. I believe for some of the reasons that A also mentioned, in terms of your position of power with regard to the resident in many ways, I believe that the pedagogic role and the therapeutic role should be distinct and clear and separate as much as possible. Obviously in either instance, as a pedagog or as a therapist, you always have to act like a human being and not tell somebody to go away, that you don't want to talk with him. At the same time I think there should be some clarity in the resident's mind as to your being his teacher, his advisor if necessary, but not his physician. If he needs any kind of formal therapeutic work with some problem of his own, then the pedagogic relationship is not the one that would be most suitable for that, in fact it might be contraindicated. You get into all kinds of transference and countertransference problems which become so incredibly complex that it's really almost impossible. . . .

B: I dont' necessarily buy that—that you get into incredibly complex transferences and countertransferences. I would assume that if you had problems, and you went and talked to one of your colleagues about it—a friend let's say—that you wouldn't say "I better not do this. I'm going to get into incredibly complex transference. . . ."

Dr. Schuster: Yes, but your colleague or friend isn't trying to be your teacher.

Dr. Thaler: Or your therapist.

B: But he's trying to be your friend.

Dr. Schuster: Why that's a different role. There is another role—teacher, friend, therapist—these are all different roles having different responsibilities.

Dr. Thaler: Look, B, I come to you as my friend and say, "B, I'm having terrible problems with my wife," and you say, "Okay, I'd be interested to hear about them," and I tell you about the problems with my wife. As I tell you about the problems with my wife, it becomes fairly clear to you that these problems involve a considerable neurotic element on my part. Now, would you then proceed as my friend and say, "Okay, come to see me once a week or twice a week, and I'll be your therapist, and we'll work out these neurotic problems of yours." Or would you say, "Look,

Otto, it seems to me that maybe you need—I know how you feel about going to a colleague for therapy at your age, but I think it might be wise. Maybe you should do that." That would be the help I would expect from a friend, but I wouldn't expect my friend to say to me, "Okay, tell me everything that comes to your mind."

B: I wouldn't say that to anybody—friend or foe.

Dr. Sandt: But you know, it seems that what you might be doing is falling into a seduction from each other's demands. The resident says to you, "Be everything to me," and you say, "I'll try," in effect when you say, "I'll take on whatever you want to say." You, in a sense, seduce the resident into talking about the sorts of things that Otto has just been bringing up as an illustration. So it ends up that the two of you are ignoring the patient, in the service of what the resident really wants.

Dr. Schuster: I guess that would be the most objectionable reason.

Dr. Sandt: That's my logic—why not get into it. Also, there's a tone you can take with the resident. Each of us certainly has had someone come up with a personal issue and say, "By the way, one of the reasons I had a tough time with this patient was that last night I was drunk, or last night I had difficulty, or these days I'm having problems with the authoritative personality." That seems to be a common trend with the residents. And your response to that could be, "Well, tell me more about that," in which case you know you're to get into some kind of childhood and associated pattern. Or you can say, "How does that relate to the patient?" And at that point you can focus and divert the resident. It seems to me this is seductive. I would never push it into that kind of willingness to have him elaborate in that direction (his own problem).

Dr. Thaler: Yet I have no hesitation in pointing out certain aspects of his personality that I perceive are interfering with him.

Dr. Sandt: Here and now.

Dr. Thaler: "It seems to me, with this particular patient you are always angry. Let's look at what this is all about." But, I would not then try to find out why he is angry in terms of his own psychodynamic structure, but rather that he sees how this interferes with his work. We can deal with that, and if it continues to interfere, then he ought to get some therapy.

Dr. Schuster: Well, I think you can use that illustration to point out the basic difference between the teacher role and the therapist's role. If the resident is in a learning situation and you're trying to teach him something you would say to him, "I notice that you're angry with that patient." If he's in therapy you might say, "*Why* are you angry?" I don't think the supervisor needs to get into the "why" part of it.

Dr. Thaler: As a supervisor I really don't care why.

B: I wouldn't agree with that because nothing is more. . . .

Dr. Thaler: Unless he's angry with me, then we've got to find it out, or the supervision goes to pot. That may happen, too, and this is why. . . .

Dr. Schuster: One thing B is overlooking, I think, is that sometimes people say more than they wish they had. I've had that experience personally—with people who came running with their troubles and I, like a good mother—all embracing—listened and then I found out later they regretted they had said all these things. Then they turn on you, and you lose a friend. So don't overlook that possibility that later the person is overwhelmed with shame and guilt and asks himself, "Why did I say these things? I should have talked to somebody 'more objective,' my doctor-therapist who's in a different role, who doesn't make any demands on me as does my teacher." This is just one more example, I think, of why the difference should be recognized.

A: If the whole system was different, B, and we didn't evaluate each other, and there was much more openness between people—faculty and residents, if you worked in a T-group environment with people, very open and candid and honest. I think that could be great if it worked. Then I would say, yes, that's part of the trust. But in terms of the system we have, what you're doing is devious and I think would be abused. It wouldn't work. So I'll say in principle, I like your approach. It's humanitarian, and it's open and it's helpful. But it seems this system can be bad, because it could be used for manipulation.

B: How? Why?

A: Well, the fact that you have to evaluate the resident—that you have to grade him, that he writes an evaluation on you, you should never do that to a therapist.

B: Why? I don't understand why. What's the problem?

A: Well, because his drive to please you and let you see the good side of him would be paramount, and the risk in letting him reveal his inadequacies to you is incredibly difficult. It's hard enough in therapy but if you, if you're still going to evaluate him, he puts you in the bind. And I think this would destroy it.

B: I think he would have to trust that what I wrote in the evaluation would be what I felt, how he functioned as a psychiatrist. It would have nothing to do with how he felt about himself.

Dr. Thaler: I think that's impossible for him.

Dr. Schuster: Yes, I would object mainly to A's point. I don't think it's in the *system*. I think it's in people. How open can people be with each other? We can't live in a world of a T-group. I think most people couldn't tolerate that. Secondly I think B's implication here is that it's kind of mean or lacking in humanity if we don't respond in this way. I don't agree with that.

B: I didn't say that. I don't necessarily feel that. I think it's just a matter of opinion. And I'm arguing on the basis of what I think is reasonable, not on the basis of . . .

Dr. Schuster: I may be incorrect, but I get that feeling.

B: And this idea that we'd be a mother figure by doing this, I don't agree with either.

Dr. Schuster: Why do you think we've all gone into this field if we didn't have strong maternal instincts. That goes without saying, I think. The need to succor or rescue, comfort and so on—that's true in all of medicine, all of the helping professions, in my opinion.

B: Well, I would say, as far as I'm concerned, that may have been why I started out, but I feel very differently than that now—in the sense that what matters to me now is that I do what I do well. Not that somebody else gets better from it.

E: If you have an individual patient, you have a certain kind of relationship with him but when you have that same patient in a group in which you don't have any other member as an individual patient, you have a different kind of relationship. In other words, you have sort of two contracts, and you can separate out your relationship in two different ways. I'm wondering if that's what you're not saying, "I have one relationship as the teacher, but when we have to step over into a different kind, we have to renegotiate." I remember in the old days they used to caution you not to take your own individual patients into group, and now the last I heard, that is not valid. As long as everybody understands what's going on. I'm wondering if that's what you're not saying, "I step out of my role, renegoti-ate—and then we—then we'll get back into the first role better."

B: Exactly.

Dr. Sandt: In other words, a great deal of the demand of the residents here might be met if there were some kind of arrangement which was built into our residency for allowing group therapy to be tolerated, at least. I was in a residency where for 18 months we were in group therapy one and a half hours a week.

Dr. Thaler: This was compulsory?

Dr. Sandt: No. It was optional. It was available for those who wished it, and the previous year people had been quite taken with group therapy, so they sort of wedged it out of the chairman. In our year we had the option, pretty much, thanks to them. And this was quite a debate—whether we were going to do it or not. Having done that I think that a great many of the issues that were brought to B in the individual tutorials were avoided, because we dealt with the kinds of things you're after—how you present yourself to the other person, how you're perceived in your public stance. That sort of thing came up in the group and took a great deal of the stress out of the individual tutorials, so that you were able to be less demanding of your tutor, less interested in discussing the personal issues.

F: The general feeling here has been that personal therapy during the course of the residency is the exception and frowned upon. So then the only place for this (a resident's problems) to come up is in the tutorial relationship, under the guise of teaching. Maybe it would come out anyway, but I have a feeling that part of the reason why it comes up here (in the tutorial) is that it's introduced under the role of teaching, but it's also the point at which, maybe the only point for many residents, where some conflicted material can ever be discussed.

G: Well, I've heard of some residencies that offer things like six months of intensive therapy on a four hour a week basis as an elective. As an elective it would be like going on a cafeteria system. The point is, though, that a lot of residents do have needs, and these needs, I think, are expressed somewhere in the tutorial system. The relationship of the pedagogue and therapist has no confluence at all for the resident. And he doesn't see it that way if he's hurting. And that tends to a lot of angry feelings I suspect.

B: The status of psychiatry is such that even though all of us have problems, if you see a psychiatrist, that means that there's something different about you. That makes it seem like all these people who aren't seeing psychiatrists don't have problems, or if they do have problems they relate differently to someone about them.

Dr. Schuster: Well, B, what you're saying I think is that being a physician there is the folklore that you aren't supposed to be sick. Everybody—the layman, the man in the streets—says, "You're sick? You're a doctor. You're not supposed to be sick." And in the doctor's mind there is the unresolved problem of infantile omnipotence also, that he can do anything. He's invulnerable, and why should he need a doctor. I'll bet if you took a random sample of anybody, people in this department, they wouldn't even have, most of them, annual physical examinations.

Dr. Thaler: I'll go with that.

B: Then I'd say, wouldn't our talking to each other more about our problems break that down?

Dr. Schuster: I doubt it. I think it might drive some things underground. There's no guarantee that if we all had to get in a T-group that anybody's problems would come to the surface. I think we'd all be so defensive, most of us, that we would, on the contrary, entrench our problems.

B: But if a resident says, "Look, I want to talk to you about something." I certainly wouldn't say that we, as tutors, should encourage them to talk about their problems. I don't mean that. I just mean we should be ready and willing, within a limited degree. I wouldn't as you said, Otto, sit down and say come every week and we'll work on all your problems, but I don't think that all problems need to be solved on a regular weekly basis for a certain period of time. They can often be resolved through a conversation —through argument—through a contrasting point of view. You question what you believe.

Dr. Sandt: I'm more worried about the tacit invitation and the tone that you take. That's what troubles me. The implication that you're willing to hear anything in the tutorial, like the kind of thing you've talked about.

Dr. Thaler: There are, I think, two conflicting opinions here about the role of the pedagogue versus the role of the therapist and whether there is even a difference between these two roles, and I don't think we're going to convince each other one way or the other. I think the positions are fairly distinct, and I wonder whether we ought to go on.

B: Otto, I'd agree with that but I, I mean, I would agree with going on, but I don't call that resolving the problem by saying that there are two points of view, and we'll never come to an agreement about them. I think at some point we ought to try and argue it until we come to some kind of resolution.

Dr. Thaler: That may be. My view would be that by using this specific example as an illustration we can come back to the argument at a later point. The argument at this moment sort of bogged down in that I was saying I feel this way, the other one was saying I feel that way, and we're not—making any progress.

Dr. Schuster: Also some problems are incapable of resolution.

F: Can I add one more historical complexity?

Dr. Thaler: Well, I don't know why not.

F: The other thing that may make this even more complicated is that maybe 10 or 15 years ago it was much more common for junior faculty to go into analysis after they had finished their residency. That was, I would guess, more the rule than the exception. Now more people have opted to waive analysis or analytic training, and the residents see this. They see that some people are going into analysis and some people are not. My guess is that introduces much more of a perplexity in their own minds.

Dr. Schuster: You mean, what is the thing to do at any particular given moment in history?

F: Yes, because of the fact that there are more people now whom they see on the faculty who have not been in analysis or who've not had any kind of treatment, it raises the question, well, maybe it's not necessary, or maybe you can deny problems or get over them, or because you had such a marvelous child rearing experience, you never needed it. My guess is that that adds an extra note of confusion.

Dr. Thaler: Also, there is always the thought that, "I know I have problems, but as soon as I finish the residency, then I'll really get to this. They'll resolve, so they can wait."

G: I think, an important point, though, is that the resident who develops a relaionship for his tutor isn't aware of the difference between a pedagogue and a therapist.

Dr. Schuster: He's not?

G: No. He's not. And I don't think he sees it that way, and I think for all the reasons that people hurt that he's driven at times so that this kind of a division we, as faculty, make doesn't have the same validity for the people we are training.

Dr. Thaler: One last thing would be to involve some residents in this kind of a discussion to find out how they feel about it—their perceptions of what's going on. That might be very interesting.

A: One thing that seems to happen in this discussion is that in a kind of peripheral way something else has kind of sneaked in. We've gotten into it and then discarded it, and I'm disturbed that we discarded it. And that is the question of being more open amongst ourselves, and I think that's terribly threatening. I think what concerns me is residents who do therapy, group therapy, and individual therapy which I've supervised, often expect patients to do what they can't do. I think that's unfair. It's very risky for any human being to expose himself. We keep forgetting that. We get out of it by labeling the patient as sick, and he's got this problem, and there's a very subtle judgment. It happened right here. I perceive you as a very neutral person in terms of judging, and yet when you talk about this as possibly neurotic, there's a very subtle judgment about this. It really hit me, because I think this is what's behind the binds that psychiatry gets itself into. How can we say, "We are sick"? People see, not sickness, but problems with life which everybody has in one way or the other; and I think that the T-group movement is very healthy, because it's saying people are people and people have problems in living. We need each other to get through life, and I think that's very sane. I think that if we can at least experience how hard it is to be open with each other, we'll have a little more respect for patients.

Dr. Sandt: I think we've been missing this.

A: And I think we do miss this. I think it's pertinent to this conference, because we are dealing with supervisors' problems. I think playing the saint is risky for me. It makes me anxious. I'm revealing personal things about myself. Here I had an interaction with the resident. I would rather present some academic issue that he did this, and he did that. I think that it does raise the question of why so much fear of having a model of openness—it"s much more important than just didactic teaching in psychiatry, because I think that's where it's at—all of therapy.

Dr. Schuster: Well, A, I agree with many of the things you've said, that we do tend to be judgmental and pejorative. For example, there's a hierarchy of mental illness, isn't there? I mean, it's more respectable to, let's say, have one kind of illness than another. A neurosis is not so bad, but if you're schizophrenic, that's something else again. But well—that just represents how the majority feels.

Dr. Sandt: But it's not right either.

Dr. Schuster: However, I think when you say that to ameliorate that situation we should move to the psycho-social view, that this is an evasion also. Then we say the illness isn't in us, but it's in society, and that can be an evasion of recognizing the unconscious in my opinion. That doesn't derogate, let's say, external reality or social issues, but I think we have to somehow place the problem where it is, and at the same time struggle not to be judgmental. Of course, like all other human beings we're frail, and we're all lost sheep in one way or another in this life. But that doesn't mean that we're prepared to expose this to all the rest of our fellow men. That's where the problem comes in. Why it's so hard for us to be really open with each other. Now, around this table we can be open about professional issues which is very good, and we can have a frank, at times, passionate exchange of opinions; but it doesn't involve exposing our own problems, except indirectly as they can be seen by each one of us as we listen and watch the other person talking.

B: That's okay. I mean, no one is asking you to go to the root of one's deepest problems.

Dr. Schuster: No, but A is pleading for more openness, and I understand what he's saying, but I'm saying there are limitations that aren't entirely rational.

B: I would agree also.

Dr. Thaler: I'd like to respond with a footnote maybe to A's point about using the word neurotic. I tend to sort of agree with him, but the point, I think, remains a familiar one. I wonder what other language to use to take the sting out of it. If the resident brings you a problem which you recognize as based on an unconscious conflict, then you have to decide whether to address that unconscious conflict with certain specialized therapeutic techniques in which you are skillful, and the application of which requires a certain specific set on both your parts, or whether to address yourself to the conscious problem. Namely, you have a problem and these are some of the things you can do about the problem in terms of taking it to somebody who will work with you therapeutically. That's it.

A: Yes.

Dr. Thaler: I mean, between the problem that the pedagogue can deal with at the conscious, realistic, rational level and the problem that can only be dealt with by addressing himself to the resolution of unconscious conflict.

B: What's unconscious one minute can be conscious another.

Dr. Thaler: That's clinical. That's a matter of clinical judgment.

Dr. Schuster: I think A points out another—a very important point which we don't talk about very often—the possibility that any one of us can be contemptuous of the patient, and that's something we don't like to talk about. And often we are, and that is something we should face. It's the defensive nature of the contemptuous attitude—protect ourselves, maintain the illusion that we are perfect, and he, the patient, is different. This is something we should think about.

RESIDENTS' VIEWS OF SUPERVISION

During this conference discussion we began with some of the residents' views of our "tutorial" program and continued into a discussion of some aspects of their experience in the Clinic. There was some controversy about whether or not residents are encouraged to work with marital couples which raised more general issues about the residents' professional development.

Dr. Thaler: I met with the first-year residents in our regular weekly meeting and asked them their general response so far to their psychotherapy tutorial which started on January 1. I asked them how they felt about the supervision, and what came out was interesting. First of all the sort of thing that we've heard over and over again, namely, that their tutorial hour is the most prized hour of the week. That one-to-one session with the psychotherapy supervisor they see as their golden hour, and they treasure it. However, it is also invested with no end of fantasies, some of which they recognize and some of which they don't. A number of them said they would never dare question anything that the supervisor said or does, because this is so precious to them they are afraid that anything they might say would irritate him or might put him off. For the most part they're very satisfied with their supervision. They are very satisfied with their supervisors, except for some who occasionally come late or change their hours. Then it's almost like a therapy situation. They say, well, we can accept that, but they would never dare show their anger. Now interestingly enough, they don't feel this way, or not as strongly, about their clinical director, with whom they also have a weekly supervisory session. They see this as a totally different situation, and they feel freer, more at ease, much more capable of interacting with him on a more equal level. First of all they have a lot more contact with him than the tutors. I have a feeling too that the clinical directors, for the most part, are younger than their supervisors. The psychotherapy supervisors are for the most part somewhat more senior.

D: Well whatever awe they feel in January, I think they lose pretty rapidly, because six months later they're entirely different people. It must be their first patient also, that first psychotherapy patient.

Dr. Thaler: Right, it's that first psychotherapy patient. They have all sorts of fantasies in terms of their own view of that patient, whom they see as tremendously different from the ones they deal with on the floors. They see their own ignorance very starkly at that particular point. They've gained some confidence in dealing with psychotic patients and taking histories and doing the managerial tasks of the floor, prescribing drugs and what not; but they see themselves as practically totally ignorant of psychotherapeutic skills, particularly with an ambulatory patient. They have all kinds of concerns and fears that anything they say or do might ruin the whole thing.

E: There are two dimensions of this. One is the mythical expectation about the ideal patient, which is always elusive. Where is that ideal patient that they keep depriving me of; or they keep saying that there must be such patients, but where are they? Then there's the mythical escalation of expectations about the tutor.

Dr. Thaler: When I assigned tutors and patients around January 1, there was some kind of a scheduling difficulty which prompted me to make a switch. I said to one tutee that I'd like him to work with this man (tutor) instead of that guy. This produced a really intense resentment on the part of the person that I asked to do this. "This is very disappointing to me, and I feel very badly about it," and he went on and on.

Dr. Schuster: It was like he was being sent to a foster home.

Dr. Thaler: Yeah, right. It was a tremendously intense reaction before anything had even transpired between the two of them. Fortunately, I was able to recoup this thing and to keep it with the man he had been assigned to initially. I think there must have been certain myths about that certain tutor, that he's especially helpful. The other thing is that Dr. Z who's coming back to us as a second-year resident next year has been practically deluging me with letters. The first person he saw when he returned here was me, to make sure that he would have a tutor, and who it would be, could he request one, and so forth. This is just one hour a week, and yet to him that was the most crucial thing that he had to settle before he returned to us. He was going to have a psychotherapy tutor to help him and work with him when he returns here. These are the kinds of attitudes that you meet. I think, aside from all the fantasy aspects of this, it also indicates how highly important to the resident psychotherapeutic skills are. We see that again and again.

Dr. Schuster: I was wondering why they invest it so heavily.

B: I think the myth is that one tutor is outstanding. We're all closer together than they fantasy us to be. We're all close together in our abilities.

E: If they were in treatment themselves, though, I wonder if this hour with the supervisor would be as valuable.

Dr. Thaler: I think to be in treatment oneself of necessity further enhances one's views of the values of psychotherapy. It really must be terribly good, if I undertake it myself, and if I hope to get some help from it myself. Therefore, the model of one's own therapist becomes a source of identification.

D: But we're still talking about the first-year residents. How do second-year residents fit in, and how would a third-year resident view this same experience? Would it be overvalued, valued, devalued?

Dr. Thaler: I have little data about this; However, the second-year residents, from what I've seen of them this year, view this a little bit more realistically, but in terms of what they haven't been getting and what they think they ought to be getting. They feel almost unanimously that their education in psychotherapy has been deficient, so that even though they have this valued tutorial hour, it hasn't been enough. I think as a consequence that they are more critical. They speak of the lack of didactic work and generally their lack of skill as they enter the second year. I think that's fairly evident, because they asked for elective and other help with this. As far as the third-year residents are concerned, my very impressionistic view is that they're sort of shaken down, and there are some who are interested in psychotherapy and there are some who are simply not. I'd say about 50% would welcome a more intensive third-year experience in psychotherapeutic work, and the other half would either not be interested nor talented for it. My feeling is that in the third year any kind of formal teaching exercises in psychotherapy ought certainly to be elective. In the first and second year, there should be something specific and obligatory.

F: That's like saying the surgical residents shouldn't be in the operating room.

Dr. Sandt: Some surgical residents aren't. They're in the dog lab where they belong or in surgical pathology.

Dr. Schuster: If they *are* in the OR there are certain limitations as to what they do. Their interventions are very carefully defined.

E: Otto was talking about aspirations. There are a number of residents now who don't particularly want this (training in psychotherapy), and I can see them in other roles—in community psychiatry.

Dr. Thaler: For example, somebody like Dr. X who has decided that clinical psychiatry isn't for him at all and that he will go into research. We're a house of many mansions now.

Dr. Sandt: There was a double track system that perhaps did exist 10 or 15 years ago—you were an analyst or analytically oriented and had long-term cases, or you weren't. Now the thing is all blurred. You can do 5 things and still be a virtuoso in psychiatry.

Dr. Schuster: Sort of a jack of all trades, and a master of none.

A: I have a problem that might be of some interest. I got a call at home yesterday from a former day hospital patient who is married and has one child. She is sort of bored with life, a very bright girl. For months she's been complaining about problems with her husband, and he seems very cautious about coming in for help. He talked about coming in once, and the resident was going to put him in a group and said he was going to call him back. He never did, and used this as the reason. It seemed that every time she would suggest they both come in for help, he would block that. Finally he agreed. What they want to know is, if they come to OPD can they see a resident who will see them as a couple? This is a problem that is coming up more now as people hear there is a family program. I am wondering if this would be worth discussing for a little while, because it *is* a problem when people come in and say they don't want to be seen individually. We give a kind of mental set of the resident in the OPD and that's how they work (one to one).

Dr. Schuster: As far as I am concerned there is no restriction about being seen as couples. The problem in this kind of situation is whether the message about both of them being seen gets through from the screener to the supervisor of the diagnostic study.

A: It's a bit misleading, because the screener may not have time to decide things like that, and because he may have been taught to do individual work, and nothing else. In this case they convince a patient that he shouldn't be seen with his wife or husband. The resident doesn't have any experience with couples.

B: Yes, but the supervisor is there to help make some of these decisions.

Dr. Thaler: Suppose the patient is saying the two of us want to be seen together. Should they be seen together in screening to begin with, and then some kind of determination made as to whether they will continue to be seen together?

Dr. Schuster: But if just one comes for screening, you can't see them together, or if a patient wants to be seen with his or her spouse but doesn't mention that during the screening session. If the message is clear, then I would recommend, I often do, that they should be seen together, or that one should be seen first and then the other. If there are clear indications for a couple to be seen together, I always encourage that. Maybe the residents are sometimes reluctant.

D: No, I think the residents do see them as couples. Many of them have worked very long and diligently with couples. I don't think they are reluctant to take on couples.

Dr. Thaler: In my experience the set is that you see the patient who presents, even if the wife is there. You wouldn't even ask them how they want to be seen. I am called all the time, "Should I bring my husband?"

Dr. Schuster: You direct your attention to the one who is the declared patient, because sometimes it is impossible to do otherwise, even though you suspect the spouse may be the sicker. You direct your attention to the one who comes as the patient; but if you were to discover in the course of the screening or the diagnostic study that it would appear to be a marital problem, you wouldn't be disinclined to recommend that they be seen together, would you? As I look back over the experiences I've had in screening, most couples who come together don't both consider themselves patients. One is usually the patient in both their minds. Occasionally some couples come and say we have a problem we want to both talk about. We feel we are both contributing to this, and we want to talk together and solve it. But that's not the majority.

B: After our meetings here are terminated, there ought to be an ongoing seminar specifically devoted to therapy and not taught by just two people (as was the case at this time). We're in work where there are a lot of varied opinions, and the more the residents get exposed to different points of view, and the more *we* get exposed to different points of view of our colleagues, the more likely some kind of a reasonable denominator of teaching is going to emerge.

Dr. Schuster: For what group of residents?

B: I would think it ought to begin probably at the second year, and that the third year could then be more elective as Otto suggests, and then they could elect to have certain . . .

A: I like the idea, but I'm conflicted, because I feel that we haven't closed the issue. From my experience most residents will not see a couple. What they do in the diagnostic studies is remain deaf to an obvious family or couple situation, and I can understand this, because the set is against that. They don't know whether their supervisor or tutor will be interested in that. I think one thing that might be helpful is to identify residents who are interested in seeing couples and supervisors who'd be interested in supervising them. Residents I've supervised are constantly amazed when I suggest what about bringing in the wife that he keeps talking about. They say, "Well I never thought of that." When they talk about not knowing whether their tutors would be interested, I can understand that. Why should they have to make all these decisions?

B: All tutors should be accepting this.

A: But it doesn't work this way.

G: I don't see though that they need to be so constrained about asking for such things.

D: My guess is that if they would ask their tutors more often, they would get involved in other treatment modalities.

Dr. Thaler: I have the feeling that from what I heard the other day that the first-year resident is scared to death to ask any kind of question. I think the second-year resident is very, very different. Many of the third-year residents, I think, would really like to be in business on their own altogether. I've seen again and again the tutorial hour that the third-year residents have is often not utilized.

Dr. Schuster: I don't think we answered the point about residents seeing couples. I can see where there might be a neglect in this area, and I think it's been natural enough. I don't think it's been deliberate neglect, nor do I think it's necessarily that we want to be more comfortable. I think it's a natural thing to direct our attention to the patient. That's the whole medical tradition. That the rest of the family might be neglected I can understand. I don't think that there is an active exclusion of the rest of the family. Maybe we wouldn't agree on how many patients are suitable for this, I don't know. You, A, with your interest in family work probably see more possibilities for this than I do.

A: I don't think it's an active exclusion. I think that most of the tutors the residents look up to are reasonably skilled and trained in psychotherapy, and what they will say is, "I'll see the family as a couple if you supervise me." I can't do it, and then I have to think, "Well, who could?" and I don't know. What I'm asking is for more visibility—not just for the resident but for myself. I think it would be appropriate to designate a number of tutors who would be interested in family work and make them known to residents.

B: It's not just an emphasis on general therapy. I think tied in with that is the general influence of psychodynamics—one's past is the primary reason for discomfort in the present. The training program says that people are unhappy now because of what happened to them in their development.

Dr. Thaler: That's not so. I think what we've talked about mostly is the concept of multiple determining factors in psychopathology, and that one of the important determining factors is past life experience. But that certainly is not *the* one.

Dr. Schuster: I think the emphasis on ontogeny or development is, of course, an important emphasis.

B: I agree, of course, but that ties in with the concept of an emphasis also on individual treatment. You work out your problems with your own development. That emphasis maybe could be modified some.

Dr. Thaler: Well, I don't know. I think actually from what I've seen of residents and their psychotherapeutic work and the kinds of depth that they get to, which is usually very shallow, that the ontogenetic factors are hardly ever brought in. We may use them in our attempts at explaining to the residents what seems to be going on with a patient. But very rarely do I find a resident who deals with his patients in any depth as far as ontogenetic determinants are concerned. Most of what the resident does has to do with the "here and now," and sometimes with current events, and very rarely do they make connections to the past.

A: One resident was seeing a woman who was very hysterical and came in with a complaint of frigidity. He saw her and the husband, interestingly enough, and described the husband as very concerned about it. He started working with this woman alone. He obviously didn't feel comfortable working with both of them, and that was fine. When I said, "When she's better, what are you going to do about the husband?" He said, "What do you mean, her husband will be delighted?" So, of course, as she got better, the husband started sabotaging the treatment, because his own difficulties with sexuality became obvious as she became more capable. The resident was amazed at this. He never thought of it, and he wasn't a fool.

D: Since we no longer have had the regular weekly meetings with all the second-year residents, you were not there to represent family tratment. I wasn't there, and I had no contact with them in either tandem or marital work. I've never had a resident come to me and say, "My tutor wont' let me work with the spouse, or my tutor won't allow this, because we're working on individuals." Usually the resident himself gets kind of stopped, and then he will get terribly involved in the marital relationship. Let me give you an example of one that came through, and I think this is what happens with some of them. The first-year resident will pick up a patient on the floor, and when he's ready to be discharged, will come down to me and ask about doing marital work. One resident asked me if I'd work with him. I said I'd be glad to be his co-therapist. We worked with this woman, who was the patient, and the husband weekly. In the meantime, two of the children were involved in therapy at a local clinic.

A: I can deal better with somebody like Dr. —— (one of the faculty) who says he believes in individual therapy, and he doesn't do this other stuff; so I know, and the resident will know, that that's not his cup of tea. I'm not saying this is wrong. It would be good if three or four of the faculty said, I'm interested in family work. Then the residents would know that. They don't know it now.

Dr. Schuster: You see there were many complaints by the residents in the past about divergent opinions of participating members (faculty) of the OPD conference. You may remember that that was a very constant theme. Personally, I didn't feel so strongly about that point. I thought, "So what? Their minds are not so fragile that differences of opinion are going to shatter them."

E: That's one of the strengths of the tutorial hour. Residents recognize a certain arbitrariness to this, but when you're trying to learn something it helps so much to have a consistent point of view, even if you feel like you're going to outgrow it.

Dr. Thaler: Again this is also a matter of what level of growth they are at. For a first-year resident to be exposed to the same patient with five different opinions about him is confusing. For the second- or third-year resident it may be easier to take.

Dr. Schuster: Their identity may be well enough established at the second-year level to tolerate this sort of thing.

B: I think a good course in psychotherapy should be taught in the first year. They would then have a foundation with which to enter into supervision of their individual cases and be able to tolerate conflicting opinions of the staff over management of cases.

GOALS AND STANDARDS OF TRAINING

Dr. Thaler initiated the discussion of this meeting by summarizing some impressions he had gained from several meetings he had had with residents from all three years concerning their views of our training program. They commented that they felt a lack of structure in our teaching about psychotherapy, although they regarded highly their individual supervision. They expressed the need for a more organized presentation of a number of topics, including psychodynamics, and indicated their dissatisfaction with teaching in the family and group areas. Here, too, they were satisfied with their supervision but not the formal presentation of subject matter such as rationale, indications, and theoretical considerations. This introduction led to a discussion by Dr. Thaler of the first-year residents' initial experience with group work on an in-patient floor.

Dr. Thaler: The whole business of groups is very confusing to the residents, because in the very first year one of the first things that happens to them on the floor is to be thrown into certain kinds of group activities. They are terribly puzzled about what that's all about. There was also an almost uniformly negative feeling about the patient-staff meetings on the floor. They all felt that they didn't know what they were supposed to do; they felt unable to be openly critical about it in the floor setting. Most of them felt frustrated and angry, because they didn't feel they did anything. They felt at times that it was even harmful to the patient, and that the whole setting was inappropriate to that sort of regular ongoing meeting.

As Are these first-year residents?

Dr. Thaler: Yeah, they were first year, but the others felt the same way, too.

Dr. Schuster: You mean they were still talking about that in the second year?

Dr. Thaler: Yeah. Now the group experiences on the floor that they did feel were useful were on a couple of floors where it was finally arranged that a group would be chosen who were felt to be suitable to participate in a group therapeutic experience. A resident would take a turn over a number of weeks, which was contracted for with the group, to do the group therapy with observation and supervision. The members of the group, when they were discharged from the hospital, agreed to come back to continue with the group. This they felt was useful, and also the supervision they felt adequate. Where they were just sort of thrown into a group and each resident had to run the group every week or twice a week with only his patients, they felt for the most part was useless. They might find themselves with three or four patients having ECT and a couple of senile patients sitting around for the hour. Generally speaking they felt that there was a lack of any kind of structure or a didactic program. Maybe we could spend a little time today talking about our own supervisory ideas and how to go about it.

Dr. Sandt: I wish I'd taped Dr. Z. He's a lovely one to parallel. You want a fellow you have to talk about gestures with.

Dr. Thaler: Here again Z doesn't gesture at all, he's like paralyzed. The interesting thing about this is there are times when we are too critical. When I first got with his manner I said, "My God, this is awful," because he was so quiet.

Dr. Schuster: He doesn't put his foot in his mouth.

Dr. Thaler: That's exactly it. After I'd listened to five or six or seven of the things he did, I concluded, he's all right. It's his style, and it's not the greatest, but he does all right. He pops the questions just at the right moment, and he gets the material that he needs, and he doesn't overlook much.

Dr. Sandt: Our response to these things shows you that we accept them almost as if they're permanent fixtures of the resident's style. From the way the resident comes to you on day one, it's very hard to say that he is at stage so and so, and what he has been doing.

Dr. Thaler: We automatically assume that the resident's style ought to be like ours, and if it isn't like ours the first response is that it isn't good. If you listen a little more you find that there's more than one road to Rome but. . . . I wonder whether we could say something about a formulated approach to the supervisory relationship. Do we have a curriculum in our mind that we want to cover in the first year, the second year and the third year tutorial? Is there a syllabus of some sort, either vague or specific? What are our goals, what are we trying to get across to the residents?

A: Rather than answer that, because that goes back to the beginning of our getting together, what might be helpful would be to extract what we have as a group discussed or what are the crucial issues for us from your presentation. That will give a sense of achievement. Otherwise we're going to play tapes over many weeks, talk and then go back to day one and talk about what we each think supervision should be, and then play a new tape. Many issues have come up which I never put into words myself. I'd like to see them noted, some of the issues that come up in supervision for all of us, such as the tenuous boundary between being a therapist and a supervisor. And I'd like to see us come up with some agreement on this. To me that would be achieving something from all the weeks we've been listening to tapes.

Dr. Thaler: How shall we go about this A?

A: I think we can try and recollect some of these issues and see if we can reach agreement. I'd like to see us generate some principles of supervision here as a group.

Dr. Sandt: The first issue has to do with what's the end product that we're after. Having decided what it is we're after in some nice general terms, what do you do individually to attain this?

Dr. Schuster: To get back to the central point of what is the knowledge that we consider necessary for the resident to acquire. My feeling is that at the present time we're dealing with a very difficult situation, because there's a great impatience in the minds of many people about "helping" psychiatric patients. Mental health workers of all kinds with great diversity of background and training are involved in the community mental health movement. There is a great tendency to dismiss the details of intrapsychic considerations and an impatience with spending too much time on individual patients. Many people are rushing, without proper preparation, into dealing with groups before they know anything about individuals. This is one of the points that Ned Freeman and I made in our paper on supervision of the initial interview. The fact is that to learn anything about intrapsychic considerations requires a fairly painstaking approach over a period of time. It involves seeing a lot of patients with proper supervision, doing some reading and understanding a little about one's self.

Dr. Thaler: So I think to get back to our resident—what are the principles?

Dr. Schuster: I've fought to see that the residents have some decent experience for the six months they spend in OPD, with thoughtful consideration of a number of individual patients, with experienced clinicians helping them. I think that's one of the first principles. There is no substitute for that kind of experience. A correlary to it is the opportunity to follow, hopefully more than one but at the very least, one patient in some kind of continual psychotherapy. Patients they can see more than once a week, over a period of some months in order to gain some feeling about continuity, something about psychic determinism, something about the unconscious transference.

Dr. Thaler: Earlier we talked about the way we set up our diagnostic studies, the time available for them, the things they are supposed to accomplish. I think we commented that there seems to be inadequate time available after the patient is seen to discuss fully the outcome of the interview and all the things that the resident should learn, because the interview goes for an hour. Here again, I think two things we might try to specify more precisely are: what should be the goal of the diagnostic study, and how much time ideally might be required for full discussion of the diagnostic interview? This would include the resident's way of entering the problem. That's the diagnostic end of it. The other thing would be what about the treatment end of it, and how much help is he getting with that. One of the glaring things that I've noticed is that the resident sees a lot of very interesting patients whom he wants to follow; but once he's out of the diagnostic phase he has to get his supervision in a "catch as catch can" fashion, because he has only one hour of tutorial a week. My hunch is that there's no time during that one hour to attend to all these follow up things that should be done.

A: Something comes to mind which we've never talked about, but it might be interesting. I think it's very threatening to talk about. We never look at our standards for judging a good psychotherapist (I'm using the word psychotherapist as a broad term), and I think we don't look at them for very good reasons. If I looked back at all the people I've supervised, let's say there have been 15, I think perhaps two had a talent for psychotherapy. The rest are mediocre, and hopefully they won't be destructive. I hope they'll know enough to be fairly competent, and they'll dodder along and at times do quite well, and some will be compassionate and some won't. Talent in my estimate would vary. Psychotherapy is so complex, it's such a fine art. You can indoctrinate people for 30 years in psychodynamics and psychoanalysis, and they can be clods. We know that. The residents have this war cry that nobody gives us structure. A talented resident who learns the same as his colleague can do a good job. I see this in the second year already. Some of them just have that sensitivity. They may not have knowledge enough but they know what's going on in the patient, because they're open to the patient. Those who are very closed will hold out for structure, because they're defending against something much more basic. I think maybe we could look at standards we use, and if we accept this reasoning that very few people make outstanding therapists, we look in the whole community and find maybe half a dozen outstanding therapists. If we accept that our goals are somewhat more modest: namely, to provide people with enough knowledge and to get them to focus on themselves to some extent so they're not too destructive.

Dr. Thaler: I wonder, though, whether that point of view is a little too extreme. I agree with you that there are few outstanding psychotherapists; however, I think there are a lot of competent psychotherapists. In terms of our resident population, obviously with each group there may be one or two who will make very good therapists. The rest of them, for the most part, will make competent therapists, and there are a few who are obviously lost souls. Our efforts, I guess, should be toward the very good ones and the middle group. In addition to that the need for structuring and the cry for structure comes from different motivations. I think you're right, and those who aren't very apt at interacting with another human being want the treatment to be in mechanical terms. The talented ones also want a kind of structure and knowledge, because they know that they will be able to exercise their talent more effectively and more subtly and with greater precision if they have what they feel is lacking in their knowledge and training. I've noticed, for instance, a group will come to me and say, "We want to do some reading." I meet now with the third-year group periodically and do some basic reading on psychotherapy. Out of that group we have about 5 or 6 who come regularly, and they are the ones that are more capable.

Dr. Schuster: I'd like to comment on your views too, A. It may be that you're taking a little extreme view to make a point, but we needn't argue about that. We certainly can't disagree that talent in whatever field it may be is a rare commodity.

B: What are we talking about? What's talent?

Dr. Schuster: Well, we'll come back and let A define that if he wishes to, but I think the implication is that everybody should be a consummate psychotherapist at the end of three years. In the first place, that's impossible, and we should disabuse ourselves of the notion that we are going to turn out psychotherapists. . . .

Dr. Sandt: The first assessment you make is where the resident is, given the goal which I guess is something we can identify fairly well. There is a pattern to the way you have to judge this. What kind of issue confronts him, and how much does he stumble over himself? Then can you leave that alone, or does it get right in the middle of things? All these are influenced by the kind of case he has.

A: A minor issue I recall from many weeks back was the question of the merits or demerits of using the resident's office as opposed to our own office. These are minor things, but they're interesting.

Dr. Thaler: We picked that up early on in our discussion, and I think it had to do more basically really with what should be the ideal relationship between the supervisor and the resident. What are their positions vis-à-vis each other? How should they optimally perceive each other in terms of what sort of pedagogic relationship this is. I have another thing that occurs to me, one of the things we talked about a great deal, the resident's attitude toward the patient before he has even seen the patient.

A: In other words, people form a set before meeting the patient by virtue of the little data they get.

Dr. Thaler: I think we were also getting into some of the problems about what sort of a model is the most appropriate one to use, and we had some discussion about the so-called medical model. I think some of us wondered is there such a thing?

Dr. Sandt: Does anybody here know Matarazzo's interaction chronograph? This research involved the comparative study of three interview styles: structured, unstructured and a combination of these. They felt that the composite style was most comfortable for the patient, but they were primarily interested in discovering the effectiveness of patient-therapist "fit" in terms of style. The patient, of course, was most negatively affected by the shifts in style of the interviewer. The beginning second-year resident often heavy-handedly mixes styles based on "medical," structured interview technique and on open-ended techniques. If you say that the resident should have his own style, and all roads lead to Rome, that still leaves the issue of how this has impact on particular styles of the patient. The hysteric is not going to be like an obsessive, so there has to be some flexibility.

Dr. Thaler: The problem is how to teach and also how to perceive in the resident the rigidities of his style which are counterproductive in terms of the interview, and conversely how to teach skill in interviewing within the constraints of the resident's individual style. Finally if his style is totally inappropriate, we must teach some alteration in his style, some modification of it.

B: Don't you think, too, that if you could say that the goal of every person was to establish some identity, some concept of himself which he is free to assert, that then in the supervision of a resident part of the goal would be that we teach him certain things as well as support his development as a person? So that in the teaching of a resident as in the treatment of a patient, the goals are essentially the same—that he develops a sense of what he believes to be right for himslf as a person, a psychiatrist.

Dr. Thaler: Aside from what he thinks is right for him, are there certain basic common aspects of skill and knowledge which are necessary to be an adequate therapist and a teacher? What are the basic skills and knowledge, particularly in terms of today's ambience?

Dr. Schuster: Is it necessary that a graduate of a residency program be a psychotherapist? That's controversial, of course. I'd like also to express some concern about continuing education, particularly in the area of psychotherapy, of the graduate resident. Because our work is so private, he can't, as the young surgeon, hang over a senior surgeon's shoulder in the operating room and learn more about what he's doing. He has very few opportunities once he gets out in the world to talk with colleagues seriously or in any continuous way about the work he's doing; so there is a tendency to have his work become rather restricted and constricted. He can drift through life unchallenged and uninspired to look into what he's doing. It's very simple to fall into that sort of life. I think we should direct some of our concern and future deliberation to some devices for continuing education for at least a couple of years beyond the residency program. I'd also be interested in what you regard as talent, if you can define that. Also need a graduate of a residency program be considered a psychotherapist?

A: I don't know what talent is, and I think it's a subjective matter. I think in principle that we agree that the outstanding therapist is not common statistically, just as the outstanding lawyer is not common. What I'm trying to say is, let's look at what are reasonable goals for three years' supervision. In other words, what should be our goal of supervision in terms of expectation? What can we reasonably expect from the average resident? I don't think we've ever clarified that, because I think we all have different levels of expectation. Many residents tell me the supervisor just sits there and nods at them. One supervisor who comes to mind never says anything, he just agrees with everything the resident does. That's very nice in a way, because the resident is never threatened, but he learns nothing either. I think the message the resident is picking up is that this supervisor feels that the level he's at is what is expected of him. "He doesn't expect me to be different." If I look at a resident walking in, I have to think how much should I confront him, how much should I point out, how much should I expect of him?

Dr. Thaler: In other words, how much does each of us feel it is necessary, and at what level, to intervene in what the resident tells us about the patients he's dealing with. There are some supervisors who just nod their head, and I think I'm probably at the other end of the thing, because I talk my head off every time I meet with the resident. I don't know whether that's good either.

A: Well, let's be more specific and take Dr. X, for example, because we have so much data on him. I think what we have to ask ourselves is, what reasonably could we expect from him? We could sit back and say, well he's got personality problems, and he may have to go into therapy, or he's still learning, so why make such a fuss? Therefore, I shouldn't have intervened so much. Or could we say we expect this from a second-year resident?

Dr. Thaler: Maybe expectation isn't really enough. Even if he does what we expect him to do at a certain level, that's still no reason to keep my mouth shut.

Dr. Schuster: Well I think A touches on a very important point: We have not defined our task very carefully, and it's part of the vagueness of our field which I always say need not be as vague as we allow it to be. It's lazy on our part not to define things more carefully.

Dr. Thaler: If a resident does do what I expect him to do at the level he's at, I say, "Hooray for you," and then I try to tell him how to do more than what I would expect him to do. For instance, I supervised Dr. V last year, and she was superb, one of the most stimulating people I've ever worked with. It was a joy for both of us. I didn't talk any less, because she would do not only what I expected but usually a lot more. Yet I felt that I could stimulate her to do even more than that.

Dr. Schuster: Are you saying then that you talk the same amount for somebody who is very talented?

Dr. Thaler: As long as I feel that I have something to add to make it richer, then I do. Most people who come to be supervised don't expect you to just sit there and say nothing.

A: This is interesting, because I was the supervisor for Dr. V, and that's true. One could say she's very talented, and because she's talented she will respond. Then go to the other extreme where you get somebody like Dr. Q who will never make a psychotherapist. We have this delusion going where this resident is supposedly being supervised and supposedly dealing with patients therapeutically. It's a game. He will probably turn out to be competent in a different area, but not as a therapist.

Dr. Thaler: I also feel very strongly, as far as supervision is concerned, that any two people at the same level of experience can supervise each other. In other words, I could benefit from being supervised by anyone around this table, because you never hear all the things that somebody else hears. I doubt that I could benefit a great deal by being supervised by somebody who has a lot less experience than I, because he probably wouldn't hear the same things that I heard.

Dr. Schuster: I wonder why we don't make more provision to discuss our work with each other.

Dr. Thaler: I wish I had time.

Dr. Schuster: I don't think it's a question of time. I think we don't *make* the time. It's an interesting question.

B: The idea of talent that A brings up. I don't think you can really separate that from this idea of certain funds of knowledge that every resident must have.

Dr. Thaler: There's natural talent, and there's educated talent.

Dr. Schuster: Joan Fleming said in her early papers that without talent, supervision is hopeless. With talent a person can grow and gain, so that's the differentiation between the talent and knowledge that you mention. Some people can have good intellectual knowledge about psychiatry and still not have the talent for psychotherapy. We've seen residents like that.

Dr. Sandt: Well, I think there are some other things you ought to consider—how they can be less harmful than they might be without learning a few things. There are a great many things one can at least have the resident confront by himself, so that he stays out of the areas that are difficult for him.

B: I don't really understand what talent means, but I think it has something to do with the knowledge of psychodynamics, what makes people react the way they do to both inner feelings as well as conditions of their life. To be able to help the patient overcome these influences and in a sense develop himself is what the ultimate talent or goal of psychotherapeutic experience is for a patient. Therefore, if you don't deal with that and the problems that the resident has which are interfering with this development of the patient . . . what I'm trying to say is this idea of talent has to do pretty much with the personality of the resident. Just to give him knowledge and not to deal with that personality is . . . I mean we're back to this point where you have to deal with the personality of the resident in order that he be as good a therapist as he can. Even if he had all the knowledge, I don't think. . . .

Dr. Schuster: Are you making knowledge and talent synonymous in your mind?

B: No, I would call knowledge the thing that you teach.

Dr. Schuster: It isn't the same as talent?

B: No, I would say talent is . . .

Dr. Schuster: It's not personality either?

Dr. Thaler: I think talent is sometimes what we call psychological mindedness. I think it's an ability to view human behavior in a certain way, to be able to think in psychological terms.

Dr. Schuster: Well, this also includes such things as empathic capacity.

Dr. Thaler: This I think is part of psychological mindedness. I don't think you can understand another human being unless you have some compassionate, empathic feeling.

Dr. Schuster: That's a very questionable thing, because I can remember some colleagues in the past who had psychological mindedness but who had very little capacity to be empathic. Some psychiatrists are very intellectual, but they turn away from the patient. They can understand the patient, but they cannot engage with the patient. I think there is more than one ingredient to talent.

Dr. Sandt: It's also the fit between the psychological stance of the patient and the therapist. This is where you find in a person what looks like empathy on one occasion and psychological mindedness on another. It's quite clear that a resident might indeed relate to another obsessive, relatively angry person magnificently, and understand him, too, but not to a passive aggressive or dependent character.

PROBLEMS OF THE FIRST-YEAR RESIDENT

This excerpt from a conference discussion followed the presentation by one of the conference members (F.) of a tutorial session with a first-year resident. This resident had presented certain difficulties in his understanding of how to elicit pertinent information from his patients. This discussion reminded us of some of the deficiencies in certain areas of our instruction, in this case in the teaching of interviewing techniques at the outset of the resident's first year with us. This led to a brief discussion of some of the problems confronting a beginning resident on the in-patient service and the various devices —such as T-group—being employed to assist him in his work and developing identity as a psychiatrist. It also stimulated our thinking about possible new approaches to supervision during this critical period of professional maturation.

Dr. Thaler: F. is continuing his presentation of a tutorial session with a first-year resident. From our discussion last time he certainly exhibits typical, classical problems of the beginning first-year resident. As we listen to the tutorial I'm impressed again with the lack of formal instruction of these guys when they first come here, as to what they are supposed to do, what is expected of them, what is the theoretical framework within which they operate, etc. I think this relates to discussions we are having in the Curriculum Committee about the renewed attempt to set up some kind of more formal instruction for the resident just as soon as he gets here, so that he'll have some idea as to what's going on.

Dr. Sandt: Didn't we teach a course earlier? Wasn't that supposed to do the sorts of thing we're talking about?

Dr. Thaler: Well, we had all kinds of didactic exercises, including one on the psychotherapeutic approach to patients which included a series on hospital treatment.

F: But that part of the course stressed aspects of other techniques like Rogerian, it's the only time I learned anything about Rogerian techniques. Part of that also was a good series on drugs. I recall the least we had was about psychotherapy. I remember Dr. R gave a couple of lectures which were so incredibly theoretical for first-year residents that they were totally lost, and so I don't remember psychotherapy being taught in a way that was particularly useful.

Dr. Thaler: I think you're right. We've had our very considerable ups and downs with regard to teaching this particular area, and the only consistently well received aspect of it has been individual tutorials.

A: Well, you know part of the problem is moving from certainty to uncertainty. It's really hard, because it's not dealt with directly in that the medical student has years of formal training, much of it concrete. He can see, he can feel, he can think. It's very concrete, and then he moves into a field that is so ambiguous, particularly psychotherapy. And it's almost like he's got to learn an attitude rather than facts. It's like being open, using yourself, not clinging to concrete, simple facts or being arbitrary and controlling. At another center where I've had experience, a fairly supportive T-group led by a very sensitive psychiatrist really helped the first-year residents. They said they were very frightened at first, but it helped them because they were allowed to open up a little and see that they weren't such bad people and they didn't need to hide from themselves or from their colleagues. They found they had many mutually similar problems, and it really helped them and gave them emotional support and made them more open to their patients. The experience was helpful, because it gave them some attitudes. Without something like this they feel they're unique and what they do is they become aggressive and defensive and controlling in order to hide their own difficulties.

Dr. Thaler: I suppose inadvertently, although I didn't call it a T-group, that's pretty much what I've done this year with the first-year residents.

A: You meet with all the first-year residents?

Dr. Thaler: Yes. They articulated what they share in terms of concerns and seemed reassured to find that everybody else felt the same way. I indicated that often indeed there are problems of uncertainty—not precisely knowing what to do, that continue to be with you no matter how much experience you have had. That seemed to be helpful. I didn't call it a T-group. I focused it primarily on clinical vignettes which they presented and from which we then derived certain judgments.

Dr. Sandt: Do you see any shift in them?

Dr. Thaler: Well, it's hard to know. Currently I'm focusing on their beginning experience with psychotherapy, and I'm trying to substitute for a non-existent course in psychotherapy. What we're doing is—like I've asked them, for instance, to present an initial interview, then we go over that and try to get some general form for it. Then we read Freud's papers on technique, which are really very clear and simple for beginners.

Dr. Sandt: Are they able to pick that up now, do you think, and assimilate it?

Dr. Thaler: Oh, yes.

Dr. Sandt: The way they do it in most places is to have a vehicle called a continuous case which has obviously some aspects of a T-group.

Dr. Thaler: Our present psychotherapy seminar has been moved to the second year because of demand for a formal course. It's essentially a continuous case seminar that goes on in the second year.

Dr. Sandt: That not only incorporates elements like a T-group, the sharing of concerns, but also involves turnings in the ways he (the resident) deals with his specific case.

F: It's also helpful to know something—so that the exercise is both a group experience but also you can defend it in terms of the fact that you're presenting a tape of a patient ostensibly in treatment. It also helps to have some sort of background.

Dr. Thaler: I tend to be fairly didactic. I like to talk, and I free associate to their comments from my experience, reading and so on. I feel it is a fairly didactically oriented exercise rather than ostensibly a therapeutic one, although I have no doubt that it has therapeutic value. There does seem to be early on in the year for first-year residents some sort of a dichotomy. It's a problem, because on the one hand they're supposed to act therapeutically with patients, and nowadays it's different from say 10-15 years ago. They have some very potent vehicles with which to do this; namely, the phenothiazines and other drugs and ECT. But at the same time they're also supposed to develop an attitude which, as you point out, is quite different from that of intervening with major chemical modifiers—and that is very difficult.

F: And the other thing is not only the issue of phenothiazine, and ECT, but they're also asked, at least on some of the floors, to begin to get some notion of other treatment modalities, as on our floor they're expected to conduct a small group. So they're expected to learn something about group principles. Dr. K has a seminar for them in group process, and we're also putting more and more emphasis on families, particularly at least family interviewing. It's relevant here because as I pressed this resident (first year) to become more engaged with the patient, one of the things that he did was to see the patient and her husband together with a nurse on the floor. The nurse is somebody who happens to be very quiet but very effective, she doesn't challenge him directly. He's seen the couple together now about four times, and it's going very well. I supervised one of their interviews last week between the husband and the wife. The couple is being helped by it. In fact at the end of the interview they're asking, "When is our next one, we want to continue this." It's been helpful to the resident also in the sense that he has this fairly sensitive nurse who doesn't threaten his leadership. He opens and closes the session, but she makes some of the more sensitive comments through the course of the session, so in a sense that's helpful to him. But also it's asking him to deal in one more psychological treatment modality; we're adding one more burden. One justification I would offer for doing that is that I think that unless you introduce somebody to this in the first year, as a group, it's going to be difficult to introduce them to it later on.

Dr. Thaler: That stimulates me to think of a new kind of supervisory set. We've talked here about group supervision where one supervisor supervises more than one resident at the same time. This has certain advantages and disadvantages, obviously, in terms of the residents getting more exposure to different clinical material. Also, however, this is a less private thing. As you were talking, it occurred to me that it might be an interesting exercise to have a supervisory panel to attempt a supervisory situation in which there would be somebody who's primarily interested and skilled in individual therapy, somebody else who's interested in family, and somebody else who's interested in group, all of whom might supervise the same resident or the same group of residents. Each could provide the input from his own somewhat slightly different stance and view of the patient's problem.

F: I don't understand how that works.

Dr. Thaler: Well, let's take, for instance, this situation where he starts with an individual patient and presents this material to the supervisory panel. One supervisor would chime in and comment on the patient's immediate transference response related to some comment the patient had made, another supervisor would say, "Shouldn't you be seeing the husband?" Then the supervisors would jointly focus on determining the meaning of what is going on from the point of view of the husband, the point of view of the family, the point of view of the individual as well. It might be interesting.

Dr. Sandt: I have a label for it called "Supervision by Assault." It's been described in literature. One of the difficulties is that the input is a bit overwhelming for the stage where the resident is in the first year, but I think he probably could absorb this in rounds.

F: I think they need priority, even if it's the pseudo-priority of only having to deal with one supervisor.

Dr. Sandt: One person at a time. I think you have to sort out when you have multiple supervisors . . .

Dr. Thaler: I think we all do it for ourselves.

Dr. Sandt: That's what I'm thinking. A panel discussion would be more for the panel than for the resident, which may not be a bad thing. Obviously everybody is selectively attending to certain aspects of the interaction.

F: Things are better when you do something like this in the second or third year.

Dr. Thaler: What I'm trying to think about is how best to help the resident when he first comes to the floor, when he has to deal with at least four kinds of different treatment modalities; he has to deal with the conventional in-patient treatment problems; he has to deal with individual psychotherapy; he has to deal with group psycho-therapy; and he has to deal with families.

F: And he has to relate to the floor staff also.

Dr. Thaler: Yes, and besides that he has to have administrative duties. How do we best provide a somewhat structured didactic teaching experience that will encompass these various approaches early in his training, so that he doesn't feel thrown into many different and strange modalities which he's supposed to master from day one?

A: An example that illustrates this is when the Family Group was invited to do rounds on the floor. The patient was a 20-year-old music student, male, admitted to the floor. I can't remember exactly why, but the resident felt there were family problems and asked for consultation from the Family Group. It was unusual in that there were something like 13 people in the family, but it was interesting because although he is having supervision of this patient, and there are administrative and management issues involving the rest of the staff, the family approach threw a new light on it. He suddenly saw how in that family set-up a lot of things made sense which didn't seem earlier, such as the fact that the parents saw this kid as a genius, which he wasn't. He's struggling to try and prove that to them, and this hadn't come out in individual sessions. There was also a conflict concerning his separation from the home—this kid kept talking about going to New York. The rounds also gave the floor staff an opportunity to share their observations of the family members. So this was really helpful. So I think it is possible for first-year residents not to be overwhelmed and yet exposed to different ways of seeing the same patient. This is what it really amounts to.

Dr. Thaler: Well should we perhaps plan in a somewhat more deliberate manner than we have so far to make sure that each of the first-year residents within their first few weeks has an experience like this. Take a patient, let's say, that a resident is seeing and present this patient in three different modalities: present the patient as the resident deals with him individually; have the family in and present that point of view; and then look at another aspect, how that patient operates in a group. This might be a very interesting exercise, and it could extend over a period of several weeks for the whole group.

Dr. Sandt: You mean include all the residents in this? All the first-year residents?

Dr. Thaler: Yes, have this like a grand rounds except only for resident staff. It might work out very well.

A: I think what is important is that with some of the faculty there is a tendency to categorize each other, and in turn the work we do— he's a group man or a family man. But those who do group and family work also do individual therapy. This tendency to categorize each other gets to the resident, and then they're forced with choices. For example, if the resident knew that a faculty member known for his group work also did a fair amount of individual work, he wouldn't feel he needed to choose this method or that method, but could be open to a variety of approaches.

Dr. Sandt: That's one of the problems with setting it up this way. You are indeed fragmenting the identity that we'd like to make synthetic. I don't know why one person . . .

Dr. Thaler: You know I have the reputation of being opposed to group therapy, which I'm not. I'm opposed to unsupervised, unskilled, wild kinds of adventures.

Dr. Sandt: I believe it's worse, more dangerous to be wild in individual work than it is in group, if you want to talk about which of those two is more dangerous. When you think back over our meetings, individual supervision is what we're after.

A: There are only two kinds of therapy—good and bad, and we've had them both.

Dr. Sandt: Well, I think that's one of the difficulties about setting up this kind of a panel approach. It does indeed dichotomize and fragment, unless the same person can present all of the modes.

Dr. Thaler: Unless it becomes evident, as from a group like ours who know each other fairly well, that though one may be a family expert, another a group expert and someone else an individual expert, we all have a certain agreement. We may view the same clinical problem from different vantages, but we're not diametrically opposed and we understand what each other is talking about. We're simply dealing with a group of people who have more experience in one area than another.

A: It's like that Japanese movie, Right From Wrong, where there are many aspects of truth, but the truth is that none of them is wrong and none is right. It's just many facets. This is where we keep slipping. I think it's we who do it. We convey to the residents that it must be either this or that, and then they really get anxious, because they don't want to displease us.

Dr. Sandt: It's very hard to have a linear statement which by selecting details from the student point of view doesn't have bias and devotion. Marshall McLuhan just encompassed everybody in some kind of total gestalt. A good trick. That's what I think we're trying to do in fact by having multiple input.

Dr. Thaler: Well, no. I wouldn't see it that way. I would see it as an opportunity to see different facets of the same problem.

Dr. Sandt: It sounds like a good experiment. It could be tried.

F: We could do it during the summer in successive sessions, and then in the fall edit one video tape each—edit out segments and make that into one grand rounds package. That would be an economical use of the time.

Dr. Thaler: One thing about grand rounds, if you look at the grand rounds over this past year I dont' think any of them have talked about treatment—none of them. Well, aside from drugs we haven't talked about therapy.

F: We never do.

Dr. Thaler: It's a very difficult subject to deal with. So often the focus is on diagnosis. Is this organic? Is it schizophrenic? Well, I was thinking it might just be possible to transcend that by talking about the problems of the interview. I think in the meantime I'll talk with the first-year residents. Maybe we can do something like this one of these days.

Dr. Sandt: There's a developmental process involved here. Everybody's read that Schlessinger paper which reviews modes of supervision. He talks about the differences in supervision—ultimately it's a question of whether you want to focus more or less on the patient or more or less on the resident. Whatever is going on internally, to focus on the interaction between the supervisor and the resident being supervised. Well now, it seems to me in the first year you're after issues of identity, and so it's natural, of course, to focus much more away from the anxiety of the resident onto the specific issue of diagnosis. What's going on with the patient? So with a first-year resident I should ask, "What's going on with the patient? What kind of person is this? What sort of viewpoint does he have? What sorts of issues is he contending with?" That sort of thing. What's the setting for this patient? And you can distance it a great deal away from the resident as an instrument to the patient. And as you go on, the resident's identity becomes more comfortable. By the third year you're probably seeing much more of the supervision of what's going on with the resident, what's going on with the subtleties of the transference, rather than what's the matter with the patient. The bridge is the second year. You really see this if you listen to tapes from the OPD. You really don't know where you are at first, because the resident has yet to make that switch, to talk and to be comfortable with himself.

A: I've sort of got an example, quite a humorous one which really clarifies this. There's an analyst I knew who used to do a continuous case conference—a weekly thing. This resident was presenting a girl, a hysterical nurse in her 20's, and she kept telling him about her sexual problems. This went on and on for some weeks, and progressively her dress got more and more revealing. It occurred to me that she was talking about this to please him—to interest him, rather than getting to her basic problem. I mentioned this, and the analyst dismissed it and continued to talk about her sexual problem. Afterwards he called me and said he'd like to terminate this case.

DISCUSSION OF A TUTORIAL HOUR

In Chapter IV we discussed our "tutorial" program, an integral part of our supervisory program. We have also pointed out earlier that the tutorial "hour" is prized by the resident as far more valuable than any other of the seminars and conferences we have described. In this final excerpt from our supervisory conference dialogue we had chosen to listen to a recording of one such tutorial hour. The resident, Dr. W., was presenting (playing sections from a tape-recording of one of his own patient interviews) a history of a young woman he had recently seen in the Crisis Clinic. We begin with his opening comments to his tutor, also a member of the conference (B). He gave some of the patient's presenting problem which led to a discussion by the conference members of why the resident brought this particular problem to his tutor, as well as the difficulties this patient afforded the resident. We spent considerable time in assessing the nature of the clinical problem and the type and timing of interventions we felt were indicated. Eventually we focused on the transference aspects of this case, how they made particular demands on the resident, and how we could help him understand these issues. Later on we discussed various technical considerations involved in assessing and treating this particular patient and finally the outcome of a short course of psychotherapy with her.

> *Dr. W:* This is a young girl who appeared in Crisis Clinic a week ago. She is 19. She's been married for 2½ years. She has no children and she has worked in a variety of jobs. She's been an Avon girl and various sorts of things like that. She sounds as though she's probably a socially competent girl. She came along with the complaint that she thought she was going crazy and there was something happening to her, and she didn't know what it was. She said she thought she should see a psychiatrist, and that was just about all she could say when she was seen in ED. And that's about all she talked about in Crisis Clinic. At times she was pressured and worried about something going on, that she was on the verge of some serious illness. I can't get her in DS (diagnostic study) for a month or so, so I decided to keep on seeing her and then decide what to do—to refer her for DS or keep her myself. To cut a long story short, it turns out in this interview that for the first quarter of an hour or so she tests me to find out whether she can trust me by asking me questions that would ordinarily get a reply of yes or no. I tried to stay away from that, and then it came out what the problem was. Two months ago when she was with a girlfriend, on Halloween, the girlfriend touched her and that

set off the latent homosexual things in this girl. Ever
since then she's being torn between staying with this girl
and becoming a lesbian or living with her husband. She
hasn't indulged in any sexual relationship with the girl
yet, but she's thinking of it. It seems that she comes
along to make a decision one way or the other. My
difficulty is knowing how to handle it and try and work
things out with her. I'm just not sure of where to go
with it.

Dr. Thaler: Before we hear what B says, should we stop a minute
and examine what is the patient's problem? Does anybody want to
comment on that? What are we hearing? I'm sure each of us hears
something different.

Dr. Schuster: I want to understand the situation more clearly.
I have a predilection for wanting to start at the beginning, so I'm
interested in the patient's complaint. What brought the patient to
the clinic? I'm confused because Dr. W first said she didn't seem
certain about what her specific complaint was. She appeared at the
Crisis Clinic at whose prompting, or do we know that?

B: This comes out later in the interview.

Dr. Schuster: What did she present with when she first saw Dr. W?

B: With feelings of anxiety and tension based on being . . . well
the way it comes out, this girl touched her in October, and she didn't
come in until December because her husband hadn't really begun
to be much of a problem until then. She had spent too much time
over at the other girl's house, and the husband had asked about it, and
they got into some kind of discussion. Although the husband doesn't
know what the nature of the relationship is, he does feel she's spending too much time over there, and this created added problems for
the girl. It isn't clear just yet why she is here, but it has to do with
pressures from family, pressure from her husband, pressure from
this girlfriend and her feeling caught in all this.

Dr. Schuster: Well, we don't know all the factors, but at this point
what we do know then is that the patient views the problem as one
of not being certain whether she should stay with her husband or
live as a lesbian with this girl. That's how she presents it. Now what
does it mean that on Halloween some girl touched her? Do we know
any more about that?

B: This girl is a known lesbian.

Dr. Schuster: Yeah, but what does it mean touched?

B: I asked him the same thing. It was a pass, because this girl is a known lesbian.

Dr. Thaler: From these first few minutes in a patient interview, which often are so instructive and crucial in terms of understanding the patient's problem, can we understand the resident's problem? What is his problem here? What is he coming to us for? One thing he's saying is that he could have intervened more directively but by using non-directive techniques this girl told him what the real problem is—namely the lesbian conflict. Then he says he doesn't know what to do. What is his dilemma? He's asking B, "What should I do? Should I tell her what to do or not, how should I pursue it?"

B: In answer to your question, Otto, there's an element sometimes in the tutorial that is like an apprenticeship, in which the resident is presented with a problem, and he comes and asks, "How do you do this thing?"

Dr. Thaler: Yeah, like coming to the master craftsman for advice.

B: Lots of residents do not do that, they just present something without asking a question. They seem to be wanting verification of what they've already done, rather than seeking to learn something.

Dr. Thaler: So there are two things: one is the resident may come to you primarily to have you say, "You're doing okay, go ahead" or he may come to you like Dr. W here did with a specific problem and ask, "How would you tackle this?"

A: I don't quite understand this. He saw this girl, because he was on duty in the emergency room?

Dr. Schuster: No, the Crisis Clinic.

A: That's what's important, because I hear him also not being clear about which option to adopt.

Dr. Schuster: I think what he's saying, and I work in the Crisis Clinic so I understand what he's talking about, is that there was no DS appointment available until January, so what should he do with this patient? I sense that he wishes to maintain his responsibility with this patient and not just pass her off to someone else, so he has a choice of seeing her later on in January when he comes to OPD or seeing her now, There's an understanding in Crisis Clinic that you see nobody more than 6 times, and then some other disposition has to be made. There are other possible dispositions.

Dr. Sandt: He was giving a pretty clear indication of the dilemma, either he stays with her, or he doesn't. He puts her on the waiting list, or he doesn't. Either he keeps continuing with her . . . he's asking you, should he keep her?

Dr. Thaler: He's made a choice.

Dr. Sandt: He made a choice to maintain a firm relationship, but the interesting underlying thing is whether this is going to be a longer term case than an immediate crisis handling? He says maybe, I'll stay with her, but should I keep her after this crisis?

A: Will you please explain how a patient comes to the Crisis Clinic?

Dr. Schuster: They're referred from the Emergency. The Crisis Clinic is operated conjointly between the ED (Emergency Division) and the OPD. It meets in the OPD three times a week, and these patients come from the Emergency, are referred by the residents. They're patients who usually present some acute situation, and they can be then seen within one to three days.

A: Well with that background, my first question is what's the emergency? She's been waiting for months, so what does that say about her?

Dr. Sandt: The crisis is there's no DS available.

Dr. Schuster: The crisis can be other things, too. It can be in the resident's mind, you know.

Dr. Sandt: She may have looked more upset if she were in the ED.

Dr. Thaler: Was she acutely anxious, is that what comes through?

B: Not in the interview.

Dr. Thaler: So one thing that comes through here is that the resident is interested in this young woman because of the particular problem which she presents, which is slightly unusual. We've seen a lot of young men in OPD who have either overt or not so overt homosexual problems. We don't see very many women who come with that complaint. Another question that occurs to me, do we now find out what this resident knows about female homosexuality and do we use the tutorial to instruct him, to refer him to reading about it? To say before we do anything about this patient, should you not find out something for yourself about this particular syndrome?

A: That could be premature, because it seems that the hardest thing for the new second-year resident to do is to learn to listen to what a patient is saying. They often buy whatever the patient says. If the patient says "I'm a lesbian" they take it literally. Very often that's not the reason the person is there, and that's why I'm raising the question, what's the emergency? I think it's so easy for the resident to go wrong and read tomes about homosexuality, when in fact it's got little or nothing to do with why the person's there.

Dr. Thaler: So you're saying that a didactic intervention here is premature, and one should wait until the problem becomes clearer, and then perhaps at some later point introduce the more didactic approach to whatever the problem turns out to be.

Dr. Sandt: At this point in the interview you don't give him a set of references.

Dr. Thaler: It seems to me that's an important point about how we conduct the supervisory tutorial relationship. I think it could be a grave error, for instance, to say, "Now we will read 3 books on lesbianism, then come back to me." What we're dealing with here is a patient we don't really know that much about.

Dr. Schuster: Well, first of all I would guess that the crisis was the patient's anxiety as she presented in the Emergency Room. We can't recreate that situation at this point. We have to hear more, but I would suspect that's what it was.

B: I don't know, I didn't ask him about the ED note. I don't know how anxious she was when she first appeared.

F: She also presents in a way that some male homosexuals do, that this is a decision point, my marriage is at stake. If you intervene properly, you may be able to save my marriage and keep me from life as a lesbian. I think that's part of what he's responding to.

Dr. Schuster: This certainly stirs rescue fantasies in the therapist, this sort of appeal, and we have to bear that in mind. The other matter that's of great interest to me is the matter of touching. Being a clinician he should be interested in the details no matter what they are, so when somebody makes this abstract or disguised reference that someone touched me, we want to find out what that means. Of course, in a broad sense it concerns the whole field of medicine. Hippocrates realized this when he stated that the physician must eschew any libidinal interest in the patient. One of the primary issues between the physician and patient, of course, is the touching of the body. It occurs to me that there is a sort of polarity between those who do touch the body, like the surgeon or particularly the obstetrician who examines the genitals, and the psychiatrist who does not generally. The body can be touched or examined only if the affects, the emotional life of the examiner can be curtailed and controlled.

The psychiatrist can more easily talk about the emotional life of the patient, because he doesn't touch the body. One of the interesting things that occurred to me about touching may be related to her religion. Remember Christ said after he was crucified and seen by one of the disciples, "Touch me not," because he had not as yet ascended to His Father. What does touching mean in the religious sense? Also Halloween, you know, is All Saints Eve, a religious holiday. I don't know what religious connotation this has. Why was this so anxiety-provoking to the patient?

A: It also has such a connotation of passivity. It's a way of saying I had nothing to do with it. *She* touched me.

Dr. Schuster: She touched me, and now what can I do?

Dr. Thaler: One might even analogize again in terms of what the patient is asking. This is already a transference phenomenon which one might need to point out to the resident. In other words the patient really was asking the interviewer to touch her in some way, to make it good, to undo the harm that has been done. In other words, she says to him in an equally passive way, now do something, help me make this decision as to where I should go.

F: And *he* turns to you. Here's a good resident. He summarized his problem well, and yet he's surprisingly sort of passive. He's now asking you to touch him in a sense and make it all come out good.

B: We've certainly made quite a thing out of this. Returning to that point you were making, Otto, in the beginning about the role of the tutor. In a sense we might need to discuss at some point further this idea that part of the contract, I hate that word, part of the agreement let's say between the resident and the tutor is that the resident has a need in him to do something different, to change just like the patient has to have that with the doctor. I always feel frustrated with a resident who doesn't present, and with a patient who is using the relationship for something other than what it's supposed to be.

Dr. Schuster: Which relationship are you talking about?

B: Patient-doctor or the tutorial.

Dr. Thaler: I think there's a point we might like to note. We're analogizing from the therapeutic contract to the tutorial. As a consequence we're saying that in a similar fashion in therapy the patient has a goal for treatment, and the therapist has a goal for treatment which may or may not coincide. It's useful often to articulate this with a patient to make sure that you both are compatible at least, if not identical. Similarly the resident may have a goal in his supervisory relationship with you, and you may have a goal—the two of which may not necessarily coincide. It might be useful when you start with a resident to talk with him about what is this about, what are we trying to accomplish and what does he want from you, and what do you want from him.

Dr. Schuster: You mean before you see the patient?

Dr. Thaler: At the beginning of the tutorial relationship.

B: To make it more complicated the resident in a sense intellectualizes his way into it, looking as though he's trying to solve problems; but I think all of us must have sensed the experience where the resident, although he talks about doing that, really doesn't ask questions. He just talks, and I think he's either looking for confirmation or he's trying to avoid being wrong with what he's done.

Dr. Schuster: B, I agree with you. I don't like the term contract either, but why do you object to it?

B: Because it sounds static. It doesn't change as you go along although you're both committed to it. It doesn't sound personal, it should be like an agreement.

Dr. Schuster: You don't mind the word agreement?

B: I never really thought of any substitute word, I just rebelled against contract.

Dr. Schuster: Well I agree. I don't like the term either. It's too legalistic, and I don't think really precise in terms of what you're trying to describe in the relationship between the therapist and the patient.

Dr. Thaler: I do like the term, although I agree with you. I wish we had another one that had fewer economic, legal and other kinds of connotations; but the reason I like the term is that it implies a number of things which I think are important. It implies an equal status between the two participants. It implies a mutual responsibility. Each of the participants has responsibility for the process and not just one, or one more than the other. Often with patients I've found it useful sooner or later to point out that he is responsible for what goes on here just as much as I am.

Dr. Schuster: I don't think equality is the correct issue involved here. If you were equal, what reason would the patient have for consulting you? The patient consults you because he assumes, rightly or wrongly, that you know something more about the problem than he does. It's not a position of equality at all. A contract isn't a matter of equality either. A contract is a legal document which expresses certain rights or issues and states the position of both parties, and I think it's simple enough just to say you have an understanding with a patient or an agreement which means that it's a loose agreement, too. The patient understands that you're going to try to help him and that he in turn has to pay for your time. Beyond that, there may be precise delineation of what constitutes the agreement.

F: You may be talking about something that feels right to you in terms of where you are at in terms of your professional career. I think in terms of the needs of beginning residents or beginning psychotherapists, and just the hardness of the word has certain advantages.

Dr. Schuster: You mean it helps them get a handle on something?

F: Yeah. I think this came out of the psychotherapy study that was done on the teaching of psychotherapy a few years ago. There's a disinclination to look at that whole area, that you're the rescuer, you're the helper and that's all there is to it. That's one of the unfortunate aspects of the first year, that they're thrown contractless into these relationships with the people on the ward. In terms of the needs of the residents and their resistance to face that, I think it's a good word even though it might not be for you.

Dr. Schuster: Well, I'm being too fussy about this, but I bring it up merely to examine what we mean by the term.

Dr. Thaler: I would like to come back to the equality thing, because I think that bugs us all. I agree with you certainly that there are certain inequalities. There are other aspects I think where the patient and the therapist in both instances should have an equal status as human beings in some way and in terms of certain kinds of decisions. The patient certainly should be as free as the therapist to terminate the contract. They should have equal rights with regard to that.

A: I was just thinking what happens if General DeGaulle goes to see his physician. Does the physician feel superior to him or not?

Dr. Thaler: That's the problem with the VIP patient.

A: What I'm asking is when going for help is there a change in the hierarchy because of that fact?

Dr. Thaler: A long time ago I happened to get involved in seeing someone connected with a very high official, and I was very junior and very much impressed by the status of that particular individual. Something came up where that individual was to consult me about the other person, and I was ill at ease as to whether I go to him or would he come to me? He solved this tactfully by coming to me. I didn't have to confront that. He just said I'll be over, and he came to my office, thereby indicating his perception of the situation. As it turned out that was a good thing and also the intervention that resulted was useful, and it made me feel more confident that I was in a position where I could tell him what the score was.

Dr. Schuster: I think F's position is very important, that the resident is searching for some kind of precision and structure and organization of his thinking and approach to patients, and we should help supply that. I am very much in favor of making as precise as we can the concepts we use and talk about all the time. They should not be loose. But I don't want concepts to become sort of encrusted or calcified or become clichés. This term contract is bandied about thoughtlessly by many people. I know that, and that's why I attack it as an example of why we should not be mindless about the way we use words or slogans. The equality business raises my ire, because I know I'm accused of being doctrinaire and traditional and an old fogey. But I'm disturbed, because I think the pseudoegalitarianism which is sweeping the mental health field, if unchanged, will result in the annihilation of the clinician. The idea that everybody can do what everybody else can do, whether he's a well meaning housewife from the inner city or a psychologist or psychiatrist or social worker or whatever, that we're all brothers under the skin and we're all buddies and, we all can do the same thing is utter nonsense.

B: Well the first one was right, but all the others weren't. We *are* brothers under the skin, but we can't all do the same things.

Dr. Schuster: The fact that we're brothers under the skin has nothing to do with our professional competence. I might go to somebody who's competent whom I do not admire as an individual or whom I don't regard as a brother or a comrade, but I go because I know he's competent. There is also a great disinterest in the intrapsychic, in the one-to-one study of patients, and this is becoming a national problem. Ned and I made this statement in our recent paper, because we believe so strongly about it. Now I hear disquieting news from a colleague, who has been visiting a number of medical

schools throughout the country, and from my own visit of two
schools recently, that the importance of the clinician is diminishing.
His role of teaching students to make careful observations of patients is under tremendous pressure by those who want to eliminate
the internship, eliminate one year of medical school, reduce the
number of patients a resident studies, make things shorter and easier.
There is a strong tendency to dilute quality of medical education.
We have to preserve this important role of the clinician.

Dr. Thaler: Now should we go on with B's tape for a little bit?

> *Dr. W*: There are indications that she had a good
> heterosexual adjustment in the past—no previous homo-
> sexual contacts, this is the first one.

> *B*: You said the girl touched her.

> *Dr. W*: Touched her hand.

> *B*: In an affectionate way?

> *Dr. W*: The other girl is a known lesbian and she knew
> that.

> *B*: She knew it before she went there. She'd known all
> along that this girl is a known lesbian. If this happened
> on Halloween how come she appeared at the Crisis
> Clinic, was it as a crisis?

> *Dr. W*: Yeah. She wrestled with it for a week or two
> and then decided to come in because she wasn't sleep-
> ing. She's eating up to 9 meals a day, there's friction
> with her husband. She kept herself physically isolated
> from the husband ever since then. She barely stays in
> the same room as he, she talks very little to him. So
> much so that the husband was getting a little sick
> of the way things were going on. As a matter of fact
> they had some arguments which kind of border on. . . .

> *B*: Is she saying or did it say on the tape why just
> because this girl touched her she changed her attitude
> then towards her husband? Why this issue became such
> a cause for this?

Dr. W: The way she puts it is that she'd like to live with the girl's parents because she would take care of her and she said not that my husband didn't take care of me, he's good to me, but she feels that would be much better.

Dr. Thaler: One of the things that occurs to me listening to the transference sequence is that the patient is saying to W: "This is what I want you to do for me." In other words, "I want you to take care of me. I'm coming here. I have a choice. Either it's this girl or it's you. I want you to do this, so my husband isn't, etc." W, on the other hand, is coming to you, B, to ask you to take care of him, just like she is asking him to take care of her. Would you point out to him at this particular juncture the possible transference meanings of this comment on her part and then try to pursue with him as part of your didactic plan which way to go with this? Now should he just keep this in mind as information for himself that this is what seems to be developing, namely, her demands on him? Should he make an intervention in terms of trying to point this out to her, or should he use it in some other way?

Dr. Schuster: Well, I think ideally it should be pointed out to the resident. Whatever way one may chose to do that—pointed out as one of the possible expectations of the patient in coming in to treatment, the set you might say the patient has on entering the door. It is not that he is supposed to say to the patient "Aha, that's what you want," but he bears that in mind in terms of observing what dependent demands she may make on him in subsequent encounters.

Dr. Sandt: A great deal depends on what you want to be doing with this resident. By the time you reach this point in this session, I'm sure B has a pretty solid idea about what he's going to be dealing with W about, and since the parallel you're making is not going to be restricted to this case around this particular resident, I think you have to be very delicate about the way you bring up that kind of issue. Pointing it out too confrontationally has negative aspects. I think I wouldn't bring up that issue at this point with that patient. It's not a question of what is she after, let him discover that issue.

B: If you were pursuing that issue wouldn't you lead into why is she coming? What is she after?

Dr. Sandt: Yes. Right. You do it more that way than coming in directly. . . .

Dr. Thaler: Then, you see, the negative question the resident will ask is, "Okay, now I know that or I suspect that there may be a transference issue involved in this woman's describing how this girl will take care of her, etc. What do I do now?" So then the next job of the teacher would be to tackle the question of intervention. Do you tell the resident? Do you give him choices? There are a number of things one can do to accomplish this kind of an insight. Just tell him what the possibilities are—the options are and then let him choose. Or do you say to him "Now I would do this or that."

Dr. Sandt: When that comes up—a question of options—I usually try not to do the listing and force "some orientation" on the part of the resident toward that kind of listing. As a matter of fact that's pretty much I guess what we all do. The very term options comes up early in the game.

Dr. Thaler: What I asked is that knowing this, now what would you do?

Dr. Sandt: Provide him with a set.

B: By knowing this you mean knowing . . .

Dr. Thaler: Knowing that the resident is making a covert plea for dependent gratification.

D: But this is true of all patients when they come, so why would you single it out now unless you wanted to use it in a clinical way of asking the resident what other people has this patient made demands on, such as the husband or a mother or a friend or an aunt, to see what diagnostic material you've gotten.

Dr. Thaler: The reason I singled out here is because of the way she does it. Other patients may do it more directly saying, "Look, doc, I need your help and I want to tell you my problems so you can tell me what to do."

Dr. Schuster: Well, you could remove it from the realm of the transference if you wanted to and approach it from another angle, as a commentary on the patient's character style. How she relates to others—these other women. That would be worth emphasizing to the resident I think.

B: My feeling about that is that in general the use of the transference tends to be overstated, it tends to make the resident ask questions about the patient's feelings about the resident before the patient is anywhere near ready to . . .

Dr. Schuster: Premature understanding.

B: Yes. So in answer to your question, I would be inclined to stay away from anything about the transference until it is in some way an important issue in the eyes of the patient.

Dr. Schuster: Well, then you get into another problem, and I'm not disagreeing with that. That certainly is a point of view that's worth discussing—keeping away from it so to speak—but then it involves another issue—prediction. In other words, if you feel confident that you can avoid any acting out of the transference by the patient—that you can see it in time to do something about it—then I wouldn't object to your waiting. What you're saying is wait until the transference is a little more obvious issue before talking about it.

B: Or it's a problem in some way.

Dr. Schuster: Yes, but sometimes it becomes a problem very quickly, and then you're not on top of it. Then the patient acts out, or some unfortunate direction takes place.

B: That's true, I can see how that could happen, except that I don't think that's as likely to happen as this other problem, that is, talking with the patient about problems that he's not aware of or ready to talk about.

Dr. Thaler: Wouldn't this be a good chance to make the point very clear to the resident that what he hears and knows from the patient's communication doesn't necessarily mean that he has to in turn talk about it with the patient? In other words I think it's very important to make sure that the resident knows that his knowledge of the patient's dynamics doesn't necessarily mean that he has to make any interpretation. As a matter of fact it often tells him what *not* to do.

Dr. Schuster: There are two aspects to the transference issue, one is knowing what's going on in the transference, and two is the use of this material with the patient in an interpretive intervention.

Dr. Thaler: Or the non-use of this.

Dr. Schuster: Yes, right, and so the resident then has to be helped in some detail as to what he should and shouldn't say about what he knows.

B: Well: I've heard residents say "I felt I should say something about my awareness that the patient is talking about me" and so they've gone ahead and done it (interpreted the transference to the patient) and then told me later they wished they hadn't.

Dr. Thaler: Part of the instruction then should be to emphasize the matter of timing.

B: Isn't there some way of being able to say in general when the time is right?

Dr. Schuster: Well, Freud mentioned this in his papers on technique that you don't talk about the transference until the resistance appears. It's a matter of time, a matter of the presentation, type of presentation, how it's worded.

B: It would seem to me that it's awfully important when you make such an interpretation that the patient see it not as something that just is between you and the patient, but as another example of the thing that happens in his relationship to others. Then the intensity is somewhat taken away from the actual interaction. But too often the resident just makes the interpretation. . . .

Dr. Schuster: Well, I think the usual consequence of that is an intellectual evasion on the part of the patient, and so the transference does not assume the quality of immediacy, the affective aspect of the transference. If it's prematurely interpreted, it's an intellectualized concept, so it's no use to the patient or to the therapist.

Dr. Sandt: You know this is the sort of thing that I think you've got to tell the resident along the way. What we're talking about now is much further down the trail of therapy than we are at this particular session.

Dr. Schuster: I err on the side of overstating because it is a natural phenomenon, we all have an unconscious mind, we all have resistance operating, and so the tendency is to overlook the transference. I've seen too many examples of difficulties developing later on because not enough was understood about the transference as one went along. Now I agree with B that premature use of this with the patient is not helpful, but somehow we have to demonstrate the transference to the resident and help him in using or not using it as is appropriate. I quite agree that there are some patients with whom you do not mention the transference at any time throughout the course of psychotherapy, for example in supportive psychotherapy.

Dr. Thaler: But in a sense to be able to do that, not to mention it, you have to know that it's there, otherwise you might inadvertently do something that enhances or further facilitates transference when you don't want this to happen.

B: May I draw an example. Let's suppose a man comes in who's having marital problems, and over a course of say 5 or 10 sessions with the psychiatrist comes to see that he has always had difficulty expressing feeling to women, that he's afraid that they are too fragile or they have to be held on a pedestal or something like that. Through talking about this he is able to speak more directly to his wife, to deal with her more directly and improves his relationship to his wife and feels much better and leaves thinking that the therapist is just terrific. Here he's really helped him resolve this issue. And now I wouldn't exactly call that supportive psychotherapy, even though any kind of relationship between the patient and the psychiatrist is never discussed. I think what I'm trying to illustrate here is that Freud said we all have transference to everybody. I think in all our relationships to everybody, things other than the reality of the relationship, the reality of that person, affects our feelings about them. So the concept of the use of transference is only pertinent when it is in the service of the patient's feeling like "I'm unhappy with myself. I want to make some changes in myself." If they make changes, and they're happy even though they use these certain transference things, I don't see that it ever needs to be discussed at all.

Dr. Thaler: I agree with that.

B: And yet I wouldn't call that supportive psychotherapy.

Dr. Schuster: Well, I think I've erred in implying that it's just supportive psychotherapy where one does not speak of the transference with the patient. I think there are other varieties of psychotherapy along the continuum between supportive and uncovering. There are all kinds of variations, which I've sometimes called focal psychotherapy or sector psychotherapy where we make a brief sortie into some particular area of character, let's say, or the conflict situation, I quite agree you don't need to mention the transference. I think you have to be aware of it though. That's my point and it's part of understanding what's going on in the patient.

Dr. Sandt: You weren't talking about a resident, you're talking about you and the patient, but if you put a resident in between there. . . .

Dr. Schuster: He might not see what you're saying.

Dr. Sandt: He may not see it at all, and you can't put him in the same position as the patient.

Dr. Schuster: He might not understand, for example, that the patient is using borrowed strength from you, identification with you to meet his problems that you've discussed, and so the resident should understand some of this, too.

Dr. Sandt: Yes.

B: You mean it shouldn't all just go on without anybody saying anything about it.

Dr. Thaler: Now the resident might say, "Well now this guy has changed, but really there isn't enough insight. Maybe we ought to pursue further why he changed, and what his feelings were towards me, etc." And you could say, "Well, look, from our understanding of the transference situation at this instance, stay away from that. Don't tell the patient 'I think the reason you got better is because I'm your father who's permitted to screw your wife, and you feel better about that because you used to be afraid of castration' and all the rest of it with any speculation you might want to make about that." Instead you tell the resident, "Look, now this may be what has been a factor in the patient's improvement, but he's fine, he's had enough. The result is good, so keep your mouth shut."

Dr. Schuster: I think one other reason that it's important to stress the transference and its corollary, the countertransference, which is little written about in the literature, is that the resident must somehow get a feeling for the strength of the unconscious and its potential, particularly the potential for destructiveness. One way he can get a feeling for this is through the transference, especially when the patient acts it out. The resident has to learn that the therapeutic situation utilizes some powerful tools, including transference-counter-transference operations, which can open up areas of the patient's personality and lead to hopefully good things. But it can also lead, if mismanaged, to bad things. The older I get, the more I realize the destructive possibilities, particularly when the therapist is not sufficiently aware of some of the irrational elements in the patient and in himself and not in sufficient control to avoid an unfavorable outcome.

D: I think this is interesting, because in the training of social workers the emphasis is always on countertransference. Very little about transference, assuming that that's going to be the good part of it. But the countertransference is really kind of stepped on, watched and hovered over.

Dr. Schuster: To put it in caricature form, it's as if your profession has been holding itself in check very carefully over the years. I know that supervision has always been a very prominent feature of social work training. The emphasis has been on very careful, detailed supervision and an attempt not to intervene too much with the patient. So it is an interesting difference between your profession and ours which has been much more adventuresome.

B: In teaching if you emphasize the unconscious, I think that the resident then will think that that's the most important part and will think only about that when he's listening to the patient's realistic problems, his environmental situation.

Dr. Schuster: I wish that were so, but I've usually not found that they are as aware of the irrational side of things as I would like them to be.

Dr. Sandt: We might well focus some time on how we assess the resident's situation prior to this. All these things that we're talking about today are secondary to a basic analysis of the resident's situation. Because you're not going to say the same kind of thing to each one. How do you go about that?

Dr. Thaler: You mean in other words that you *do* manage the transference problems in this particular instance, but would you do this the same way with the first-year, second-year and third-year resident? How do you introduce the resident to that concept in the first place? Where is the best place to do that?

Dr. Schuster: Speaking developmentally, which I think is what Jack is emphasizing, in the first year there's no better way to demonstrate the unconscious than by presenting a caricature, a gross mental mechanism, like projection, at work.

Dr. Thaler: For instance, when I started meeting with first year residents one of them brought up an incident of a patient just admitted. He went in with the patient, a woman who looked at him and said, "Now, it's not me who's crazy, it's you who are crazy, and you're the one who ought to have a psychiatrist. Not me. Let me out." He was just totally stumped—"What do I do now?" he asked. "What is this all about?" Aside from which he felt maybe she's right. This led to a discussion as to what the patient actually meant by this statement and what the patient was really trying to communicate.

Dr. Sandt: And the response of the resident at that point is very appropriate. There you're not treading on the kind of thin ice that B is trying to avoid in the second-year situation. It's all so blatant, as you said, and it's not too personally invidious to make a confrontation with the first-year resident such as, "How did you feel when you were with this patient?" Not in the second year, it's very touchy. Well it's an out-patient, and they're much less understandably in a position to feel free to say, "I felt like this about this lady."

Dr. Thaler: I think we ought to listen to a little more.

> *Dr. W*: I went to the waiting room to get her first. She was sitting on the floor playing with the children's blocks with a little baby that turned out to be Janice, the lesbian's daughter, and I couldn't believe it. She looked younger in many ways than 19. I couldn't believe this, here she was playing with blocks and "gooing" and "ahing." This is essentially one of the kind of positive things that this girl sees in this relationship; as a mother-daughter relationship I think. She wants to be looked at, and she can't say that. She also indicates that that's more important to her than sexual aspects. I think there are pluses on her side for not becoming a homosexual.

> *B*: Is this a tape of the first interview?

> *Dr. W*: No. The first interview was in Crisis Clinic only for a few minutes. This was last Wednesday, and I was seeing her again this morning. Yet the girlfriend wants to talk to me, too.

Dr. Schuster: That raises the issue as to what we should do about demands that are made on us like this, the girlfriend wants to talk to him. Is that worth discussing briefly?

Dr. Thaler: Well, yes, in terms of how does one deal with that kind of demand on the resident.

Dr. Schuster: Right.

A: I think that's a very important thing in the OPD, because in the in-patient floor the residents usually cop out of any contact with family members by leaving it in the hands of the nurses. But when they're in the OPD, they get calls from husbands and wives and brothers-in-law and cousins, and they don't know what to do. Some of them respond and get tied up in inappropriate relationships, often losing the patient that way. Some ignore them. I think it's important because it's a specific new factor in OPD work.

Dr. Thaler: I don't know whether your perception of in-patient work is entirely correct, at least in my experience. We used to not only encourage, but insist that the resident see the family of the patient, and they would do that. They rarely were reluctant to do that.

Dr. Schuster: I think that varies on different floors, Otto.

Dr. Thaler: This may be so, but certainly on my floor it was a routine to set up special times to meet with the family. It isn't always appropriate to do it in the same way, and one has to use special precautions in terms of what the patient knows about what you're doing.

A: The in-patients are relating to an institution not just to a person.

Dr. Thaler: The resident has the protection of the institution, but also he doesn't often leave the family out of it.

Dr. Sandt: The Out-patient Department is an institution, too, and the hospital setting in which this Out-patient Department is located —people come to Strong Memorial Hospital, they always phrase it that way.

Dr. Schuster: On the floors they've got the nurses, they've got the other residents, they've got the Activities personnel, social workers, psychologists. The transference is distributed and diluted.

Dr. Thaler: What's the crucial issue that you need to deal with? And maybe each one of us has a different issue in mind.

Dr. Schuster: Well, presumably this Janice called W, didn't she? Because he said, "She wants to speak to me." You mean you'd wait until you saw the patient. Do you tell him to wait until he sees the patient and then ask her, "Janice called. What should I tell her?" or "Why is she calling?" or something like that? This has happened to me on occasion, and then the other person who called said, "Oh I didn't want you to tell the patient that I called."

Dr. Thaler: Well, I think one has to make sure on the telephone with another person that you set the ground rules. In other words, somebody calls and says I want to talk to you about Miss X. So you say, wait a minute before you start talking, I'd like you to know that

I will communicate this to Miss X. I'll have to ask her whether she wants me to talk with you further, or not. Also, anything that you say to me I have to share with her. Then the other person can make the judgment as to whether he wants to go on.

Dr. Schuster: And usually there's a deadly silence.

Dr. Thaler: Right.

Dr. Sandt: Well so much depends on the situation of Miss X. If you have a suicidal patient, you're not going to turn off the other party so abruptly. You might say, "I don't think it's appropriate for you to be talking to me."

Dr. Schuster: There are exceptions as you point out; for example, Federn is quoted as saying that there should always be one person in the home, an ally, that you are in touch with when dealing with a schizophrenic patient, particularly an adolescent. But there again, most of the time I think the patient can and should know about this arrangement. Now there are some rare times when it's awkward for the patient to know about this.

Dr. Sandt: If they're very descompensated then you're not going to . . .

Dr. Thaler: I have one lady who decompensates periodically, maybe once every other year or so, and there is a friend who calls me when this happens.

Dr. Schuster: So that you know what's happened.

Dr. Thaler: Yes. Then I usually get in touch with the patient and say, "Miss So and So called me and says that you're upset again. I want you to come in and see me."

A: What about the validity of doing that without a patient knowing about it?

Dr. Thaler: To not tell the patient? I've very rarely found that to be helpful. I don't really recall any time that I've felt that I couldn't or shouldn't tell the patient.

B: I can't either.

Dr. Thaler: Unless the patient's so totally out of it that they wouldn't even know what I was talking about.

D: The patient is in communication anyway with all of these people who would be calling. I don't think its' that secretive.

Dr. Sandt: I had a call this morning from a patient who's very paranoid. I've seen her about three or four times over the course of two years, and she keeps worrying about where the records are, and who knows it and that sort of thing. She had come home just for Christmas vacation, was going back to Washington and left a message to call back. I called back, and I know that from the tone it had to be her mother. She said, "Who's this?" and I thought, "Should I really tell her who this is?" The patient is insistent on her family not knowing whom she's seeing, and yet I gave my name and said she asked me to call back. The patient needed to know that I cared enough to call back.

Dr. Thaler: I wonder whether I would do that.

Dr. Sandt: Well, she left this number, and she knew that she was going to be gone some time today. She knew that I would call back and who would answer the phone.

Dr. Schuster: Did the patient's mother know that she is seeing you?

Dr. Sandt: She knows she's seeing someone.

Dr. Schuster: But doesn't know the name.

Dr. Sandt: Right. The patient takes care of the bills. She's older, about 27. She poses an interesting problem by leaving that phone number and knowing she won't be there. Instead of cancelling the call, she's that paranoid. If she didn't want me to do this, she would have called back. I know her well enough. She'd say, "Do not call that number after such and such." But the thing that comes up really critically with that sort of patient is where they don't want anyone to know they have bills from you. I think you owe the patient that much consideration certainly. But with this girl, when she decompensates very badly, I've got her phone number in my desk. That's where her relatives are.

Dr. Thaler: However, one could say that maybe the reason she arranged it so that you would call and her mother would answer was because she wants her mother to know who you are. So I might say, "Look, I called, I can't disguise my name. I don't do that."

Dr. Sandt: The way the mother responded to my name indicated that she must have heard it before. This is what I needed to know. These tricks about telephone calls strike me as a very important issue for the resident to learn.

Dr. Thaler: There's a whole area of teaching about how to use the telephone.

A: To talk about external people influencing your therapeutic relationship, what happened with a resident recently is illuminating, and he was really in a bind. The patient was a very tense ex-marine, a paranoid guy who really took to the resident and began to trust him more and more. What happened was that a member of the faculty called the resident and said, "Your patient has been pestering the wife of a doctor in the community, and you've got to set him right." What do you do? There's an ethical question involved—a tremendous ethical question.

Dr. Schuster: Yes, that involves another issue in this case, because I heard about it. The cheerful bearer of ill tidings involved in this, the doctor's wife, had her own grudge.

A: Well, this is why it becomes an ethical question.

Dr. Schuster: Yes. Let's evaluate what she's trying to do. Knowing that she's a destructive person, what is she up to, and how accurate is the report?

Dr. Thaler: Well, what can one do about it? I think one's obliged to try to tell the patient precisely what happened.

Dr. Sandt: Would you?

Dr. Thaler: Yes.

Dr. Schuster: In other words, tell the patient, "This has been brought to my attention. I don't know anything about it, but I tell it to you because you should know."

Dr. Thaler: Right. That's the reality.

A: In other words, who told you that?

Dr. Thaler: I'd tell him. absolutely. The patient then knows something about your own reality, which particularly in a paranoid patient may be very important.

Dr. Schuster: But there's a matter of honesty too. I always find patients somewhat surprised when you deal with them in this direct manner.

Dr. Sandt: They see that you operate in the same reality system that they're going to have to learn to deal with somewhere.

F: W wants to know what to do.

B: But what do I do here? This girl kind of came in in a very urgent sense.

Dr. Thaler: We talked about the girl's asking D what to do. Now he's asking B what to do and how he should handle this.

B: I'm asking you what to do.

(We return to the patient and Dr. W. We learn now that it was the patient who asked Dr. W to "meet Jan" rather than the latter contacting Dr. W.)

> *Pt.*: You may turn out to be bored or something. I'd like to have you meet Jan.

> *Dr. W*: She wants to talk to me? You already talked with her?

> *Pt.*: Yes. I want you to talk to her.

B: He's talking about arranging for an appointment with Jan.

> *Dr. W*: What does she think about meeting me? Do you think she'd want to talk to me about something that is . . .

> *Pt.*: Yes. She probably wants to talk to you. Some of it you know.

B: They're talking about whether they ought to meet together, all three of them, or separately.

Dr. Schuster: W now is caught up in the details of whether they should meet this way or that way instead of finding out why this patient wants him to meet Jan. Does he get to that? I'm curious why she wants W to meet Jan.

> *Pt.*: She might say something alone that she might not say in front of me. I don't know. I'm shy and she's shy.

> *Dr. W*: Sounds as if you'd be shy too.

> *Pt.*: Not as shy as Jan, but I am mixed up. I don't know which way is up.

> *Dr. W*: (*Speaking to B*) She hadn't told me at this stage that it's a lesbian relationship. I guessed it by now. That's what she was building up to. That's what I was doing. Trying to find out definitely.

> *Dr. W*: You said a little while ago that your family wouldn't like it with you living there together with Jan.

Pt.: It's crazy. I don't see why they can't accept me. If they could it would be so much easier. I have so many people upset.

Dr. W: What do you think they feel? Just knowing you're living together?

Pt.: They'd think it was wrong.

B: It's still unclear to me what she means when she says things like "I'd like you to meet her." There's an implication there that either she's already made you part of the problem or she's going to.

Dr. W: What she wants is for me to make the decision for her on whether she should leave her husband and all that, or whether she should have a homosexual relationship. I'm sure that's what she wants. I think this is anxiety because it was helped considerably by Valium, 5 mgs. t.i.d.

B: Anxiety about what?

Dr. W: Anxiety about her sexual role, about the future. It's a very important decision.

B: Well, what do you see as the dynamics of her problem as causing that, I mean? What are the dynamics of the anxiety? What kind of life does she want? Does she want to go with this woman? Why was she lured off in that direction?

Dr. W: Her husband is much older than she is. This woman is much older than she is, and the other thing now is that she perceives both relationships as ones in which she was taken care of, looked after. I think actually I said it's sort of like a mother-daughter relationship, and she said yes only different. I think the needs that are being fulfilled are dependency needs, but I think the sexual gratification is very secondary with her. Just being looked after and cared for. I guess where all the conflict arises is that this woman is very much like her mother. The mother is the sort of person who says that if you do something against me, I'll kill myself and you'll be to blame. From what I've seen of Jan, I think she's the same sort of manipulative demanding person.

B: Jan is the lesbian.

Dr. W: Yes.

B: If you don't come with me . . .

Dr. W: I think that sort of threat is being applied. If you don't have a sexual relationship, this has to all end, and you can't come any more. I think that's probably in the background. The girl doesn't really want to have a sexual relationship, she wants a dependency relationship.

B: Well, I don't understand it all but I would—the first thought that comes to my mind is some kind of moratorium should be declared for her about making no decisions until she understands herself better. That is the part of all this anxiety and excitement that comes from the tension. She's deeply involved emotionally and is afraid in relationship to her mother, I suppose, guilt about her husband—both you could say—total perfect mother satisfaction and/or sexual gratification. Doing something illicit is intriguing her. It's all complicated and stimulating and for her to make a decision or for you to push her to make a decision, she'd like to think at this point that she would act out against it.

Dr. W: What about if I push her to make a decision not to make a decision? I think that's what we would hope for, to give it time to let things cool and see things more clearly.

B: What do you think?

Dr. Sandt: After that it's for you to say what you think. To that business of the dilemma of no decision equals a decision.

B: Oh yes. Say, that's right?

Dr. Sandt: He's pushing you into the same kind of dilemma the patient's pushing *him* into.

Dr. Thaler: We are making in our own minds a decision whether to do this, that or the other thing. Even when you don't do something it makes a difference.

Dr. Sandt: In the data gathering process this is also a means of postponing decision making. What you're doing is saying, "I don't quite understand yet." That's what he says to the patient. Most residents would be saying to the patient "I don't quite understand yet," and that postponement makes for a decision-making delay anyway, so in effect you get a "moratorium" just by saying "I don't understand all of this yet" and taking time so that the "more data" strategy is a postponement.

Dr. Thaler: She impressed the resident with the idea that this is not the time to say anything.

Dr. Sandt: But the postponed process isn't just a passive Hamlet-like delay.

B: No, it's for a reason.

Dr. Sandt: There is a payoff because you don't rush into silly actions, but there's also the virtue of finding some more so he can make some structural interpretations.

Dr. Schuster: I feel the resident could have gotten at this problem at the point where the patient started pressing him about seeing Jan. I think at that point he should have tried to find out what she wanted him to see her for. What do you expect to happen? Why do you want me to do that? That would have immediately put the patient into the position of having to think about what she is really requesting, demanding.

Dr. Thaler: There are patients who come to you with a dilemma— they want confirmation of a decision they've already made. This patient impresses me that she doesn't want that. She wants somebody to support her in delaying a decision, and here again, I think the resident is doing the right thing.

Dr. Schuster: Well, now which decision are you speaking about? Her marriage?

Dr. Thaler: No. The decision as to whether she should move with Jan or stay with her husband. Now this woman doesn't yet know what she wants to do. We saw a patient with Dr. X early on. A woman with a marital problem, having an affair with her husband's best friend. At the beginning of the interview she felt indecisive and said she wanted to know whether she should stay with her husband or whether she should go with the friend and get a divorce. Well, as the interview progressed, it became very evident that she actually wanted to get support to stay with her husband. She'd already made up her mind and didn't want to go with this man, but now she saw this as a grave injury to this guy that she had an affair with who's already divorced his own wife in order to get married to her. But she got cold feet for a number of reasons, and she decided she'd rather stay with her husband so she wanted support in not doing anything at this point.

Dr. Sandt: Doesn't it strike you, too, that this woman certainly is not acting out in terms of homosexuality, so that she's gone in terms of what direction she's more likely to decide in. It seems away from the homosexual relationship, although there is this pressure at the moment.

Dr. Thaler: She's sort of playing with the idea.

Dr. Sandt: Yes. I think what she wants from W is to point out the fact that she's not a lifelong homosexual, and W is supposed to say something to cure her. We don't know that at this point, but I'm saying there are certainly some hypotheses you can make from the history.

Dr. Schuster: Well I find the history obscure at this point in this regard. We don't know her lifelong history, and we don't know the state of her marriage. She presents this as though having met this person a short time before and having this encounter—the touching, and so on—following that her marriage falls to pieces. Now I don't believe that, but that's the way it's presented. So we again come back to your admonition about cool it until we find out some more facts, because we don't even know what the facts are at this point. We must know them before we get involved with Jan or anybody else, I would think.

B: I think I was trying to say that in the end we want this girl to be able to make her own decisions, and she can't do this now because she's all in a turmoil. Also she probably can't do it, because she never has done it, and so before she could do something like this she would have to understand herself better and develop further —mature further. Then W says, "Well, if that's your goal to have her make her own decisions, then what about this idea of telling her not to do anything? Isn't that making a decision for her?" And I think I've tried to answer that a little later. It comes up here, but it is a kind of philosophical—I mean in a sense he asks a good question. He's saying I can do one thing, but I'm not supposed to do the other.

Dr. Schuster: He ought to know better. You're asking him to do something which is constructive, and this kind of an intervention is a somewhat neutral one and in the interest of the patient. He knows. He likes to joust.

Dr. Thaler: The difference is between these two decisions. One not to do anything at all, and the other either she must go with her husband or go with the girl. The second one is an irreversible decision. If she goes with the girl she's had it with the husband, and vice versa. To say now, "Don't do anything for the moment," still leaves her open to option. The decision you help the patient make is that which offers the patient the most options.

B: Maybe I did something like this. I think that's part of the point.

> *B*: Before a commitment of herself with me. Well, now you're saying to push her into that, she's likely to rebel against that.

> *Dr. W*: If she's still saying I'm pushing her to go back with her husband and that might cause her to sort of act out and do contrary things. By the same token it's quite possible that you're saying don't make a decision about it, and I don't know how to deal with her.

> *B*: You're frustrating her from having what she wants.

> *Dr. W*: Yes.

> *B*: Well, except that she is very ambivalent about it. That's why she has this anxiety, and I think that you're not saying no, you're not being authoritarian. You're just saying—you're appealing to her, that part of her that feels distressed by this whole bit, and what you're saying is, "Let's understand it better." That's what you're saying. "I think you should grow up a bit before you make big decisions about your life."

Dr. Thaler: I think these are very interesting issues because we never really formulate as clearly as we can here the things that are involved in supervision, and it occurs to me there are three things that one can respond to: Number 1, What is it the patient wants most? That's one reason why you chose one way of doing it rather than another. I would feel the patient wants most not to do anything, so you support that. Number 2, What gives the patient the most options? Again not to do anything at the moment. Number 3,

What would cause the patient more anxiety? And I think to suggest to the patient either to go with Jan or to stay with the husband would cause a great deal more anxiety for her and hence would encourage her acting out, more than to say to her don't do anything now. This is another reason to pursue the course that you recommend.

B: Well, I think there's an issue here with—you all seem to feel that he's jousting there with me.

Dr. Thaler: Yes, there's sort of a talmudic quality involved.

B: Yes, that's true. I know that, and he does that, although he never seems to hurt or do it in a hostile way. The other thing is I think he actually does have a point. If you could answer that question that he poses I think you have to agree with . . .

Dr. Sandt: The point that the supervisory strategy could be aimed at the manifest rather than the latent. Yes. In fact it better be, it seems to me in this particular case.

Dr. Thaler: Yes, when somebody asks a hostile question like that, I just point it out rather than attack him.

B: You ask why are you doing this?

Dr. Thaler: Yes. I use the response, "That's a good question," then I tell him why.

A: Actually it must be frustrating for the residents, too, because there's no consistent model of whether you advise a patient or not. On the in-patient floors, typically they do—don't go home this weekend, don't visit your mother or whatever. I find there are differences between us, and they have to deal with each of us and our own biases, and this is hard for them. I note for one thing that my own belief is you never advise a patient. That's my bias, and somebody else will have a different bias. We also say that this is a chronic schizophrenic, therefore you structure and advise, whereas this is more an intensive therapy patient, and you don't. The poor residents listen to this and are unsure, and then they ask is there a model, and the answer is no. W is also faced with the dilemma that all the residents are faced with, do I advise this patient or don't I?

Dr. Schuster: Well, there are occasions when there's genuine confusion and frustration as you say. I don't feel it's quite as critical an issue as apparently you do, A. I think the resident is accustomed to different models, and he realizes he is in a field that's somewhat more ambiguous, and where you tolerate more uncertainty than in lots of other fields.

F: That only makes it hurt more.

Dr. Schuster: On the other hand, another way to look at it is to say that all roads lead to Rome, by which I mean if you try to inculcate certain principles in the course of the supervision of the resident, he will be able to make allowances for differences in style. Now if he meets too many clashing and opposing opinions about how to handle a specific problem, then that's a serious problem. I don't know how often that occurs. That there are different styles he should accept without too much agony, or else he should go into engineering. If he really receives too many conflicting opinions about how to handle a specific problem, then it is a problem.

Dr. Thaler: It happens occasionally and I think it happens more on the floors than any place else. The most outstanding case I can recall was one in which I was involved where one attending was intent on doing aversive behavioral therapy with a young woman who had lost her voice. He was giving her rather intense amounts of electrical stimulation in order to bring back her voice, to the point where she was in agony. I intervened, and the resident was in the middle. I got involved emotionally also. The resident in retrospect really got buffetted by the conflicting opinions.

B: An example of this came up this morning with W. He had started in the OPD, and he now has a diagnostic study and I'm still his general tutor. He said, "Oh, what an immense difference between the floors and the OPD." He said that his doubts about psychotherapy are completely changing. There's nothing like a little success to make you feel like there's something to this thing, and he said I've had several good cases and they are progressing and moving along well. "Also, my OPD supervisor sets up very definite criteria as to who is acceptable and who isn't acceptable. This helps me clarify things." He said, "I'm not sure that you would feel the same way he does in terms of the criteria, but . . ." We talked a bit about it, and we saw that the person who likes and treats young, severely disturbed schizophrenic patients at a place like Chestnut Lodge over a long period of time has different criteria and point of view of psychotherapy than someone who doesn't. I think his supervisor is at the other end of the spectrum, that there are certain definite criteria, and if the patients don't fit, out they go. W said, "Now I can see that the kind of cases I should discuss with you might be those that he feels are untreatable." In our talking I've said that my position is that as long as the patient is motivated to change, I personally feel it's worth working with them. To me motivation is everything, and he said, "Well, that's a different point of view."

Dr. Thaler: But is it? In a sense it sort of begs the question, because then you have to specify. I think in the end you would probably not be so far apart from his supervisor, once you try to clarify what you mean by motivation, how you recognize it, etc.

A: That's a circular argument because a patient needs ego strength to have motivation to want to change and . . .

Dr. Schuster: I would say that this was an example of different views which should not be too disturbing to the resident or to us, because in the last analysis he has to decide what are the criteria for accepting a patient in psychotherapy as he matures clinically. The fact that he receives different criteria from different people I think is good, because what one does not cover the other one will. That's part of the educational process.

B: But I think these things should be spelled out so that the resident knows and understands that if he enters into this puzzling new world of psychotherapy there will be very different points of view, although all go to Rome as you point out.

Dr. Thaler: Ruth Monroe in her book, *Schools of Psychoanalytic Thought* examines 8 or 10 psychoanalytically derived dynamic theories, and she comes to the conclusion that after looking not at what people say and what their theory is but what they do, that the experienced therapist and ethical therapist who has some dynamic principles and uses unconscious mental processes, that most of us do the same sort of thing in our actual work with patients. They do not differ as much as they do in their theoretical assertions.

Dr. Sandt: There's a book by Donald Glad called *Operational Psychotherapy*. Have any of you seen it? It has a verbatim transcript of various points of view of therapy, and it comes to a different conclusion than Ruth Monroe, because she started within a psychoanalytic framework. This thing goes across the board, taking in Rogers, etc. You can see a terrific difference in terms of operational commentary. In terms of people who are psychoanalytically based it's quite similar.

B: I agree with Otto that we are more alike than we sound when we talk to each other, because when we talk to each other we have to assert ourselves in some way.

Dr. Schuster: I don't think we should go to the other extreme and say we all think alike, even though we talk differently. I don't think we think alike, nor do I think it's necessarily conducive to a resident's development to have all his teachers think alike. That would be very convenient for stamping out certain kinds of bureaucratic minds, but not producing somebody who's going to have an interest in his work. I don't think we should be so disturbed about this, and I don't see how you can prevent it. You could say at the outset, "Here you're going to be exposed to a lot of different views and different ways of doing things, and don't be concerned—it will all work out."

F: We seem to be in a very conciliatory mood, so let me just take the other tack. There is a lot of upset in first- and second-year residents. I think part of the reason why there isn't more is that the resident reduces the cognitive distance. In other words, he begins to perceive very, very quickly what your orientation is and what you're going to like and not like. Depending on his learning style he's going to really put down to a great extent the fact that he's heard something quite different from his other tutors. This creates a flexibility. I think the fact that this seminar has not been held before now in the history of this department is an indication that it's scary for people to sit down and make explicit what it is that they supervise.

Dr. Thaler: I think part of what you say though, F, also matches the way people have to learn. In other words, if a resident is with me he will learn from me what I have to give him, and he will try to exclude what everybody else has told him. Then he goes to somebody else, and he will take that person's views and forget about me for a while. Later on he'll integrate all these things. We see this in medical students, too, when they go from one service to another. They learn a lot in psychiatry and think they are going to apply this stuff, but when they go to surgery, it's a survival mechanism for them to shut up about what they've learned in psychiatry, because the surgeons don't appreciate it. They're now focused on another area, and they're so busy trying to figure out what the layer of fascia is that they're cutting through, that they forget about the layer of mental processes that they've learned about.

F: I have a feeling that the identificatory processes early in the residency are more like introjection than identification. What we would consider more adolescent or adult-like identification comes more in the latter part of the first year and the second year. At first it's more imitation; there's no other way to operate.

Dr. Thaler: You see this also when they move from floor to floor. After the first 6 months when they come to another floor, they say, "My God, these people don't know what the hell they're doing, everything is wrong. There's only one way of treating patients."

Dr. Schuster: Well, there are all kinds of interesting and parochial points of views and rivalries among faculty members. It's all part of the gamesmanship of the residency in a sense.

B: Isn't part of the reason that we're meeting here in the first place to try and find some common ground that all of us could share in spite of our different points of view?

Dr. Thaler: Also I think what we're trying to do is to identify pedagogic problems and how we deal with these problems. Just to identify the problem, such as we've done, in itself might help all of us.

D: What do the residents say they want?

B: I would say that they want to learn how to be psychotherapists, that's one of the things I've heard them say. As though they were an apprentice, "How do you do this thing, how do you help this person?"

Dr. Thaler: I've met with each group earlier on in the year, and it's not very clear just what it is they want. I think they want all kinds of things. One of the surest things to me is that the tutorial consistently has been one of the most cherished, valued and invested experiences of the resident. His feelings run highest when he can't get the tutor that he's asking for, or when his tutorial is poor, or when something interferes with it.

Dr. Schuster: If nothing else, it confirms something I've often said in the past—that medical science, no matter how you slice it, is an applied science based essentially on the apprenticeship system. I like to say this to some of my colleagues who get too fancy about medical education. When it comes right down to it, anybody who wants to be a physician or a practitioner of some sort wants to have somebody show him and tell him how to do it.

A: The resident finds himself in a strange world of psychiatry which is hard to relate back to medical school, and he simply endures it and needs support in a very basic human way. What patients need, he needs. Supervision is one way of getting your hour of therapy, support and everything else. It's a basic human need.

Dr. Thaler: Many of us have tried group tutorials, but this has never caught on in the department. Some people still do it on occasion, but still the one-to-one with the residents is considered both by the faculty and by the residents to be a major experience in his training.

F: Somebody recently wrote a paper about three quests that residents have in the early part of their residency. One was the quest for omniscience, they wish to know everything from the deepest parts of analytic theory to the biochemistry of the nervous system. That's an initial kind of quest. Another was the quest for omnisentience, to be able to feel everything. This has to do with undoing some of the more repressive aspects of medical training. They see within psychiatry you're allowed certain kinds of feelings. Then there is the quest for omnifascience—to be able to do everything, to be the triple-threat man who can do insight therapy, ECT, drugs and all of these kinds of things. Then what happens is the gradual falling out. Like so much of life you begin to modify and. . . .

Dr. Sandt: That's the way you go through medical school, where you start out with an undifferentiated physician model, where you're total and you won't admit you can't do surgery just as well as the surgeons or deliver a baby just as well as the obstetrician. You have to fall out in the same manner through your junior and senior years.

Dr. Thaler: I was presenting a clinical vignette to the first-year class to illustrate a very general point about adaptation, and one of the students in the first row said, "Now you haven't told us enough as to what to do in this instance." I said that's not the point. "What I'm trying to do is illustrate something." The student said, "But what if I should meet somebody at a party, and they tell me about a problem, I wouldn't know what to do" I said, "Don't do anything. What if somebody came to you at a party and said I have a pain here, would you take him to the kitchen table and open him up?"

Dr. Sandt: Do you know that paper of Ernest Jones on omnipotence—the parallel between the preacher and the psychiatrist in terms of God equals omnipotence, and the scientific God equals the psychiatrist? That's our field.

Dr. Schuster: As to the question of individual versus group tutorial, I personally have always felt and have occasionally practiced having more than one person to tutor at the same time. I think there are many good points to this kind of supervision, such as the model of the continuous case seminar in the psychoanalytic institute; but I think the greatest impediment is sibling rivalry, and that's hard to get around when the resident is, so to speak, young in his work and so hungry for your approval.

D: I rather feel though that it has to do with the resident's relationship with his tutor and the model and identity that he makes with that particular psychiatrist as he is becoming a specialist as a physician. I wonder if all of this talk about who says what and when and how and where is really as important to the resident's learning as this group feels.

B: I think you're right, and it pertains to what A says, too, that they want to feel that the supervisor thinks they're good. In not feeling very competent, they look towards external reassurances about this, and it's easy to say this is what you should do. But we don't talk too much about what it is you want from me, we sort of let that go and just provide what we think they need.

Dr. Sandt: The key to the residents seems to be their need for identity balance and acceptance of their process. That you understand that they're at a certain stage of development, you understand that they're an individual in that stage, and you're interested in developing them through that stage. Once you get through that, they learn a lot better, because they're not then so defensive about exposing their inadequacies and understandable naïveté about things.

Dr. Schuster: There's a difference in the whole process of establishing an identity in the process of becoming a psychiatrist, as opposed to becoming a surgeon, in that we don't have the props to help here. The whole thing is more ambiguous. The young surgeon can always hang onto a retractor—that's his identity at that point, a very concrete and simple task. This makes it easier for him. Their role is strictly defined. They watch and listen while they're holding, but they don't get their hand in the wound or tie knots at first. I think our task is much more difficult. The intervention is less clearly defined.

Dr. Sandt: The external trappings of identity aren't too many. If we didn't have any white coats, you'd know. Look how much more difficult it is on wards where they don't wear them. I know they put a great deal more stress on us in my residency, because white coats were not part of the game. As you came from internship into first year of residency you didn't wear a white coat anymore, but a suit; and everyone went around saying, "Where's my stethoscope?" In fact some of the residents in my first-year group would carry stethoscopes to maintain some security.

Dr. Thaler: We have to indicate to the resident in his uncertainty that you never finish, and that you yourself are not always sure about what to do, that you fall flat on your face periodically, etc. In other words, when he comes up and says, "Look, I'm so discouraged about this patient, etc.", he needs the support not only of your saying, "You'll learn, and it will be better," but also, "Well that's how it's going to be. It's still like that in my practice sometimes." I tell them about patients I've seen for years where nothing has happened to them. The other thing is to try to demonstrate to them that indeed there are many situations in which it is possible to learn precisely what is going on and exactly what to do, and that what you do will be effective.

Dr. Sandt: The same thing happened to me. A resident gave me a follow up on two of the patients we had seen previously, and he mentioned how reassuring it was to validate something that was predicted. He said he did such and such pretty much the way we had talked about it, and it came out that way. He said that was the best thing that had happened to him so far.

D: That's when you demonstrate your expertise, and they must have this.

B: Let's finish this up.

> *B:* Although you might not say those things to her, I think that she would respond with some relief to the fact that she's not going to have to do something right away. She's not going to give up her impulses, nor is she going to be forced to act on them and then in turn give up other things like her relationship with her husband. I don't think that she'll respond as though you were her mother, saying if you don't do this I will kill myself. In a sense you will be allying yourself with that part of her that agrees it's best to not act on it right away. As you talk with her, do you see her as try-ing to get away from things by wanting to come into the hospital?
>
> *Dr. W:* She said, "I ought to come into the hospital to get out of the mess," and I said I didn't think she needed to do that.

Dr. Sandt: That's a critical point in your supervision. Do you put somebody in the hospital or not. Are they in control enough to maintain their lives outside of a structured environment? Usually you bring that up early.

Dr. Thaler: What she wants is to get out of the mess, not to do one thing or another.

Dr. Sandt: It's an argument about the delay. You're using it at this point with W to validate and corroborate your point of view about this, like you don't really think she's so collapsible that she can't tolerate being out of the hospital. In a sense that leads on to' things, like she's capable of making decisions.

Dr. Thaler: He did say she'll act out no matter what I tell her, and this indicates that he doesn't give her credit for any kind of self-observing ego, that she can't observe her behavior in any way. You're saying, "Look, if you tell her one thing—stay with the husband or go with the friend—this will provoke anxiety which she will not be able to handle." It sounds as if her ego was intact enough to be able to do what is realistically in evidence. That's why she's here in the first place, to explore herself.

B: That's what she's really here for, and it looked like she was here for him to tell her what to do.

> *B*: There's a lot of problems to discuss about this. Why don't you see her as you're planning to do today, and then do you want to meet again? Do you feel there are reasons to meet with me again?

> *Dr. W*: Well I'll see her today, and providing things don't go too badly I'll play the tape next week for you.

> *B*: I won't be here, and that's why I want to make sure we can arrange a time if you feel you want it. This seems to be a crisis, so I thought we might meet again to see where you think you stand after talking to her another time.

B: What happened was she decided on her own to go back to her husband. A couple of sessions later she decided this was the thing to do, she didn't feel there was anything else to be done. She felt she'd resolved it, and all was settled. Then the next thing W hears is that the lesbian told the husband that his wife had been making approaches to her. With that the patient took an overdose of Valium and came into ED. They talked it over, and it seemed serious enough for admission.

Dr. Schuster: I'm beginning to see now why she asked him to see Jan. "Get her off my back."

B: She went into the hospital, and was only there a week, resolved certain things with her husband, and now they are in Florida.

Conclusion

We have attempted to assert our belief in the importance of sound clinical training for a psychiatric physician and the role supervision plays in this training. We have enunciated some principles of the clinician, reviewed the literature on this subject, pointed out some developmental aspects of psychiatric training and described our own program—including some of its defects. Finally, through the dialogue of a conference on supervision we have attempted to illustrate specific issues involved in the supervisory experience.

We were motivated to do all this by our concern that interest in and respect for the clinician and what is involved in his development and maturation have diminished recently. Psychiatry, as all of medicine, is caught in the cross-fire of demands for change, new methods and services, and answers to pressing social problems. Affluence and regressive trends in our society have insisted on instant solutions and gratifications—magic and illusion rather than hard-won, more modest gains. The loneliness of man is reflected in the fascination with groups, touching, "encounter." Under the impact of these and other forces, psychiatry has questioned itself—sometimes constructively, other times too harshly. Our professional identity has suffered accordingly.

We maintain that, regardless of fad or fashion, psychiatry remains a branch of medical science. Basically it derives from and is related to the practice of medicine. It behooves us, therefore, to continue our stance as clinicians—this is our identity. It is therefore necessary to maintain proper standards of training and not allow ourselves to be lured into abbreviating, diluting or abandoning tried methods. This is not to say that innovation should be spurned. The same interest in inquiry which is an integral part of the clinician's *modus operandi* should spur us constantly to re-examine our teaching procedures, looking for improved ways and means.

Looking broadly at what we have been doing over the years, our main criticism is that clinical teaching is more cross-sectional than longitudinal. By this we mean that many of the encounters between resident and supervisor concern a patient and his problems at a certain moment of time. The resident and his teacher do not have many opportunities to continue to view this patient and his vicissitudes over a span of weeks, months, years. The tutorial program provides a certain kind of continuity, to be sure, but we feel the need for other longitudinal approaches. This may be illustrated by contrasting the role of resident and practitioner vis-à-vis the patient. A patient coming to the Emergency Department will be examined by one or more residents; if admitted to the in-patient service he will be temporarily taken care of by the admitting doctor and later assigned to a "regular" resident. If he is referred from ED to the OPD he will be "screened" by yet another psychiatrist before being assigned to a second-year resident. Quite aside from the inconvenience and at times distress of the patient engendered by such experiences, it is obvious that each resident sees a different glimpse of the patient and has limited opportunity for follow-up information. He thus gains no longitudinal, long-term view of the life history of this patient's illness. The practitioner, on the other hand, follows his patient through these various vagaries of care and has a continuing appreciation of the clinical changes.

Somehow we must pattern our teaching more on the practitioner's role, having a resident follow a patient through the various phases of his illness and steps in his treatment. This is not easy to accomplish, as it involves an intensity and continuity of supervision difficult to comprehend. It would, for example, involve repeated views of the patient by the same resident and supervisor over perhaps the total three-year period of training—through "thick and thin," visits to Emergency, OPD, hospitalization, day care, referral to social agency, back to home and family, to employment, etc. Some of this the resident does now, but the long-term supervision is spotty and often inadequate. The patient is not often seen repeatedly over time by the supervisor, and details of behavior and symptoms are lost through the necessity of keeping abreast of a large case-load.

We regard the achieving of more longitudinal teaching as the next phase of our continuing efforts to train skilled and humane psychiatric physicians. In conclusion we wish to repeat something we said earlier.

"Only the intellectual rigor and scrutiny of the supervisory situation applied in some manner to our subsequent professional life can assure our own and our profession's advancement. Thus, we, as seasoned clinicians, are on the same continuum of maturation—of professional ontogeny—as our residents." We can—we must—learn from each other.

Index

332